WOMEN AND FAMILIES:
FEMINIST RECONSTRUCTIONS

PERSPECTIVES ON MARRIAGE AND THE FAMILY
Bert N. Adams and David M. Klein, *Editors*

WIFE BATTERING: A SYSTEMS THEORY APPROACH
Jean Giles-Sim

COMMUTER MARRIAGE: A STUDY OF WORK AND FAMILY
Naomi Gerstel and Harriet Gross

HELPING THE ELDERLY: THE COMPLEMENTARY ROLES
OF INFORMAL NETWORKS AND FORMAL SYSTEMS
Eugene Litwak

REMARRIAGE AND STEPPARENTING:
CURRENT RESEARCH AND THEORY
Kay Palsey and Marilyn Ihinger-Tallman (Eds.)

FEMINISM, CHILDREN, AND THE NEW FAMILIES
Sanford M. Dornbusch and Myta F. Strober (Eds.)

DYNAMICS OF FAMILY DEVELOPMENT:
A THEORETICAL PERSPECTIVE
James M. White

PORTRAIT OF DIVORCE: ADJUSTMENT TO MARITAL BREAKDOWN
Gay C. Kitson with William M. Holmes

WOMEN AND FAMILIES: FEMINIST RECONSTRUCTIONS
Kristine M. Baber and Katherine R. Allen

Women and Families

Feminist Reconstructions

Kristine M. Baber
Katherine R. Allen

THE GUILFORD PRESS
New York   London

© 1992 The Guilford Press
A Division of Guilford Publications, Inc.
72 Spring Street, New York, NY 10012

Printed in the United States of America

This book is printed on acid-free paper.

Last digit is print number: 9 8 7 6 5 4 3 2 1

Library of Congress Cataloging-in-Publication Data

Baber, Kristine M.
   Women and families: feminist reconstructions / Kristine M. Baber,
Katherine R. Allen.
      p.   cm. — (Perspectives on marriage and the family)
   Includes bibliographical references and index.
   ISBN 0-89862-082-1 — ISBN 0-89862-083-X (pbk.)
   1. Women—United States.   2. Family—United States.   3. Sex role—
United States.   4. Feminist theory.   I. Allen, Katherine R.
II. Title.   III. Series.
HQ1421.B33   1992
305.4—dc20   92-20561
                                                                         CIP

To our partners,
Bill Baber and Tamara J. Stone

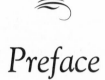

Preface

This book is a comprehensive exploration of women's experiences as members of families written from a postmodern feminist perspective. We address key topics in women's lives and examine how women shape, and are shaped by, their families and the wider society in which they live. Although much of the information we cover is relevant to women in other cultures, we limit our analyis to the United States. This in itself provides a vast challenge without introducing the complexities of dealing with the differences in women's experiences cross-nationally.

We wrote this book to make feminist ideas about women and families more accessible to ourselves, our undergraduate and graduate students, our colleagues within family studies, and our colleagues across disciplines in women's studies. We have attempted to communicate clearly and in plain language about the struggles women face in trying to fulfill societal expectations while carving out lives that reflect their own needs, interests, and choices.

We hope the book can be read on many levels. The postmodern feminist perspective guiding our work is complex, but we believe it is the most appropriate for our topic. Chapter 1 provides an introduction to the theory that should be understandable to most readers. We locate our arguments in multidisciplinary assessments about women, families, society, and change and draw from a multiplicity of resources. The extensive bibliography itself should be a useful resource to those interested in theory and research about women and their experiences in families.

A particular contribution that this book makes is the inclusion of the experiences of lesbians and their families. Although diversity has claimed both popular and scholarly attention, family diversity has usually meant that consideration is expanded only to single-parent families, stepfamilies, African-American families, or heterosexual cohabitants. Lesbians and their families have been virtually invisible in the family studies literature.

No book can do it all. We cannot do complete justice to the diversity we see around us, nor can we fully describe situations and processes that we do not experience. Our perspectives, choice of topics, and choice of examples are limited by our own personal and intellectual heritages. We are both white, middle-class, educated, feminist women who were trained in the early 1980s in family studies programs, and we teach in similar academic departments at state universities. Our differences in perspective about women and families come from our personal histories and marital and parental careers. These differences have contributed to a rich exchange of ideas and possibilities regarding what women's lives are and what they can become. One of us (Baber) is in a long-term marriage and is child free; the other (Allen) has been married and divorced and is now coparenting a young child in a committed relationship with another woman. We have learned about the feminist project of solidarity and diversity through our own association and through constantly encouraging each other to represent diversity more accurately. We have learned that we cannot simply lament the lack of diversity between us; rather, we have worked closely to understand just what we mean by women's solidarity in the context of their diversity so that we do not treat diversity as just a mark on a demographic checklist.

We have attempted to locate our own perspective as honestly as possible in terms of our areas of expertise and to help each other with our particular blind spots. We have been frustrated by the limitations of our similarities, even as we are buoyed by the strength of our shared experience and standpoint. We worked together intensely for three years learning to share and to challenge each other's ideas without valorizing or attacking. This work together has brought home the feminist commitment to solidarity in an intellectual sense and to sisterhood in a personal sense.

Our project, although comprehensive, is not complete. We see this book as contributing to the dialogue about women, families, and inequality in our society. We hope our approach encourages others to enter the discussion by offering their experiences and speaking from their own perspectives.

We are not just placing "society" or "the individual woman" in the center of our vision. We are placing "women as members of families" in the center. The boundaries immediately become blurred between the integrity of the individual and the holism of the group. The family we envision is not a clearly identifiable entity. Contrary to the sociological and psychological theories of our century, we do not posit the family to be a unity of interacting personalities, nor do we adhere to the textbook definition that a family consists of those related by blood, marriage, or adoption.

Our view of what constitutes a family has become more and more open-ended as we consider the variety of ways women define families for themselves. We deconstruct the unitary view of the family as consisting of a husband who is the male head of household, his supportive wife, and their biological, dependent children. We work back and forth between structural definitions of families and emergent definitions of families that include an aspect of personal choice. Historians of the family have long recognized that the affective experience of the family must be separated from the physical composition and the economic cooperation of members of a household. Feminists argue, as well, for the deconstruction of family, household, and affective ties.

In addition to self-definition, we see the family as a major context in which sexism, heterosexism, classism, ageism, and racism are fostered and reinforced. We work back and forth between the microsystems of women's families and the broader macrostructure to determine factors that perpetuate and those that resist biases and the resulting inequities. Our analysis of women's lives is complicated by the "talk" about families, because families are loosely bounded units filled with affective and con- flictual associations. Our work is a process of clarifying, critiquing, and reevaluating the products of this analysis.

As we deconstruct existing ideas about women and let our own vision emerge, we realize that our work about women and their families is not just an intellectual exercise removed from our own lives and hopes, designed merely to contribute to the scholarly record. As other feminist collaborators have found, feminist work takes on a life of its own. The human enterprise of our work together deserves recognition as meaning- ful, productive labor, but this labor is easily rendered invisible by the scholarly production process.

We want to make our process and our product visible because we care about each other as people, we care about the messages contained in this book as a symbol of our work together, and we care about how we are characterizing others' arguments about real lives. This caring has taken on a dimension that is valuable in and of itself. Too often, the behind-the- scenes labor is lost, mystified, or transformed into a commodity whose worth is judged by abstract academic standards. As scholars, we welcome this discussion and critique, but we go on record for ourselves and our work to say that the process of feminist practice and scholarship has changed our lives and affirmed the value of feminism as an epistemology, ontology, and methodology. The feminist vision we construct in this work is rooted in our affective relationship with each other; it was created and modified through our labor. We hope that both the process and the product of this labor generalize beyond us as individuals. We hope that this book will be read by others and that our analyses and proposals for change will serve to improve the lives of women and their families.

Acknowledgments

We wrote this book with the support and assistance of a variety of other people. Bert Adams and David Klein, editors of the series in which this book appears, read the entire manuscript several times and provided candid, timely feedback and insightful suggestions for revision throughout the process. Sharon Panulla of The Guilford Press showed unflagging enthusiasm for the book from the beginning and guided us through the publication process with flexibility, tolerance, and understanding. We also want to acknowledge our feminist colleagues who influenced our thinking and writing in countless ways. We thank Alexis Walker, in particular, for bringing us together and suggesting our collaboration in the first place.

There are many who deserve thanks for personally supporting us during the three years we worked on this book. We want to thank our families, our friends, our coworkers, and our students for their accommodations as we labored over our book. A special thank you to Jay Mancini for his generosity in providing encouragement and resources along the way.

Most importantly, we thank our partners, Bill and T. J., for their loving support and patience which allowed us the time and energy to devote to our writing. Their wise insights and concern for our well-being often gave us the confidence to continue. We dedicate this book to them in honor of our sustaining partnerships.

Contents

Women and Families:
Our Feminist Perspective

Intricate patterns of family relationships and responsibilities characterize the lives of contemporary American women. Family life is an important arena for creative and generative expression for many women. Yet, families, particularly those based on traditional ideologies and practices, are tension-filled arenas, loci of struggle and domination between genders and across generations. Feminists have exploded the myth of the family as a safe and stable haven and pointed to ways in which women's lives are constrained by even their most intimate and caring relationships. Feminists have also identified ways that women resist domination and become innovators in the family nexus of caring and struggle.

Feminist analyses have revealed that there is no unitary family experience for women. Decades of mainstream family research, as well, have revealed that no one pattern of intimate life characterizes the experiences of all women—or men, for that matter. In the late 20th century, far-reaching socioeconomic changes are occurring at an unprecedented pace, intersecting with similar changes in intimate and emotional relationships and resulting in more complex family dynamics and configurations.

Family diversity has replaced the old idea about uniformity among the American population. On the threshold of the 21st century, it is apparent that plurality is an even more accurate concept than diversity. These pluralistic changes and the unsettling uncertainty that accompanies them require radical revisions in our ways of thinking. Postmodernism is a *new* way of thinking about people, families, and societies and thus holds great potential for guiding a discussion about the promises and risks of pluralistic approaches. A postmodern perspective critiques the philosophical underpinnings of modern theory—essentialism, universalism, and dichotomous thinking—and, instead, stresses plurality, difference, and marginality (Best & Kellner, 1991). Postmodernism offers feminists and family scholars a perspective that recognizes the problem of reducing the complexity of women's lives into dichotomies such as male/female, black/white, and gay/straight.

In this book, we combine *feminism and postmodernism* to examine the phenomena of family life from *women's perspectives.* Postmodern feminism deconstructs ideologies and practices that sustain and legitimate male domination and also challenges essentialist feminist theories that ignore differences among women related to factors such as age, race, class, or sexual orientation (Best & Kellner, 1991; Flax, 1990; Fraser & Nicholson, 1990). We struggle to go beyond dualistic approaches to thinking about women and their families and to give more than lip service to the *pluralism* that increasingly characterizes women's lives. We embed our analysis in the sociohistorical context of women's oppression and stress their active resistance against domination. Our goal is to acknowledge ways in which women are *innovators* in their own lives.

THE CONTRADICTIONS OF FAMILY LIFE FOR WOMEN

A basic dilemma for women in families is the tension created as they attempt to fulfill their own needs while effectively meeting the needs of those for whom they care. Women socialized to believe that they have the responsibility to serve the needs of others are inclined to sacrifice their own interests in the name of care and responsibility (Gilligan, 1982; Miller, 1986). The needs of others, particularly children, partners, and ill or aging parents, are often given priority in women's lives.

Neglecting one's own needs and desires, however, can lead to frustration and deprivation. Women who ignore developing and maintaining their personal abilities and skills are particularly vulnerable in today's society. Research on the consequences of divorce for women describes the long-term personal and economic costs of a woman's decision to put her family's needs ahead of her own education, training, and career (Okin, 1989; Weitzman, 1988). At the interpersonal level, most women gain a sense of satisfaction and fulfillment in caring for and attending to the needs of children and partners. However, the woman who is devoted selflessly to others may be rejected as a smothering partner or mother (Miller, 1986). A challenge for contemporary women, then, is to reach a synthesis that acknowledges and resolves the tension between commitment to others and commitment to self. One of the goals of this book is to explore the personal and social transformations that result as women individually and collectively address the internal contradictions of family life.

The family is one of the most powerful socializing institutions. It is within the family that people construct beliefs about the sexual division of labor, learn about the regulation of sexuality, and experience the effects of gender, class, and race hierarchies in personal and intimate ways (Flax, 1987; Glenn, 1987). That the family has emerged as the focus of critical analysis by both feminists and antifeminists is not surprising (Cheal, 1991; Glenn, 1987; Stacey, 1986).

Feminist scholars have contributed to our understanding of women's experiences in families by challenging existing paradigms and assumptions. Glenn (1987) asserts that this has been a more complicated task than one might imagine because of the centrality accorded women in families. If women's lives are embedded in families, it is difficult to move women to the center of analysis so that we can understand what women do in families and what families do for and to women (Bridenthal, 1982; Glenn, 1987).

This book attempts to do just that. We examine the ways that women have been dominated and oppressed in families, and, by portraying them as active agents of change, we stress the power and empowerment of women. Flax's (1987) description of the work that feminists must undertake serves as a guide to this project:

> We need to 1) articulate feminist viewpoints of/within the social worlds in which we live; 2) think about how we are affected by these worlds; 3) consider the ways in which how we think about them may be implicated in existing power/knowledge relationships; and 4) imagine ways in which these worlds ought to/can be transformed. (p. 641)

A postmodern feminist perspective guides this investigation of women's relationships, caregiving, sexuality, reproductive decisions, paid and unpaid work, and power, to reveal the dialectical nature of the choices women face in everyday family life. The use of a postmodern feminist perspective to guide the analysis and generate strategies for change may be seen as radical by most traditional family scholars and risky by many feminists. No one theory can guide current and future thinking about families, given the multiplicity of voices and experiences associated with families in postmodern life (Cheal, 1991). Multiple and even contradictory perspectives need to be examined (Harding, 1987b). Provocative though it may be, a postmodern feminist perspective provides a logical, although not final, next step in the push toward the liberation of women and other oppressed groups.

In addition to describing and elaborating women's experiences from a postmodern feminist perspective, we critically examine the consequences of these experiences. Although acknowledging the exploitation of women in families is essential, we pay special attention to processes and outcomes that promote growth and empower women and their families. An empowering synthesis can be achieved only when dichotomized positions are transcended in a way that acknowledges the interdependence and legitimacy of each conflicting position. The underlying assumptions of our approach are that women's needs and goals are equally as valid as those of men and children and that the subjugation of women in families is exploitive.

The greatest challenge we have faced was identifying ways in which gender relations and women's experiences in families can be transformed. A major task was to conceive of social relationships in ways that neither perpetuate adverse consequences of sex-related differences nor obscure their differential effect (Rhode, 1990).

A postmodern feminist perspective is useful in developing strategies for change because it can accommodate a *multiplicity* of approaches aimed at bringing about change at both personal and social levels. At the personal level, individual efforts to resolve conflicting demands and resist oppression lead to new and, ideally, more adaptive ways of being in the world. This process is not linear, however. Crises induced by conflicting demands do not occur only in one aspect of a woman's life or in one relationship. We conceptualize this progression of syntheses not as a chain but as a web. The synchronization of conflicting needs in one relationship is often tied interdependently to the coordination of needs in another. For example, as a woman tries to develop a balance between her infant daughter's need for care and her own desire to return to work, she may be considering simultaneously how her relationship with her partner will be transformed as she tries to meet the demands of work and mothering. An empowering synthesis involves an understanding of interdependence and an acknowledgment of the legitimacy of the needs of each person.

The sociohistorical context influences the individual decisions women make by affecting the real and perceived options that are available to them. The structure of everyday life is dictated, in part, by social institutions that oppress women. Sexism, racism, classism, heterosexism, and ageism have restricted women's access to material resources and positions of power and influence in the world. These limitations on women's rights and choices are played out in their relationships and the ways they resolve conflicting needs. As Hartsock (1986) stated, "Our daily lives are the materialization at a personal level of the features of the social formation as a whole" (p. 10). Part of our intent in writing this book is to make explicit the social forces, often invisible, that influence women's day-to-day experiences (Smith, 1987).

There are reciprocity and reflexivity between individual syntheses and societal change. Although societal beliefs, norms, and opportunities define women's real and perceived options, the choices that women make also influence the direction of societal change. Both individually and collectively, women's decisions may perpetuate or transform social institutions. For example, as more women make the decision to enter the work force and demand quality child care, working becomes a more legitimate option for other women, and child care becomes more available. In addition, women's participation may transform the very nature of work and the environment in which it is done.

A continuing problem for women is the lack of synchronization between micro- and macrolevel changes. Transformations in social norms and social policies occur slowly and lag behind change in individuals and families. A societal response is likely only after a significant number of people with some political power make similar choices that result in similar demands. Throughout this book, we work back and forth between the micro- and macrolevels to consider strategies for empowering women in all aspects of their lives.

This first chapter presents the central focus of the book and explains the use of a postmodern feminist perspective for organizing our ideas and generating strategies for change. Our approach reflects an integration of ideas from family studies, lifespan human development, and feminism. This is a book about women written from a feminist perspective that examines selected ways in which women, throughout their lives, shape and are shaped by their families and the society in which they live. We present women as active constructors of their own reality rather than merely as passive respondents to sociohistorical events and family socialization.

Our perspective is unique in that we incorporate feminist thinking and research from many disciplines and place *women* in the center of vision. The female world, in all its diversity, is largely unexplored (Bernard, 1981). Women are treated as if they were all the same; their experiences are flattened and portrayed as part of the monolithic family that feminists have deconstructed as a myth (Boss & Thorne, 1989; Thorne, 1982).

Also unique to our perspective is a transactional approach (Ehrhardt, 1985), examining not just unidirectional/cause-and-effect relationships or interactional/reciprocal influences, but also connections between and among women, their families, and the wider culture. The transactional approach allows a more comprehensive understanding of the complexity of the forces that shape women's experiences. It provides an opportunity to observe the ways in which women have changed society and helped shape the contours of contemporary families.

POSTMODERN AMERICAN FAMILIES

The growing diversity of household and relationship configurations challenges researchers and scholars to develop a valid and useful definition of "family." Demographic data document the relative scarcity of the traditional nuclear family in the United States, and yet this family form persists in the social consciousness as the standard against which all other families are judged (Allen & Baber, 1992b). The risks of this mythology are significant. Definitions of "family" have important consequences for policy decisions, for the way in which various family configurations are valued or devalued, and for the perpetuation of a false notion of homogeneity in American families.

The use of the plural "families" in the title of this book reflects the postmodern character of American families in the late 20th century (Cheal, 1991; Stacey, 1990). It is meant to convey acknowledgment and inclusion of all variations of intimate and committed relationships among individuals and their children. Plurality signals an attempt to move beyond a static model that opposes "the family" and "alternative lifestyles" to a higher-order construct of sexually based primary relationships in which legal, economic, residential, and parental partnership statuses are seen as variables rather than underlying assumptions (Scanzoni, Polonko, Teachman, & Thompson, 1989). Such a model allows us to analyze women's relationships as they actually exist in contemporary society and to acknowledge and savor their diversity rather than trying to fit them into a rigid notion of family.

HOW OPPRESSION CONSTRAINS WOMEN'S LIVES

Racism, classism, sexism, ageism, and heterosexism are interlocking biases of a dominant culture that stratify and objectify individuals in society. Stratification and domination lead to oppression of groups defined as subordinate by those with greater control over their own lives and the lives of others. The greater power of these elites includes differential access to resources, opportunities, and rewards as well as the power to name and define phenomena and experience (Collins, 1990; Ferguson, 1991; Ferree, 1990).

Systems of oppression are linked to personal meanings and structural aspects of race, class, gender, and sexuality. These systems justify the "right" of certain groups to have greater authority to define, govern, and control others. Typically, this authority accrues to those who are white, elite, heterosexual, and/or male. This racist, capitalist, and patriarchal macrostructure interacts dialectically with microprocesses that place greater value on that which is associated with a privileged group (Ferguson, 1991).

Women's oppression refers to the beliefs, attitudes, and acts that exclude women in general from experiences and activities that enhance their growth and development, their access to resources, and their access to positions of power (Lott, 1987). The oppression of women results from a complex system of structures, processes, relations, and ideologies, not just from men's control over women (Dahlerup, 1987). Today the process of domination may be invisible and often unintended, yet it still results in men benefiting from women's service and adaptation to their needs. Dahlerup (1987) argues that the transition from personal patriarchy to structural patriarchy means that individual women may not feel deprived of power and control by any individual man or group of men and that some men may be dominated by their female partners or employers.

Women also may be oppressed by other women. In hierarchical systems, individuals who are in elite positions are always at risk of oppressing and exploiting those who are less privileged. For example, women of color claim exclusion, silencing, and the distortion of their experiences by white middle-class feminists (Dill, 1983; Hurtado, 1989; Lugones & Spelman, 1983). Rollins's (1985) work on black domestics and their white employers and Nelson's (1990) study of women who operate family day-care homes for the children of mothers who work outside the home are two examples that reveal the intersection of gender, race, and class oppression.

The exploitation of women in families is not a uniformly experienced phenomenon. Oppression varies for different women and may be manifested differently over time (Glenn, 1987). Even in a patriarchal society, women appear to dominate the family arena (Dahlerup, 1987), but in reality they may have power and control only in the areas that are of no interest or consequence to their male partners. Adams (1986) points out that the vast majority of U.S. married couples, with the exception of the more egalitarian black middle-class family, still "engaged in either traditional or neo-traditional roles" (p. 244), in which the wife is responsible for both domestic and occupational jobs but the husband is responsible for his paid position only. Part of what makes this issue problematic is the fact that for many women the very aspects of family life that oppress them also offer confirmation and fulfillment.

FEMINIST CONSCIOUSNESS

There is a pervasive tension for women surrounding decisions about commitment, caring, and balancing conflicting needs. Individual women's degree of conscious awareness of this tension and the extent to which their choices are constrained vary considerably. Our feminist approach acknowledges this tension and encourages women to explore the aspects of their own lives that constrain or empower them in making growth-promoting syntheses.

A redefinition of the self and an acceptance of the legitimacy of one's own needs affect each area of a woman's life and call into question all of her relationships (Hartsock, 1986). This disruption can be threatening, not only to those whose needs the woman has been serving, but also to the woman herself. If women are socialized to believe that they exist to meet the needs of others and that others love them *because* they are selfless, who will love them or even tolerate them if they give their own needs equal value and take on the determination of their own lives (Miller, 1986)? If one's sense of self depends primarily on others' approval and acceptance, fear of the loss of a relationship strikes at the core of a woman's identity.

Acknowledging an active role in the process of change can also make women uncomfortable as they face the burden of responsibility that accompanies *deliberate* choice. If a woman feels coerced to have an abortion because her partner does not want a child, she may feel sadness, anger, and loss but not necessarily a sense of responsibility for ending the pregnancy. However, if the woman deliberately chooses to abort, particularly if her partner wants to have the child, she is likely to feel a tremendous responsibility for resolving the conflict among her rights, those of her partner, and those of the developing fetus.

Regardless of the discomfort involved, women derive a sense of power and energy from the realization that they can effect change (Hartsock, 1986). This empowerment is enhanced as women break the silence and isolation in which many have lived and come together to share their experiences. This book seeks to extend these discussions of women's experiences by acknowledging and making explicit the tension between constraint and opportunity in women's lives.

OUR FEMINIST PERSPECTIVE: POSTMODERNISM AND BEYOND

Although feminist perspectives range from liberal to socialist to radical, three common feminist themes regarding women and their experiences are stressed in this book: (1) a belief that women are exploited and oppressed as subordinates in a hierarchical system that affords privilege to more valued groups, particularly elite white males; (2) a commitment to empower women and change the conditions of their lives; and (3) an acknowledgment of women's experiences, values, and activities as meaningful and important (Acker, Barry, & Esseveld, 1983).

Generally, feminist inquiries are guided by a belief system about the nature of reality—what we know and how we come to know it. The three models of feminist epistemology most often recognized are feminist empiricism, feminist standpoint theories, and feminist postmodernism (Flax, 1987; Hawkesworth, 1989). These theories of knowledge offer competing and sometimes contradictory strategies for understanding women's lives and addressing social inequities (Harding, 1987b).

Feminist empiricism is a revision of traditional scientific methods based on the assumption that there is an objective reality that can be revealed through the use of systematic observation, experimentation, and recording of data. Feminist empiricists maintain that the use of appropriate scientific methods to address issues of importance and relevance to women can eliminate sexist and androcentric biases and make possible a truer understanding of reality. Although feminist empiricists argue that traditional mainstream methodologies need not be incompatible with radical critiques of social life (Peplau & Conrad, 1989), alternative approaches may be necessary to locate and eradicate biases that ignore or marginalize women and their experiences (Harding, 1987b).

Feminist standpoint theories comprise a second belief system about how individuals come to know the world around them. Feminist standpoint theories reject the idea of "unmediated truth" and assert that what we know and how we know it depend on our position in the social hierarchy (Hawkesworth, 1989). Those in positions of power have a distorted understanding of reality, whereas those who are oppressed have a unique and privileged vantage point from which to understand social experience. Although there are various explanations for why oppressed individuals have more comprehensive and less distorted knowledge, the strongest argument rests on the assumption that people who are subjugated, such as women, blacks, and lesbians, live out their lives in both the dominant culture and their own subculture and must be attuned to both. As a result, they come to have a type of double vision that allows them to pierce distortions and have a clearer view of reality (Brown, 1989a; Collins, 1990; Marecek, 1989). The dominant group lacks this more complete understanding because they need not bother developing awareness of, knowledge about, or sensitivity to the subordinate group unless the power balance begins to shift.

An important but neglected aspect of standpoint theories is that the double vision that privileges subordinated groups must be acquired through education, consciousness-raising, and political struggle (Harding, 1987b; Nielsen, 1990). As a result of the intellectual and pragmatic work that women do on issues relevant to their lives, they come to have a new, shared understanding of the world and their relationships due to their particular sociohistorical location.

Feminist standpoint theories assume that women are fundamentally like one another by virtue of their sex and essentially different from men, who are the oppressors (Flax, 1987). Women are seen to have a privileged understanding because of their oppression. However, the assumption that women's ways of being or doing are better than men's is risky. What has been characterized as distinctively female behavior, responses, or reasoning may be the result rather than the cause of social inequality; centuries of oppression may have shaped women's cognitive, emotional, and physical abilities, resulting in the perceived differences between women and men (Flax, 1987; Hawkesworth, 1989; Jaggar, 1990).

Feminist empiricist and standpoint theories ignore differences among women and "falsely universalize" the experiences of those who develop the theories, usually educated, white, middle-class women (Fraser & Nicholson, 1990). Guided by a third model of feminist theory, postmodern feminists reject the notion of one privileged standpoint and the idea that women are, as a group and for whatever reason, less prone to distortion and error in their understanding of reality (Hawkesworth, 1989). From a postmodern feminist perspective, gender is not a natural fact, rooted in anatomical sex differences (Flax, 1987). Gender alone does not determine women's experiences, identity, or status; the way a woman constructs her understanding of reality is mediated by factors such as her age, class, race, physical attractiveness, sexual orientation, and family status. There is no single standpoint that captures women's experiences, nor is there a single mode of feminism or path to a feminist consciousness (Hawkesworth, 1989). At any time, "there are many 'subjugated knowledges' that conflict with, and are never reflected in, the dominant stories a culture tells about social life" (Harding, 1987b, p. 188).

The tension among the various epistemologies is apparent and lies at the heart of postmodern approaches. The challenge of competing epistemologies can be viewed as an indication of healthy intellectual ferment in feminist theory (Harding, 1987b). Postmodernism embraces the ambivalence, paradox, and heterogeneity that is generated and rejects reductionism and naive dualisms. The blending of postmodernism's sophisticated and persuasive critique of essentialism with feminism's social analysis and call to action provides a powerful tool for exploring women's experiences in families (Fraser & Nicholson, 1990). It is, however, controversial.

The Risk of a Postmodern Feminist Perspective

Feminists approach postmodernism with ambivalence. Paradoxically, "feminists can and cannot be postmodernist" (Gagnier, 1990, p. 23). The bottom line of feminism is that women's oppression as a group exists, and efforts to improve the world for women have relied on solidarity, shared values, and common goals among women. Some argue that as postmodern feminism deconstructs the category "woman" it fragments women's experiences and identities, undermines solidarity, and downplays the consequences of the long-term imbalance of power between the sexes (Harding, 1987a; Hawkesworth, 1989; Offen, 1990).

Postmodernism risks sliding into a relativism that accepts that all claims to truth may be equally valid. Because such relativism is antithetical to the feminist goal of the liberation of women, the challenge is to try to distinguish between partial views, on the one hand, and "false beliefs, superstitions, irrebuttable presumptions, willful distortions," (Hawkesworth, 1989, p. 555) on the other. All truth claims do not carry the same justificatory force. Feminists can use critical reflection and rational argument to illuminate the problems in social relations and identify the inaccuracies in opposing accounts (Hawkesworth, 1989).

We see this central paradox, rather than serving as an impediment to our work in this book, as a *corrective* for the blinders imposed by our own private experiences. To begin with a belief in the limitations of our own perspective requires us to explore critically and systematically existing social relations, contradictory viewpoints, and accepted explanations. Such an approach offers emancipatory potential without the expectation that we abandon our own experiences and constructions of reality.

The Promise of a Postmodern Feminist Perspective

As a way of thinking about self and social relations transhistorically, postmodernism provides a way to understand and construct "the self, gender, knowledge, social relations, and culture without resorting to linear, teleological, hierarchical, holistic, or binary ways of thinking and being." (Flax, 1987, p. 622). Rejecting holism and universalism, postmodernism captures the ambiguity, contradiction, and dialectics of women's lives. Because all women do not share the same past or the same needs in the present, different women's conceptions of caregiving, sexuality, work, and other experiences capture different aspects of complex and contradictory social relations (Flax, 1987).

A postmodern feminist approach allows us, as collaborators, to take a point of view, situated in our own lives, without claiming to speak for all women. Our knowledge claims are thus partial, fragmented, and incomplete (Flax, 1990). However, our feminist oppositions and our analyses of the obstacles to women's full participation in all aspects of social, political, and economic life will add to the work of others in the joint project of identifying inequity, resisting oppression, and empowering women (Harding, 1987b).

Postmodernism sensitizes us to "the embeddedness and dependence of the self upon social relations, as well as the partiality and historical specificity of this self's existence" (Flax, 1987, p. 626). The emphasis on social relations is a critique of a former way of seeing and thinking as well as a new way of looking at the self in relation to others and the world. Postmodernism is a reaction to and a revision of ideas inherited from the Enlightenment. Primary among these ideas is the belief in the existence of a stable coherent self and method (science) used to describe and understand the self and its relationship to the world (Flax, 1987). Postmodernists, by contrast, assume that one's sense of self and relations with others are constructed and reconstructed through social interaction— always changing and reconfiguring.

Gender is an important facet of self that affects how life is experienced. Feminist theory challenges the prevailing ideology that there is some universal experience of reality by showing how only one standard of experience, primarily that of males, has dominated social relations. Postmodern feminists have now begun the process of deconstructing the unquestioned belief in the gendered duality of women's and men's experience. Gender is no longer reified as two categories of experience or "an opposition of inherently different beings" (Flax, 1987, p. 641) but rather as a type of social relation that is constantly in process.

Construction and Deconstruction

The concepts of construction and deconstruction are fundamental to postmodernism and promise to be important and useful tools for feminists interested in a deeper and broader understanding of women's lives. At the heart of these concepts are the notions that infuse this book: dialectic, contradiction, paradox, debate, and difference.

Constructivism posits that perceptions of reality are invented through selecting, ordering, and organizing information; knowledge, truth, power, and social relations, therefore, are created rather than discovered or revealed (Flax, 1987; Hare-Mustin & Marecek, 1990).

Individuals are seen as actively involved in constructing their own systems of meaning and as influenced by their gender and other hierarchies of power such as race, class, and sexual orientation (cf. Blumstein & Schwartz, 1983; Collins, 1990; Ferree, 1990; Fishman, 1978; Glenn, 1987). Groups with the most power in a society control the constructions of reality that dictate distribution of resources and opportunities. By maintaining power, privileged groups can suppress belief systems that challenge their own.

These prevailing belief systems can be contested through the process of deconstruction. By methodically analyzing and decomposing concepts and constructions of reality that are accepted as natural and unchangeable, a reevaluation of existing social relations is possible. Beliefs and ideas that are taken for granted and used to legitimate existing social arrangements are called into question (Bordo, 1990; Flax, 1987; Tong, 1989).

Feminist deconstruction of the family has begun the process of exposing how "gender hierarchies and structures of subordination systematically affect interaction and definitions of reality" (Glenn, 1987, p. 356). The feminist project of deconstructing prevailing ideas about women and families addresses the mystification that the ideology of marriage and motherhood brings. The relatively unexplored dimensions of women's intimate connections in adulthood have received new attention that liberates women's lives from the perspective of "wives sociology" (Safilios-Rothschild, 1969). Feminist revisions of the family have made more visible the female world that Bernard (1981) described.

Decoding existing knowledge and asking new questions about women's lives leave little room for generalizing to universal aspects of women's experiences. It used to be enough to describe the typical scenario of women's intimate lives as following a series of developmental stages in the marital and parental career. Prevailing ideas about the "normative" developmental pathway for women included lifelong involvement in childrearing and caregiving, finding and moving through life with a husband, and attending to the kinship network (Duvall, 1971; Glick, 1977). This scenario captured the stereotype and cultural ideology of woman's essence as that of a natural caregiver, but it masks the diversity across women's experiences, as many revisions of family development have described (Allen, 1989; Elder, 1977; Hareven, 1987, 1991; Lopata, 1987; Mattessich & Hill, 1987).

The deconstruction process reveals the plurality of women's beliefs and experiences in arenas such as sexuality, caregiving, and work. This exposure offers a rich and complex picture of these aspects of women's lives and challenges the notion of unitary, homogeneous understandings of day-to-day life and power relations. Being open to this plurality means that discordant voices may be heard. Although the suppression of differences may be necessary to present a coherent, unified front to address oppression, it may also explain why many women have difficulty identifying with feminist agendas (Flax, 1987; Fraser & Nicholson, 1990).

The Social Construction of Difference

The issue of difference is another controversial topic in feminist discourse. For most feminists, the compelling aspects of gender relations have been the continuing examination of sex differences and the related prescriptions for gender justice. There is no consensus about whether true gender differences exist. Many feminists believe that there are basic, undeniable differences between women and men. Other vocal proponents claim that women and men are more similar than different and that any differences that do exist are socially constructed as the result of differential opportunities and experiences.

Hare-Mustin and Marecek (1990) have problemized gender dichotomies in their postmodern feminist rethinking of family therapy and psychology. They identify a central paradox embedded within ideas about gender by using an alpha–beta scheme that is similar to type I and type II errors in scientific hypothesis testing. The alpha and beta concepts are called "biases" to emphasize the belief that all ideas about difference are social constructions. Alpha bias exaggerates the differences between women and men by characterizing them as having essentially opposite natures. Beta bias is the inclination to ignore and minimize differences. Beta bias occurs when the social context and actual differences between women and men are overlooked.

Alpha and beta biases present both utility and risk for gender analyses. Although alpha bias has fostered solidarity among women and an appreciation for "feminine qualities," it also sets women apart from men and provides the impetus for depictions of them as less valued or deviant (Hare-Mustin & Marecek, 1990). Women are seen as "other" in relation to men. Man is the standard bearer, and woman is defined as "not-man."

Psychoanalytic theories are the prototypical examples of alpha bias. These theories hypothesize women and men as occupying inherently different roles in society that are predicated on their essentially different natures. Feminist revisions of the classic psychodynamic theories of Freud, Erikson, and Kohlberg are a corrective for the ways in which women's lives have been ignored or distorted but still assume basic differences between women and men. Thus, Gilligan's (1982) theory of an ethic of care emphasizes ways in which women tend to think about morality in relational terms, juxtaposing women's and men's styles as rooted in their differential natures. Similarly, Chodorow (1978) roots her theory of early childrearing and parenting arrangements in the fact that women mother and men are shadowy figures in a child's life, which leads to the creation of oppositional personalities for women and men. Women become capable of fusing with another, whereas men, early in life, learn to separate and become autonomous.

Alpha bias springs from locating the cause of these differential outcomes in women's body and internal makeup. As a consequence of alpha bias, women are seen as somehow deficient in comparison to men, and sex differences are portrayed as relatively stable and unchanging (Kahn & Yoder, 1989). At its feminist extreme, women's linkage to caregiving concerns and institutions sets them up as morally superior. In this way, feminists fall into the essentialism trap they originally sought to avoid.

Beta bias minimizes differences. Because it is manifested in gender-neutral laws, beta bias has been responsible for many of the advances that women have made in gaining greater access to educational and occupational opportunities (Hare-Mustin & Marecek, 1990). Psychologists such as Maccoby and Jacklin (1974) have attempted to deemphasize difference by distinguishing allegedly real differences between women and men from stereotypes. Ignoring differences can be problematic because some differences *do* make a difference in everyday life. Minimizing differences often means that power dynamics and control are obscured. For example, in family systems theory and therapy, gender is disregarded as a way in which families are ordered (Hare-Mustin & Marecek, 1990). Yet, mothers and wives generally have less access to power and resources both within and outside the family. Even Bem (1987) has rethought her original proposal of psychological androgyny because it conflated masculine traits with androgynous ones and thus ignored the unequal and devalued ways in which so-called feminine traits are treated.

To some extent, the polarization of these competing ideologies is rooted in different epistemologies and different methodologies. Hare-Mustin and Marecek (1990) point out that alpha bias seems to be associated with qualitative investigations and beta bias with quantitative ones. Alpha bias appears related to biological explanations of sex differences, whereas beta bias seems to have sociocultural origins. Both perspectives, however, contribute to reified stances that keep feminists involved in arguing with each other, with the unfortunate result of maintaining the status quo of women's devalued situation and men's domination (Flax, 1987).

A third approach to addressing the "difference dilemma" is to reject the categorical opposition of male/female and refuse to ignore or embrace difference as it is normatively constituted. Scott (1990) proposes that deconstructing gender difference is necessary and shows it to be an opposition that is socially constructed for particular purposes in particular contexts. The goal is to unmask the power relationship that first constructed the duality and subsequently claimed that, given the difference, there can be no equality. Gender distinctions are not denied but are seen in the context of the variety of within-gender differences that "confound, disrupt, and render ambiguous the meaning of any fixed binary opposition" (Scott, 1990, p. 146).

This third approach to construing difference is consistent with a postmodern feminist perspective. It introduces a metalevel that transcends the polarization of difference versus similarity and critiques the very process of creating the opposition. Paradox and multiple consciousness are embraced. The discordance and contradiction of opposing ideologies and competing strategies for change are accommodated (Harding, 1987b). As Hare-Mustin and Marecek (1988) claim, "there is no one right view of gender, but various views that present certain paradoxes" (p. 462).

A focus on difference perpetuates the perception of gender as an individual characteristic rather than a social construction (Hare-Mustin & Marecek, 1988). Therefore, it is important to be skeptical about this approach despite its usefulness. Postmodern feminism problemizes gender without ignoring the differences among women and men, takes a critical stance toward prevailing assumptions about the uniqueness or similarity of female and male, and considers the implications of the perspectives that are used to generate strategies for change.

The promise of postmodern feminism, then, is that gender can be construed in previously unimagined ways (Flax, 1987; Hare-Mustin & Marecek, 1988). For this book, it means no longer taking as given women's key roles and identities as strictly wives and mothers. Deconstruction of the concept "family" reveals the diversity of contemporary relationship configurations and expands our understanding of families by insisting on the incorporation of missing voices. It means, for example, taking issue with a central distortion in family social science: the exclusion of lesbians. Writing about lesbian existence and experience at once uncovers the invisibility of lesbians and acknowledges ways of life that are less male dominated. Thus, the choice to include the experiences of lesbians as mothers, workers, childbearers, and lovers has both a corrective purpose (adding certain female experience to our knowledge base) and a vision of change (lesbian pathways are mystified by the dominant culture as deviant, punishable, and despised).

In a similar way, motherhood is deconstructed as a defining role for women. The emphasis is shifted away from compulsory motherhood and toward an empowering range of options in regard to children. This approach is again corrective (acknowledging the pluralism in women's thinking and desires regarding caregiving) and visionary (caregiving as a choice and parenting as a project that is entered into willingly and knowingly).

Men and their roles in women's lives are construed in ways that are less distorted by dualistic thinking and more accepting of the complexities of female–male relationships. Obviously, men are important players in most women's family lives. One cannot comprehensively explore intimate relationships, reproductive issues, heterosexuality, or many other relevant topics without discussing men and their roles and activities. However, our goal in writing this book is to move women and their experiences in families to the center of attention. A postmodern feminist perspective that conceives of group alliances not as identities but rather as affinities and coalitions (Gagnier, 1990) means that supportive men can work with women as allies in achieving the feminist goal of equality and in constructing new understandings of gender relations, class relations, and race relations. Thus, men have a secondary place in our writing. In the tradition of sociologist Jessie Bernard (1981), we are participating in "a kind of intellectual affirmative action" (p. 14). Women's lives and experiences are important and worthy of study and analysis in and of themselves.

OUR FEMINIST METHOD

Feminist research embraces women's subjective knowledge of their own lives and thereby expands understanding of the actual experiences of women to replace what has been distorted and falsely constructed in the past with a grounded understanding of women's everyday existence (Smith, 1987; Thompson, 1992). In this book, we write about women in both concrete and analytic ways. Our perspective is both informed and limited by our own unique life experiences. What we know and how we know it derive from our "historical locus and our position in the social hierarchy" (Marecek, 1989, p. 372). We operate with a double consciousness. We have been trained and socialized in a privileged society of scholars, but we are critical of the ways in which our experiences and knowledge as women have been devalued and distorted. We are both insider and outsider, a perspective that provides a rich knowledge and insight but one that is tempered by self-criticism and doubt (Westkott, 1979). Dual loyalties push us to analyze critically traditional and feminist research in an attempt to provide a more complex picture of women's experiences in families.

Sensitivity to exclusion from socially valued practices and institutions lends a "detective's eye" (Thorne, 1985) to the process of renaming women's experience. Feminist scholars are like archeologists; as we begin to uncover and chart the realities of women's lives, we recognize how hidden, inaccessible, suppressed, distorted, misunderstood, and ignored the facts about women's lives have been (Du Bois, 1983). This archeological endeavor of learning to see anew proceeds communally, not in an isolated, abstract, individual way. Rather, it is mostly a collaborative effort, as we work together to enhance our critical eye (Bograd, 1988a). As authors of this book, we maintained a dialogue about our understanding of the knowledge we incorporated. We describe our method to demystify the construction of knowledge for this book and to make our process of collaboration accessible. By doing so, we attempt to put ourselves on the same critical plane as our subject matter and place ourselves "within the frame of the picture we are trying to paint" (Harding, 1987a, p. 9) so that our beliefs and values become open to critical scrutiny.

Feminist practice requires that the "description of what we see needs to be careful, detailed, rigorous. . . . Our work needs to generate words, concepts that refer to, that spring from, that are firmly and richly grounded in the actual experiences of women" (Du Bois, 1983, p. 110). A core component of feminist research is its social relevance (Acker et al., 1983). Feminist scholarship is for women, not simply about women (Smith, 1987; Walker, Martin, & Thompson, 1988; Westkott, 1979). We seek to provide information about women's experiences in families that will be useful to women in making choices in their own lives. Because we believe that action is critical to bringing about change that will be advantageous to women, we give priority to issues that have a liberatory purpose.

Feminists attempt to do more than describe oppressive conditions. Knowledge must not stop at "a doleful catalogue of the facts of patriarchy" (Westkott, 1979, p. 428) but must provide imaginative alternatives that suggest how women themselves have changed and how they have resisted or neutralized the forces that control their lives and constrain their options.

In writing this book, we have selected resources from a woman's perspective that place women in the center of vision as unique subjects of study themselves (Westkott, 1979), that view their everyday lives as problematic (Smith, 1987), and that employ consciousness-raising as the primary practice in transforming personal awareness into political action (MacKinnon, 1982). Interdisciplinary in the selection of evidence we bring to bear on a particular topic, we draw from traditional research journals; radical, socialist, and liberal feminist writings; and current news reports to explore the subject from a variety of perspectives. We sometimes juxtapose quantitative and qualitative research to provide both the broad strokes of the larger issue and the detail and texture of the in-depth study.

Respecting Multiple Voices

Women are not a homogeneous group. Speaking of them as though they are obscures the richness of their thinking, experiences, and contributions and oppresses women who are not allowed to speak in their own voices. In keeping with a postmodern feminist perspective, we make the point that there is no *woman's* voice, no *woman's* story, but rather a multitude of voices that sometimes speak together but often must speak separately. What is oppressive for one group of women may not be perceived as oppressive by another group; what is meaningful and salient for some may not be for others. Feminist theories must not reflect only our own values or make prescriptions for social change based on our own experiences and perceptions of what is wrong in family life (Lugones & Spelman, 1983).

Hurtado (1989) provides an eloquent example of the ethnocentricity and classism of white feminist theory in her critique of the public/private distinction that has been at the heart of white feminist discourse. She asserts that the notion of "the personal is political"—the idea that what happens in the privacy of the family is not exempt from political forces in society—is relevant only for white middle and upper classes because of the history of intervention by the State in the lives of working-class families: "Women of color have not had the benefit of economic conditions that underlie the public/private distinction. Instead, the political consciousness of women of color stems from an awareness that the public is *personally* political" (p. 849). This distinction results in different political groundings and consciousness, as well as different skills for dealing with oppression.

In an attempt to acknowledge multiplicity in women's lives, we try, in each chapter of this book, to attend to variations related to age, life phase, sexual orientation, social class, and race. Where appropriate, we use narratives from our own and others' qualitative studies of women's lives to illustrate key themes. We allow women to speak for themselves, as much as possible, to avoid homogenization of women's experiences from our own perspectives as two white, professional, middle-class women (Lugones & Spelman, 1983). However, to appeal to a wide and diverse audience and to facilitate an integrated "voice" throughout the book, we also emphasize the commonality in women's experiences. Our approach is informed by Runyan's (1984) three levels of generality: what is universal for all members of a society (in this case women), what is particular to groups (i.e., by race, class, generation, sexual orientation, marital status, etc.), and what is unique to individuals.

Feminists have long been critical of traditional family arrangements (Flax, 1982; Thorne & Yalom, 1982). Yet, in the process of reconstructing the family as a center of abuse and violence as well as intimacy and nurturance, the family has been depreciated as a focus of study. We are especially attuned to the double risk of this topic. Not only are women devalued as members of families, but also the discipline of family studies is marginalized, particularly because it is seen as primarily a study of women. Here, as feminist family scholars, we oppose ourselves: We oppose feminists who devalue families, and we oppose family scholars who devalue women. This dialectical tension assists in presenting ideas and research about women's lives with a goal toward uncovering mystifications of women's experiences in their families and their own efforts toward emancipation.

An illustration of this process of redefining reality comes from the work of feminist scholars in the area of wife abuse. Although male sociologists such as Gelles and Strauss (1988) have done pioneering work in the area of family violence, it is feminist activists who acknowledged the extensive abuse that many women and girls experience in their homes (Kelly, 1988). Childhood sexual abuse, incest, and marital rape were not even conceptualized as problems, except in pathological and idiosyncratic ways, until women working in shelters and cooperatives began to recognize the pattern of abuse. Undertaking a study to allow definitions of violence to emerge from women themselves, Kelly (1988) asked questions, such as "Have you ever been forced to have sex?" as opposed to stereotypical inquiries, such as "Have you ever been raped?" By interviewing women on subsequent occasions and sharing the interview transcriptions, the women achieved a greater consciousness of their own abuse histories. As women acknowledged their abuse, they had a forum for examining it, coping with it, and developing precautionary ways to prevent future abuse. Remembering and redefining experiences of violence were facilitated through this research process. Many women became empowered by feeling and expressing anger for the first time and by reassigning responsibility for their abuse from themselves to the perpetrators. These experiences led to increased efforts to take control over their own lives. Through a feminist research study, women participated in their own liberation. The researcher and the respondents worked collaboratively to politicize what was formerly considered a private experience.

A book for and about women and their families from a feminist perspective is, indeed, not simply a review of literature. This book reveals ways in which women not only cope with oppression but also empower themselves to create ways to survive and live in contemporary society. We also identify family issues that may become salient for women in the future in order to be proactive rather than merely reactive in advocating for women.

All aspects of women's experiences in families cannot be addressed in one book. Therefore, we address those that seem to be most salient for most women, many of which involve political struggles. Some of the most controversial issues in our society today revolve around social policies that have the power to limit women's opportunities to act in their own best interests. In light of this, we have made a special effort to include analyses of relevant social policies.

Strategies for Change

Women must make personal and social choices about how they will address the political struggle necessary for their growth and development. Some women have chosen to work within existing social institutions to enhance women's opportunities and acknowledge their accomplishments. Others have directly challenged and struggled against these institutions, resisted coercion, and attempted to replace oppressive institutions with alternatives more responsive to women's needs and experiences. An additional group of women have made the more radical choice to separate themselves from individuals and institutions that oppress and exploit them. Although proponents of each strategy may argue for the greater effectiveness of their tactics, each of these approaches can be credited with changing and improving the status of women. Rather than devaluing strategies that women have used by suggesting that they are not the right tactics, we present a variety of responses that are representative of contemporary women's attempts to bring about change.

A postmodern feminist approach to change suggests the utility of creating coalitions with others who are oppressed. Such alliances would not be limited by gender identity but might cut across other axes to create groups characterized by fluidity in their ability to mobilize and disperse as necessary (Gagnier, 1990). Coalitions need to be built among groups who share a marginalized status. Otherwise, each group's particularistic commitment to "identity politics" can lead to cultural separatism, cooptation, or repression by the dominant culture (Ferguson, 1991). To make an effective effort toward changing the economic, political, and social structures of the status quo, countercultural movements must not become static, self-enclosed subcultures in which each new group pursues its own self-affirmation or validates its own reality. The problem in asserting difference is the slide into relativism and the eventual endorsement of the very status quo that marginalized groups first questioned and attempted to change. Such groups must work together so that individual efforts toward self-validation will not dilute each other or the bigger project of human liberation, justice, and pluralism. Thus, overlapping groups of feminists, lesbians, African-Americans, and activist youth, to name just a few, must work simultaneously from their own particular standpoint and toward solidarity so that these combined coalitions will be an effective affront to the status quo (Ferguson, 1991).

In keeping with this goal, Ferguson (1991) sketched a "new vision of an ideal society" in contrast to the racist, capitalist, and patriarchal reality that exists in postindustrial, late-20th-century America. This new vision is based on decentralized democratic socialism and sexual democracy in which privileges are redistributed among all people and no longer held in the hands of a few powerful elite males. Pluralism in how people choose to live on a personal basis is tolerated and respected.

To achieve the new reality and revolutionize the dominant culture of today, Ferguson (1991) calls for a "transitional morality of appropriate ways to live our lives in the process of struggling" (p. 245) for democratic pluralism. The new values she advocates are respect, self-determination, and pluralism. These values are "bottom-line ways" (p. 246) of treating others who are engaged in the struggle for building a populist, antiracist, and antisexist politics. Members of the new social movements seek a new definition and enactment of justice in Western industrialized societies; they include women's movements, antinuclear movements, radical ecologists, ethnic movements, lesbian and gay rights movements, and counter-cultural groups in general (White, 1991).

We view this book as an effort toward social change that will benefit women and, by doing so, enhance the lives of their partners, children, and other loved ones. Each chapter addresses an arena of women's lives that is central to their experiences in families. We begin by exploring women's intimate relationships and their centrality to other aspects of their lives. Sexuality and childbearing issues are dealt with in separate chapters to emphasize that, although they are deeply intertwined, women's sexuality and their reproductive decisions deserve individual consideration and study. Next, a chapter on caregiving and its role in women's lives more specifically identifies the dialectical aspects of caring that are a central theme of the book as a whole. A sixth chapter investigates the tensions in women's paid and unpaid work, another critical arena in women's family lives.

The real opportunity for disrupting the integrated forces that oppress women lies in bringing about change in many arenas of their lives simultaneously (Dahlerup, 1987). The last chapter of this book considers approaches to doing this. We synthesize the key ideas in this book, taking stock of the feminist project to deconstruct and reconstruct families from the perspective of women. Our goal is not to reiterate solutions but to suggest strategies and highlight approaches that seem to hold the greatest promise for enriching and empowering women and their families.

Women's Intimate Adult Relationships

A desire for reciprocity in close relationships is an integral theme woven through women's lives. Females learn the value of connectedness early and find intense meaning in loving interactions. A female's first primary relationship, typically, is with her mother (Chodorow, 1978), providing early socialization toward homosociality and creating the potential for fusion in relationships with other women. Paradoxically, by early adulthood women are expected to turn their intimacy needs toward a male partner (Rubin, 1983). Using skills developed primarily in interaction with other females, women attempt to build close relationships with adult partners and expect to find happiness and security in a close and committed partnership.

What most women seek are mutuality and a commitment to involvement in the depth and breadth of a loving relationship with another adult. Mutuality involves reciprocal empathy and concern and requires flexibility, emotional availability, and interaction (Jordan, 1991). Intense mutual interest and involvement provide a foundation for ongoing interdependence between partners.

Mutuality is difficult to achieve, however, if a sense of equity and reciprocal self-disclosure is missing from the relationship. Differential socialization of females and males, combined with social inequality between women and men, makes it difficult for heterosexual couples to achieve true intimacy and mutuality. Women are taught to be self-sacrificing, to cultivate their emotional lives, and to discuss their feelings. Men learn to compete for what they want and "to camouflage their feelings under cover of an exterior of calm, strength, and rationality" (Rubin, 1983, p. 71). Paradoxically, women and men are then expected to live together, communicate clearly their needs and concerns, and negotiate economic, sexual, reproductive, parental, and social demands in their day-to-day lives together.

Traditional ideology about the family equates women with the roles of wife and mother. Yet, marriage is only one way that women meet their intimacy needs (Bernard, 1972, 1977, 1981; Blumstein & Schwartz, 1983; Cuber & Harroff, 1965; Rubin, 1976). Although most women eventually marry, a significant proportion of women forgo marriage altogether; not all women remain married, and many do not marry again after divorce (Cherlin, 1981). Furthermore, as evidence on extramarital relationships, women's friendships, and lesbian relationships suggests, being married does not mean necessarily that a woman's primary emotional or sexual attachment is to her husband (Faderman, 1981; Rubin, 1983). Acknowledging the diversity of women's relationships requires that marriage and motherhood not be depicted as the exclusive or only normal way to live (Taggart, 1989).

A postmodern feminist analysis of women's experiences in families demands a critical reconsideration of marriage as a context for women's social health and well-being. Traditional marriage has served the interests of women, but often not well, and there have been significant costs— some hidden, some obvious and deeply felt. What is the current status of marriage in women's lives? How viable is marriage as a life choice for women? What types of marriages have women and their partners constructed? How are women changing their marriages to enhance their lives and maximize the likelihood of achieving greater intimacy and mutuality?

Feminist decomposition of the family suggests that intimate relationships are not static, fixed, or experienced in a universal way (Thorne, 1982). Attachments change and are transformed over the life course (Lopata, 1987). As women age, and as the sociohistorical context shifts, there is greater variation in how women meet their intimacy needs than is reflected in the role and status of wife.

Heterosexual cohabitation without marriage is becoming an increasingly popular option in the United States. During the last decade, the number of cohabiting, unmarried heterosexual couples increased 80% to stand at 2.9 million in 1990 (Saluter, 1991). Although some cohabitants may live together to test their compatibility before marriage (Bumpass, Sweet, & Cherlin, 1991), others choose cohabitation without marriage as a lifestyle alternative. Cohabitation allows freedom and flexibility for both partners, and termination costs are low relative to legal marriage. However, living together requires little overt commitment and provides minimal long-term security to a partner dependent on the relationship.

Cohabitation may be seen as more advantageous to men than to women based on the stereotypical assumption that males and females are seeking different benefits in an intimate relationship. For women of the 1990s, however, this may not be so. Cohabitation offers a viable lifestyle for women who are not ready or willing to make a permanent commitment to a partner. How does cohabitation benefit women? What are the varieties of cohabitation? What are the tensions that pull women to marriage rather than cohabitation?

Although most women do seek a primary intimate, sexual relationship with a man (Stacey, 1986), many women continue to maintain their closest ties with other women. Women's intimate connections to other women, as friends and lovers, are often ignored or treated as irrelevant in the prevailing literature about families (Acker, Barry, & Esseveld, 1979; Bart, 1971; Rich, 1979). Male–female relationships traditionally are depicted as central to women's lives, and women's connections to each other are seen as incidental or peripheral.

Feminist analyses have identified for immediate attention "ideologies that serve to mystify women's experiences as wives and mothers, hierarchical divisions that generate conflict and struggle within families; and the multiple and dynamic interconnections between households and the larger political economy" (Glenn, 1987, p. 358). To this agenda, we add the once invisible qualities of women's connections to other women as friends and lovers. By reconsidering structures and processes that promote isolation and competition among women to ensure that they continue to rely on men (Acker et al., 1979; Miner & Longino, 1987), we expand the potential for asking new questions about women's relationships with each other (Voydanoff, 1988). Why are women so adept at meeting one another's emotional needs? Why have lesbian relationships been obscured? In what ways do lesbian relationships develop? What do lesbian and heterosexual relationships have in common, and how do they differ?

Women's and, by extension, families' interests are served by examining women's experiences in a variety of relationship contexts, including those that are obscured by the exclusive focus on so-called normative marital arrangements. In this chapter , we attend to the tension between ideology and the ways in which women actually construct and transmit their social worlds. We examine the dialectic between homosociality (having one's emotional needs met through intimacy with members of the same gender) and heterosociality (having one's emotional needs met through intimacy with members of the other gender).

We also explore the variety of adult connections that women forge with intimate partners. We challenge the normative model of marriage and motherhood as *the* ideal relational configurations for women, explore the contradictory nature of marriage for both heterosexual and lesbian women, and suggest new possibilities for intimate connections that enhance women's happiness and well-being. First, we approach the subject of women and their intimate friendships. The relationships of women with their friends depend mostly on emotional intimacy, although in many variations, particularly in racial/ethnic groups, friends are often converted into kin to foster economic interdependence, a pattern emulated by many other groups in the current postindustrial era.

Following a discussion of several ways in which women share emotional intimacy with friends, we turn to relationships with a sexual component. Our approach reflects growing attempts within family studies to reconstruct and reclaim family and intimacy for individuals by replacing the paradigm of the traditional, nuclear family with the more inclusive concept of primary close relationships (Scanzoni et al., 1989). Consistent with this perspective, we explore women's intimate partnerships that are in some combination emotionally, economically, and sexually interdependent, including heterosexually married, cohabiting, and lesbian relationships.

WOMEN AND THEIR FRIENDS

Women's socialization toward homosociality, or intimacy with other females, has its roots in earlier times (Bernard, 1981; Chambers-Schiller, 1984; Faderman, 1981). Smith-Rosenberg (1975) found that middle- and upper-class women in the 19th century were engaged in "a female world of love and ritual." The worlds of men and women during Victorian times were rigidly segregated. Female "relationships ranged from the supportive love of sisters, through the enthusiasms of adolescent girls, to sensual avowals of love by mature women" (Smith-Rosenberg, 1975, p. 2).

Smith-Rosenberg (1975) analyzed the letters, diaries, and account books of women from 35 families between the 1760s and the 1880s, representing a broad range of the Protestant American middle class at that time. Families from rural and urban geographic regions were included. The focus on middle-class family life is often necessary because testimony about working-class families is rarely deposited in archives (Tentler, 1979). By viewing women's same-sex relationships within a cultural, social, and historical context, Smith-Rosenberg debunked the myth that same-sex intense relationships have always been considered with the suspicion present among late-20th-century Americans. Contemporary ideology is rooted in a post-Freudian analysis that views same-sex relationships within an individual, psychopathological context. In the 20th century, love and sexuality became dichotomized as normal or deviant, platonic or genital—ideas that were foreign to those in the 19th century (Smith-Rosenberg, 1975).

Given the rigid distinctions between female and male lives, supported by the belief that women and men's spheres were determined by the immutable laws of God and nature, a "cult of true womanhood" developed among middle- and upper-class white women that confined them to the home (Welter, 1966). The prescriptions associated with this ideology established a separate sphere for women in which their activities were defined "by their supposedly natural capabilities for nurturing, caring and teaching" (Boylan, 1978, p. 62).

The beliefs and practices associated with true womanhood fostered homosocial networks comprised almost entirely of mothers, sisters, first cousins, aunts, nieces, and close friends. Close female relationships were paralleled by severe prohibitions against intimacy between young women and men (Smith-Rosenberg, 1975). Men were believed incapable of understanding women's needs and natures; men were not held accountable for the caretaking that filled women's lives. Women were present at each major event and transition in life, from the birth of a baby, through bouts of illness, to tending the dying. Marriage, birth, death, and sickness were shaped around elaborate unisex rituals. Women were emotionally central and valued as powerful participants in each other's lives. Female homosociality was fostered in the 19th century, and a great range of emotional and sexual feelings were allowed (Smith-Rosenberg, 1975).

Faderman (1981) suggests that cultural taboos around female homosociality did not develop until the 20th century, when lesbian sexuality became more overt. The term "homosexual" was not even used until 1892 (Halperin, 1989). Lesbian love relationships exist apart from male control, contributing to the perception of their subversive element (Chafetz, 1990).

Only recently has there been an exploration of gender on friendship patterns (Adams & Blieszner, 1989; Blieszner & Adams, 1992). One reason for the lack of knowledge about same-sex female relationships, at least until recently, may be that women's friendships are so little valued in patriarchal society (Bernard, 1981). Bernard recognized the problem of modern women's alienation from other women and their loss of their 19th-century power base of female connections, in part because of the professionalization of traditional caring activities and the return of women to the labor force (Voydanoff, 1988). Bernard predicted a present-day restoring of female friendships and support networks to relieve the relational deficit among women, which may be linked to their higher rates of depression (Voydanoff, 1988).

Of course, these observations about the alienation of women from other women in contemporary society reveal a class bias. Working-class women and women of color have always relied on female friends to help them survive the challenges of maintaining families from a marginalized position in the social structure (Dill, 1988). Working-class and poor women of all racial–ethnic groups have created "fictive kin," turning friends into surrogate family members in order to pool the resources necessary for family survival, as several investigations have found (e.g., Allen, 1989; Rapp, 1982; Stacey, 1990; Stack, 1974). Thus, Bernard's analysis of the loss of homosociality for white women since the 19th century may be peculiar to the isolation of middle-class housewives in the years before the reactivation of the women's movement. The "feminine mystique," referred to by Friedan (1963) as "the problem that had no name," signified this isolation.

The restoration of female friendships among contemporary women may be related to the resurgence of the women's movement in the late 1960s and early 1970s. Dissatisfied with their treatment in the new left, civil rights, and student movements, women came together to describe a developing consciousness of their own oppression. Rooted in the Chinese practice of consciousness-raising, which means to "speak pains to recall pains" (Morgan, 1970, p. xxiii), consciousness-raising (CR) groups began to form around 1966–67 and continued until about 1975, when issues between lesbian and heterosexual women about the politics of sexuality polarized the feminist movement (Zimmerman, 1984). The practice of CR groups survived in the form of lesbian personal narratives; coming out is not a one-time experience for lesbians who are constantly confronted with their place in a predominantly heterosexual world (Zimmerman, 1984). Consciousness-raising has also been reawakened among feminists in the 1980s in the painful but courageous confrontations that come from the awareness of racial and class differences among women (Lugones & Spelman, 1983; Mascia-Lees, Sharpe, & Cohen, 1989). Talking to each other, sharing differences, learning to listen without judging, and building political coalitions are aspects of feminism that support the survival of female networks (Zimmerman, 1984) and an inclusive sisterhood for all women (Collins, 1989; Dill, 1983).

The relationship of feminism to homosociality is less problematic than that of feminism to lesbianism (Smith, 1989). Relaxing the dialectical tension that sexuality brings to the discussion of feminism, it is important to examine the contributions that feminists have made to uncovering and documenting the ways in which women support each other throughout their lives.

Acker et al. (1979) conducted a longitudinal study of 28 heterosexual, white women, with a median age of 45, who were in the process of consciously changing their primary identities from housewives and mothers to be more congruent with their emerging feminist selves. Participants were recruited for the study through contacts and places where women in transition might be found, such as community colleges, vocational and educational counselors, therapists, Parents without Partners, and referrals from friends and acquaintances. The authors examined the ways in which women rely on each other through transition. In beginning to build a new identity, women typically returned to school, which put them in touch with other women. Their new relationships with women, formed outside the context of their marriages, were structured within the context of feminism. Social contacts organized within their marriages tended to be male-defined and constricted to their husbands' needs, but their new friendships with other women were much more open, self-disclosing, and intimate exchanges. These new relationships allowed them to begin to understand the relations of power and domination within marriage and to reinterpret feelings of frustration and low self-worth as related not to their own inadequacy but to women's disadvantaged position within marriage and society. The authors concluded that a sense of sisterhood among women came partially from a critique of relationships with men. The women went through a process in which they came to see intimacy with men constructed through relations of domination:

> Coming to this realization does not mean one can step outside those relations; these women were still tied to men in different and overlapping ways—economically, socially, emotionally and sexually. Thus, feminism did not remove the contradictions endemic in relations between the sexes, it raised them in new forms. (Acker et al., 1979, p. 106)

These women faced new dilemmas regarding autonomy and intimacy that required difficult choices between remaining married and becoming single. They also faced ongoing tensions between their belief systems about equality and the structure of marriage that left them with greater awareness of their disadvantaged positions. "Despite these painful gaps between ideology and reality, what feminist consciousness and relationships with other women did produce was a sense of self worth and integrity. These women no longer blamed themselves for the conditions of their lives" (Acker et al., 1979, p. 106). Friendships with other women offered support that enabled them to understand their dilemmas and make proactive choices.

The nature of women's emotional friendships with each other is all the more important as women age. One reason is the decreasing availability of men as intimate partners. Women's life expectancy is at least 7 years longer than men's. Women tend to marry older men, leaving a narrowing field of eligible partners as they age. Support networks of mostly or exclusively older women are not uncommon. Allen and Chin-Sang (1990) conducted in-depth interviews with 30 aging African-American women and found that their networks of other women like themselves were what sustained them as they aged. They were involved in their churches and senior citizen centers, so their primary affiliations were not with members of their families, but with friends and companions whom they turned into "surrogate sisters." The adoption of friends into their kin network revealed the same process Stack (1974) found in her ethnography of a low-income black community: Women turn friends into family as a way to pool resources and ensure individual and family survival in the face of incredible odds.

Relationships with female friends provide a context for women's relationships with male partners. Because women are socialized to expect to marry and to believe that it is important to have males to protect them and take care of them, concerns about developing and maintaining a relationship with a marriageable male tend to eclipse other relational interests for young heterosexual women.

WOMEN AND THEIR MARRIAGES

Traditionally, the role of wife has been "of signal importance in American society" (Lopata, 1987, p. 389). Marriage has been portrayed as not only desirable, but also necessary, as a means of achieving true womanhood and assuring women of a life of security and respectability. A woman's "good" marriage not only confirmed her worth as a human being, but also reflected well on her family.

Marriage, in its pure form, is associated with romantic love, adult status, and a lifelong devotion that ends only in the death of one partner (Blumstein & Schwartz, 1983; Duvall, 1971; Lopata, 1987). Weddings are big business; young women are indoctrinated into the role and status of wife through rituals such as bridal showers and gift giving to establish a household (Cheal, 1989).

Marriage is a rite of passage for women, signaling commitment to relationships that ostensibly will be supportive, loving, and enduring. The idea of contemporary marriage is that two people join together for the rest of their lives, regardless of the problems or prosperity that may ensue. Being married provides an opportunity to share with another one's most personal feelings, ideas, and expectations. The intimacy of the relationship allows disclosure of both positive and negative aspects of each partner's personality without fear, allegedly, of rejection or exploitation. Marriage provides legitimacy for bearing children and becoming a family in the eyes of the rest of the world. In an ideal sense, marriage offers a refuge from the demands of the world and unconditional acceptance of one's failures and successes. Within such a relationship, both individuals can continue to grow and change, but keep their love for and commitment to one another alive through ongoing communication.

The reality of marriage, however, departs significantly from the idealized version promoted in theories and the media. Marriage can be a source of frustration, despair, and hostility. Studies of mid-life marriage often reveal disappointment over the unfulfilled expectations that real married life has brought and the emotional estrangement between partners (Cuber & Harroff, 1965; Rubin, 1983). Relationship problems are exacerbated by individual partner problems of alcoholism, depression, job loss, parenting, and responsibility for aging parents, all of which tend to pile up by mid-life (Kerckhoff, 1976). A broad array of feminist research and clinical evidence reveals the battering and abuse that women suffer at the hands of their husbands and male partners (Yllo & Bograd, 1988).

Explanations of the conflicts and tensions of marriage highlight differences between men and women as important contributors to marital discord. Differences in communication styles, expression of intimacy, sexuality, and power are used to explain why husbands and wives become locked into continuing struggles that result in their becoming "intimate strangers" (Rubin, 1983). A more comprehensive explanation requires that societal factors such as pay inequities, lack of high-quality childcare, and a culture tolerant of interpersonal violence also be considered. Furthermore, the role of wife may be less salient for members of some racial ethnic groups, given historical and institutional factors associated with racism (Dill, 1988). Instead, motherhood may be the transition to adult status, because of the limited pool of eligible men to marry (McGoldrick, Garcia-Preto, Hines, & Lee, 1989; Staples, 1971, 1989; Staples & Mirande, 1980; Wilkinson, 1987; Zinn, 1990).

His and Her Marriage: Historical Artifact or Current Reality?

Bernard's (1972) conceptualization of "his and her marriage" is now a classic statement about married life. Marriage offers more rewards to men than to women. Women report lower levels of marital satisfaction than men. Married women experience higher rates of mental illness than single women or married men (Gove, 1972). Women do most of the interaction work of building and maintaining communication in heterosexual relationships (Fishman, 1978), and women are responsible for what Bernard termed the "stroking function" (Voydanoff, 1988, p. 272).

Women also do the majority of the physical maintenance of housework and child care (Pleck, 1985). Husbands may be helping more, but their family work is not likely to be the routine, daily, invisible work that women do (Dressel & Clark, 1990). In a phenomenological study of family care, Dressel and Clark (1990) found that women, but not men, did things for their partners, such as draw bathwater, hem trousers, or iron a shirt, that the partners could have done for themselves. The provision of routine personal services by women was rarely returned by their partners.

Women's lifelong socialization toward overattunement to others in relationships is a gender pattern that brings greater responsibilities for family care. Significant involvement in relationships with husbands and children should also bring the possibility for greater rewards for women, yet evidence does not support this contention. Qualitative investigations of marriage suggest that overinvolvement in caregiving and nurturing activities do not bring women the intimacy they desire (Rubin, 1976, 1983; Thompson & Walker, 1989). The difficulties men and women have in relating to each other get played out through differences in how they express their caring. The men in Rubin's (1976, 1983) studies tended to express their love by doing something for their spouses, such as washing their wife's car. The women tended to substitute nurturing their spouses as a way to meet their own dependency and intimacy needs. Each partner had difficulty accepting and appreciating the seemingly different ways their spouse expressed intimacy.

Tremendous expectations exist for marriage to satisfy intimacy needs, when, in reality, men's emotional distance overshadows their instrumental acts of caring. The women in Rubin's (1976, 1983) studies tended not to understand or appreciate their husbands' language of actions; they experienced love by the disclosure of thoughts and feelings. These wives substituted nurturance for intimacy and wound up taking care of their partners rather than truly sharing their inner lives with their husbands. The unfulfilled promises of marital expectations were very acute for working-class wives and husbands, whose occupational lives were just as precarious as their intimate lives (Rubin, 1976).

An important consequence of women's greater responsibility for and actual involvement in all dimensions of family work is that women seem much more ambivalent about their family roles than their male partners are. Dressel and Clark (1990) found that 75% of the women in their study reported emotional dissonance, which is a conflict between what one is doing and feeling (Hochschild, 1983), whereas most of the men did not report such ambivalence in their feelings and actions about family care. "It is a cruel irony if what endears women to their families also entraps them in an arrangement of subordination and provokes feelings and assessments by them that are at least partially and sometimes wholly negative" (Dressel & Clark, 1990, p. 778). Part of the search for alternatives to traditional marriage may be motivated by this cruel irony. Feminists have asked, "not what do women do for the family (an older question), but what does the family do for women? What does it do to women?" (Bridenthal, 1982, pp. 231–232).

We ask, as well, what does *marriage* do to women? Okin (1989) has argued eloquently that what contemporary gender-structured marriage does is make women vulnerable. Although marriage involves a degree of emotional vulnerability and dependence for both partners, the social expectations that wives should maintain primary responsibility for rearing children and subordinate their paid work lives to their husbands' results in asymmetric vulnerability for women. The partner whose wage work is given priority enjoys increased income and work status, which contribute to greater leverage in the family.

The disparity in power and income and the lack of equity in distribution of family work may seem reasonable *as long as the marriage endures* (Okin, 1989). However, when a relationship terminates, the true vulnerability that marriage entails for women is apparent. Divorced and separated women are usually cut off from the benefits of their ex-husbands' enhanced economic position and must rely on their own abilities and income. Also, a divorced or separated woman usually has continuing responsibility for her children, who, in turn, may suffer because of their mother's vulnerability after their father's departure.

In addition to the risks that traditional marriage carries for women if marriage ends, Okin (1989) points out that women who are economically dependent on their husbands lose effective voice during their marriages. Because they have less power in the relationship, they have less success in raising issues for negotiation and taking a firm stand on topics that are conflictual. Only when women have the potential to make a satisfactory exit from a relationship can they maintain their voice in the family and also protect themselves against economic devastation if the marriage ends.

The Evolution of Marriage

The persistently high rate of divorce confirms that the *traditional* institution of marriage is deeply, if not fatally, flawed. In 1989, Martin and Bumpass predicted that in the near future, two thirds of marriages would end in divorce. In a 1991 analysis, Glenn estimated that only one third of those who married in the early 1970s were in marriages that were both intact and satisfactory a decade later.

Divorce is so prevalent that it is becoming "accepted as a legitimate, normal, viable, nonpathological exit from marriage" (Raschke, 1987, p. 620). Remarriage, as well, is a common way of repairing marital disruption (Spanier & Furstenberg, 1987). Three of four women who divorce remarry eventually (Cherlin, 1981), although white women remarry at a much higher rate than black women (Spanier & Furstenberg, 1987). The prevalence rates of marriage, divorce, and remarriage may be one product of the complex gap between rising expectations for marital fulfillment and the reality of contemporary marriages (National Center for Health Statis-tics, 1991b, 1991c).

In spite of the high rate of separation and divorce, and despite feminist challenges to compulsory heterosexuality, male/female rela-tionships and marriage continue to retain their vitality for most women (Stacey, 1986). Dialectical tensions between "love and trouble" (Collins, 1990) do not dissuade most women from marrying at least once.

Marriage is an evolving institution (Blumstein & Schwartz, 1983). Historically an economic arrangement for the regulation of sexuality and procreation, marriage has become a primary context for intimacy. Indeed, such great expectations are now associated with marriage that its main function may be a therapeutic one. However, there is a gender imbalance embedded in the marital relationship that renders the promise of intimacy in marriage difficult to fulfill (Blumstein & Schwartz, 1983; Glenn, 1987; Rubin, 1983; Thompson & Walker, 1989).

Love became feminized with the rise of capitalism, and women became primarily responsible for the emotional management of marriage and family relationships (Cancian, 1987). Recent research on family care supports Bernard's (1972) contention that responsibility for the marital relationship falls primarily to women (Dressel & Clark, 1990). To their already significant responsibilities for emotional interaction work (Fish-man, 1978), infant and child care (LaRossa & LaRossa, 1989), and household labor (Hartmann, 1981), women have now added the role of economic provider (Gerson, 1985; Gerstel & Gross, 1987; Hertz, 1987).

The institutionalization of marriage means that "the idea of marriage is larger than any individual marriage. The role of husband or wife is greater than any individual who takes on that role" (Blumstein & Schwartz, 1983, p. 318). Married partners must negotiate between the institution, which is resistant to change, and the idiosyncratic ways in which their own lives and relationships develop. Gender complicates expectations about marriage because of the different statuses of men and women in society (Glenn, 1987). The tendency of women to marry men who are somewhat older, more educated, and more affluent reinforces power differences in the relationship.

One way in which marriage is changing is in the negotiation for greater equality between partners (Thompson, 1989). A paradox of con-temporary marriage is that as partners seek to transform the inequities of traditional marital arrangements, they generate alternatives that chal-lenge the institution of marriage itself (Blumstein & Schwartz, 1983).

How Viable Is the Institution of Marriage?

Most people in the United States marry at some point in their lives. A recent national survey of women aged 15 to 44 revealed that nearly two thirds of the sample had been married at least once (London, 1991). Of women aged 40 to 44, 94% of white women and 84% of black women had been married. This age group provides a good estimate of the percentage of all women who are likely to marry because most women who will marry have done so by that point in their lives (London, 1991).

Although most people do marry, marriage in the United States is undergoing evolutionary change. More people are postponing marriage and increasing numbers are forgoing it completely. There has been a persistent increase in the average age at which both women and men marry. From 1964 to 1988, women's age at first marriage increased from 21.4 years of age to 24.6 (National Center for Health Statistics, 1991b), the highest since the United States started keeping records more than a century ago. There was a similar increase for men, from 24 years of age in 1964 to 26.5 years in 1988. Age at first marriage is even higher for those with a college degree—27 years old for women and 28 for men.

Marriage rates cycle up and down in response to wars, the economy, and the number of unmarried individuals who reach marriageable age at any point in time (National Center for Health Statistics, 1991b). By using a rate of marriage per 1,000 unmarried women aged 15 to 44, it is possible to take these factors into consideration in the comparison of marriage rates over time. The marriage rate has shown a precipitous drop since 1972; it fell from 141 to 91 marriages per 1,000 women aged 15 to 44 between 1972 and 1988. The record high rate of 199 marriages per 1,000 women was recorded in 1946, just after World War II.

Norms and values regarding marriage are being restructured in such a way that marriage is becoming less relevant as an institution governing intimate relationships (Thornton, 1989). In an analysis of three data sets that gathered information about attitudes and values regarding family issues over a 30-year period, Thornton (1989) documented "a dramatic and pervasive weakening of the normative imperative to marry, to remain married, to have children, to restrict intimate relations to marriage, and to maintain separate roles for males and females" (p. 873).

Thornton's (1989) analysis revealed that the growing tolerance for nontraditional family patterns was not necessarily accompanied by changes in personal expectations about life choices and family patterns. For example, data from female high school students in 1976–77 indicated that 79% planned to marry. In 1980–81 and 1985–86 surveys, 81% of females reported that they would choose to marry. Fewer male students indicated a desire to marry, with 71% reporting this expectation in 1976–77, 75% in 1980–81, and 74% in 1985–86.

Glenn (1991) proposed that such continued optimism about marriage may be unrealistic because the probability of marital success is so low. "To make a strong, unqualified commitment to a marriage—and to make the investments of time, energy, and foregone opportunities that entails—is so hazardous that no totally rational person would do it" (Glenn, 1991, p. 269). Using data from 1973–1988 U.S. General Social Surveys, he challenged the notion that surviving marriages are becoming happier because unhappy ones are terminated through divorce. His results indicate a continuing decrease in the percentage of married individuals who reported their marriages were "very happy"—from 60% in 1973–77, to 54% in 1978–83, to a low of 49% in 1984–88.

Considering that people tend to overreport rather than underreport their happiness suggests that marriage, as currently configured, is not a source of significant happiness for the majority of married couples. To have a better picture of the interiors of contemporary marriages, data on the attitudes, expectations, experiences, and dynamics of marriage are needed. Little comprehensive research on marriage has been done, particularly research that focuses on women's marital experiences. Two recent studies identify factors important to women's experiences of satisfaction and pleasure in marital relationships.

In their study of 300 women between ages 35 and 55, Baruch, Barnett, and Rivers (1983) explored the aspects of women's lives that brought them rewards and pleasures. Married women expressed more satisfaction, optimism, and happiness than did single women, probably because of higher family income and better conditions for satisfying sexual relationships. Being married, however, did not affect women's sense of mastery, that is, their sense of control, self-esteem, and resistance to depression and anxiety.

Communication and support were found to be crucial to the success of marriages in this sample. The problems that caused the most concern were emotionally distant husbands, lack of companionship, and poor communication between partners. The marriages that women described as the most rewarding were like relationships between loving friends and were characterized by caring and cooperation.

The findings in Vannoy-Hiller and Philliber's (1989) study of 489 married, predominantly white couples were strikingly similar. The most important elements in the success of marriages, especially those of working and high-achieving wives, were the husband's sensitivity, supportiveness, and sense of self-worth. The most successful marriages were those in which husbands had been able to let go of the "more than" image of maleness and support their partners and their achievements. Reciprocally, wives had let go of their "less than" perceptions of themselves.

In both studies, women's paid work was critical to the success of their marriages. Women with a strong commitment to their work had two distinct sources of pleasure—work and family, each of which could offset problems and disappointments in the other (Baruch et al., 1983). When both partners worked and produced income at nearly equal levels, there was a greater likelihood of role interchangeability and sharing of responsibilities, resulting in women feeling more supported (Vannoy-Hiller & Philliber, 1989). Women who work outside the home have a higher sense of control and self-esteem. They are more likely to believe that they have a right to express their own needs and desires *and* to have them met, just as they meet the needs of others. Breadwinning encourages them to have expectations of equality and to feel confident in communicating these expectations to their partners.

Commuter Marriage

Still another course that couples have taken to negotiate the complexities and contradictions they face is commuter marriage. Gerstel and Gross (1987) refer to commuter marriage as a microcosm of the tension between work and family; it is "both a laboratory for viewing enduring issues in family life and a microcosm of changes in the larger society" (p. 431). As alternative family relationships receive wider acceptance and as women's preparations and desires for significant careers are matched by their families' needs for their incomes, commuter marriages become an option for solving the dilemmas of dual-career families. Like many other innovations, couples view commuter marriage not as a permanent lifestyle, but rather as a commitment a couple makes temporarily or for a number of years.

Commuter marriage was selected by the women in Gerstel and Gross's (1987) study because it allowed them to place significant emphasis on their careers. Established couples whose children had already left home benefited from the arrangement more than husbands and wives who were still adjusting to or balancing work, marriage, and childrearing with commuting.

Wives could focus on their professional lives when they were alone. The contrast between living within a family arrangement and living alone was stark. Perhaps for the first time in their married lives, women experienced freedom from the constant interruptions and demands of home life. As Hartmann (1981) found, having an adult male in the household increases the hours that women spend on housework more than the average hours men contribute to the household. Living on their own meant that these wives had much less home maintenance work to do. They were free to concentrate on themselves and their careers. Thus, women felt a sense of gain from commuting, whereas men felt a sense of loss because their wives were not performing the mundane daily tasks they ordinarily did for them.

Communication and Self-Disclosure

Intimacy and the sense of connection between two people intensify as partners reveal themselves to each other and communicate about deeply personal feelings, desires, and needs. Likewise, the inability to communicate in this way, or the choice not to do so, undermines attempts to establish true intimacy.

The fact that women and men have difficulty communicating is almost a truism. Tannen's (1990) work on male/female communication revealed that there is a different focus in the ways that each gender uses communication. Women speak and hear a language of connection and intimacy, whereas men speak and hear a language of status and independence. The result is that "communication between men and women can be like cross-cultural communication, prey to clash of conversational styles. Instead of different dialects, it is said that they speak different genderlects" (Tannen, 1990, p. 42). Because each sex judges the other by its own standards, women feel misunderstood, and men feel manipulated by women's indirect conversational style and personal talk. Both are dissatisfied.

Tannen (1990) notes that misunderstandings arise when women go to their male partners with a problem, seeking understanding and connection, but instead receive advice and directions about how to solve the problem. Women tend to use "trouble talk" as a rapport-building device sending a metamessage that "We're the same; you're not alone" (Tannen, 1990, p. 53). When men give advice instead of participating in the trouble talk, as another woman might do, the interaction becomes hierarchically structured, with the advice giver sending a metamessage of superiority. The woman does not get the support she sought, and her partner feels unappreciated for trying to help.

The role that power plays in communication between women and men was addressed by McGill (1985). He gathered questionnaire data from 737 women and 646 men and interviewed 90 men and 90 women. McGill concluded that the reason some men are not more self-disclosing has to do with what disclosure means to men. A partner who reveals deep personal feelings gives the other power and control. Information is power. If only one partner is self-disclosing, the one who withholds information gains power as the self-discloser becomes vulnerable. Men withhold information, mislead, or even misrepresent themselves to their partners in order to gain mastery (McGill, 1985).

Feminists Reclaiming Marriage

Feminist women and men who are married to each other struggle to create nonoppressive private relationships despite the institutional practices that

benefit men and penalize women. Couples who are committed to relational equality and feminist change are deconstructing the "traditional"
in marriage and redefining their own marriages with a feminist agenda
(Blaisure, 1992).

Blaisure (1992) conducted individual and joint intensive interviews
with ten long-term married couples. Both wives and husbands in these
partnerships were self-identified feminists before they married, and they
continued to be committed to feminist goals of liberation and equality
during marriage. Blaisure (1992) found that these women and men were
reclaiming the institution of marriage on their own terms. Both male and
female partners recognized the oppression that the women experience in
their broader social relations and used relationship processes, such as
vigilance about equity in marital roles and constant communication, to
protect wives from reinforcement of this oppression at home.

By arranging their marriages to benefit the wives as well as the
husbands and acknowledging the privileged status of men in society, these
couples could make deliberate choices to reconstruct their relationships in
ways that accommodated women and men. Feminism provided the
ideological and practical guidance for women and men to recover marriage from its oppressive conditions, making it more responsive to the
emotional needs of both partners (Blaisure, 1992).

WOMEN AND COHABITATION

The population of cohabiting couples has exploded since the 1970s, and
the number of unmarried women and men living together shows no sign
of leveling off (Spanier, 1991). Cohabitation has become a significant
variation in lifestyle choice and, for many, part of the process and
structure of intimate relationships. The circumstances that have led to its
prevalence include the resurgence of the women's movement, greater
acceptance of premarital sexuality, availability of contraceptives and legal
abortion, delayed marriages for educational and occupational opportunities, increased concern about divorce, increased costs of housing, and a
trend toward pluralism in lifestyles, leading to greater recognition of
variant family forms (Bumpass et al., 1991; Macklin, 1987; Spanier,
1991).

Information on cohabiting couples has been limited. Two recent
studies, the National Survey of Families and Households (Bumpass et al.,
1991) and the National Survey of Family Growth (London, 1991),
provide current information on cohabiting relationships. In the NSFG
study, slightly more than half of all cohabiting relationships resulted in
marriage, 37% dissolved before marriage, and 10% were ongoing at the

time of the survey. Cohabitation was less likely to lead to marriage for black women (42%) than for white women (54%).

London (1991) reported that in 1988 about 5% of women aged 15 to 44 were cohabiting prior to marriage. However, 25% of married women reported that they had cohabited at some time before their first marriage. For women aged 25 to 34, nearly half reported cohabiting at some point in time. Cohabitation is even more common among separated or divorced individuals. Sixty percent of those who remarried between 1980 and 1987 cohabited before remarriage (Bumpass & Sweet, 1989). Further, these figures underestimate the true proportion of "all couples" who cohabit because they do not include same-sex couples or couples who reside together but maintain separate residences.

The question of whether cohabiting before marriage improves the chances of marital success has been addressed in several studies. Surra (1990) reported, in a decade review of literature, that those who cohabit are more likely to experience marital breakdown, not less. The general conclusion is that those who cohabit before marriage are somehow different types of people, less traditional than those who do not cohabit and thus more likely to see divorce as an option. Most researchers, however, have not deconstructed the category "cohabitant" to reveal the variety of underlying motivations and expectations of those who choose this lifestyle. Also, there has been little attention to long-term, successful cohabiting relationships. Not enough research has been done to substantiate the advantages and disadvantages of cohabitation as (1) an experience in and of itself, (2) a relationship of convenience, or (3) a deliberate decision to enter the relationship before marriage.

In one study, more women (56%) than men (51%) indicated that an important reason for living together was to make sure that the couple was compatible before marriage (Bumpass et al., 1991). A quarter of the respondents indicated that sharing living expenses was another important reason for living together. Cohabitants voiced little concern with moral issues related to cohabiting or disapproval from family or friends. Only about a third of the women believed their economic and emotional security and overall happiness would be better if they were married.

A factor that may explain both the instability of cohabiting relationships and the disruption rate in marriages preceded by cohabitation is disagreement between partners about whether marriage is part of a long-term plan. As many as 20% of cohabiting couples may have disagreements regarding expectations about marriage (Bumpass et al., 1991). Contrary to expectations, cohabiting women were more tentative about marriage than their male partners, although men were more concerned about the effect of marriage on their freedom than were women. Women were more likely to perceive trouble in the cohabiting relationship and slightly less likely to expect that they would marry their partners than were men.

It is increasingly likely that heterosexual couples will live together before they marry. However, there are still great pressures on Americans to marry before childbearing, so cohabitation is unlikely to completely replace marriage as a lifestyle choice. In the United States, as opposed to some European countries such as Sweden, commitment is still signified by legal marriage (Macklin, 1987).

One of the ironies of cohabitation is that heterosexual couples must decide if they want to marry, whereas same-sex couples are barred, mostly by tradition, custom, and the courts, from legal marriage. The editors of *The Harvard Law Review* (1990) point out that the law denies all unmarried couples many legal and economic privileges regardless of sexual orientation, but the effect on same-sex relationships is especially troublesome. Lesbians partners are legal strangers to each other (Robson & Valentine, 1990). Legal marriage provides concrete advantages denied to gay men and lesbians: tax benefits (special exemptions, deductions, and refunds), insurance benefits (health, disability, and life insurance and pension plans), economic benefits (such as workers' compensation when the life partner dies), the right to assume a partner's housing lease upon the partner's death, ability to ensure that wills or trusts assigning property to a partner will be protected from court challenges, status as the spouse's next of kin, and rights of survivorship that avoid inheritance tax (Harvard Law Review Association, 1990). These benefits may outweigh the costs of marriage, which include those states that require courts to consider fault in determining property distribution and/or alimony when a couple divorces.

It is constitutionally invalid for *states*, the traditional regulators of marriage, to prohibit gay male and lesbian couples from marrying (Harvard Law Review Association, 1990). The Supreme Court has upheld the special status of marriage as a basic civil right of all Americans in several decisions:

> In Griswold v. Connecticut [1965], the Court declared that marriage "is an association that promotes a way of life, not causes; a harmony in living, not political faiths; a bilateral loyalty, not commercial or social projects. Yet it is an association for as noble a purpose as any involved in our prior decisions." (Harvard Law Review Association, 1990, p. 95)

Two other decisions reflect the Court's recognition of "a fundamental right to marry." In *Loving v. Virginia* (1967), the Supreme Court held that a state miscegenation law was unconstitutional (Harvard Law Review Association, 1990). In *Zablocki v. Redhail*, the Court "invalidated a statute that implicitly tied the ability to marry to a person's wealth" (Harvard Law Review Association, 1990, pp. 95–96). These Supreme Court decisions contradict the universal practice of states in denying the right to marry to same-sex couples. "Insofar as the right to marry derives from the right to privacy, it should extend to heterosexuals and homosexuals alike" (Harvard Law Review Association, 1990, p. 96).

Marriage is also protected constitutionally because it promotes familial and societal stability. Any stable and significant relationship between two consenting adults should be accorded constitutional protection (Harvard Law Review Association, 1990). The majority of lesbian and gay male unions are very stable (Macklin, 1987). Blumstein and Schwartz (1983) found that the level of commitment in same-sex relationships, in fact, may be higher than that in heterosexual relationships, given the psychological, social, and legal obstacles that gay and lesbian couples must overcome in order to stay together. It is the "irrational prejudice and fear of unconventional activities and lifestyles" (Harvard Law Review Association, 1990, p. 101) contained in state laws that is illegitimate, not same-sex relationships. Thus, state-level discrimination against lesbian and gay marriage is unconstitutional.

LESBIAN PARTNERSHIPS

Relationships between women that are emotionally, economically, and sexually interdependent are all but invisible except, perhaps, to other lesbians. About 10% of women are self-identified lesbians (Brown, 1989a), even though estimating the prevalence of lesbian partnerships is probably impossible (Blumstein & Schwartz, 1983).

Social science literature on lesbian and gay male couples was almost nonexistent until recently (Blumstein & Schwartz, 1983). Nonmoralistic discussion of same-sex couples has coincided with the emergence of gay cultural systems and the gay and lesbian liberation movement (Boxer, Cook, & Herdt, 1991; D'Emilio & Freedman, 1988; Faderman, 1991; Weston, 1991). The bulk of information on women's relationships with other women is small-scale empirical studies, clinical experiences, and literary analyses (Zimmerman, 1984). This literature differs from the typical social science literature on women and families in that it is mostly for and about women who are lesbians. What is done with research on lesbians is critical because of the subtle and overt ways they are silenced, trivialized, and harassed in contemporary society.

In the last 10 years, social science has shown a more positive social interest in lesbian relationships (Reilly & Lynch, 1990). Part of the increasing interest has to do with movement away from viewing the

family field as "marriage and the family" and moving toward an appreciation for varied forms of relationships (Peplau, 1982). In most texts and
treatments of the family, however, lesbians and their families are still
rarely mentioned. In an excellent, ground-breaking book about current
research on children and the new families from a feminist perspective
(Dornbusch & Strober, 1988), lesbians are not mentioned. Only
"homosexual rights" are discussed, in terms of family policy (p. 29) and
religion and social conservativism (p. 56). In two comprehensive family
sociology textbooks, lesbian couples or families are not indexed; only the
generic "homosexuality" is indexed. Collins (1988) devotes a paragraph
to power and equality among lesbian couples (p. 295), and briefly cites
lesbianism and gay male relationships as examples of sexual radicalism (p.
497), although the discussion collapses important distinctions between
gay men and lesbians into a single category of homosexuality. Skolnick
(1987) does not discuss lesbian existence at all; homosexuality is mentioned only as a historical phenomenon. These examples suggest that
lesbian relationships continue to be marginalized, and more work needs to
be done to bring these relationships into the center of analyses of women
and their families.

Compulsory Heterosexuality and Lesbian Existence

Rich (1980) described the ideology of compulsory heterosexuality, in
which women are defined as the adjuncts of men, and female sexuality is
the passive acquiescence to male demands. Women who choose each
other as life partners, co-workers, lovers, and passionate comrades are
suspect because lesbian existence has the potential to liberate women
from male control (Rich, 1980). Lesbian existence is often characterized
as deviant, pathological, and in need of correction because it exists
outside the dominant expectations of a patriarchal and heterosexist society (Andersen, 1988). Yet, women who choose other women as partners
are making a choice for women, not against men (Rich, 1980).

Lesbians and gay men comprise a tremendously diverse minority
group (Duberman, Vicinus, & Chauncey, 1989). Keeping in mind this
diversity, Brown (1989a) identifies three common aspects that serve as a
model for understanding lesbian existence as well as an alternative paradigm for psychological inquiry. Brown's work foreshadows a positive shift
in the scholarly attention that lesbian/gay reality is now receiving. The
first aspect, biculturalism, refers to the fact that most lesbians were raised
in heterosexual households and probably have behaved heterosexually
during their lifetimes. Biculturalism for lesbians is much like the experience of biracial existence. Lesbians are forerunners in knowing how to
"embrace what is other in oneself" (Brown, 1989a, p. 449). Second,

lesbian women and gay men both know the experience of marginality, of being outside the rituals of heterosexual culture. Being outsiders to what is considered mainstream has enabled lesbians and gay men to "be freer to see, speak and act other truths" (p. 451). One way in which lesbians have created another reality is the innovation of two women raising children together (Brown, 1989a). Third, normative creativity is part of gay and lesbian existence: "By lacking clear rules about how to be lesbian and gay in the world, we have made up the rules as we go along" (Brown, 1989a, p. 451).

Merger in Lesbian Relationships

Merger is a relationship issue for lesbian partners (Bristow & Pearn, 1984; Brown, 1989a, 1989b; Burch, 1987; Krestan & Bepko, 1980; Krieger, 1982; Pearlman, 1989; Peplau, Cochran, Rook, & Padesky, 1978; Vargo, 1987). Lesbian couples are comprised of two women, each with a probable history of socialization toward caregiving and connection. Feminist clinicians acknowledge that fusion (Krestan & Bepko, 1980) or merger (Pearlman, 1989) is a reality of lesbian existence, presenting both possibilities and challenges for relationships. In family systems theory, however, fusion is labeled "enmeshment" and seen as dysfunctional (Bograd, 1988b). Lesbians and feminist clinicians have reclaimed merger, rejecting the notion that emotional closeness with a life partner is problematic.

Pearlman (1989) defines "merger" as "a psychological state in which there is a loss of a sense of oneself as individual and separate" (p. 78). She proposes multiple meanings of merger. Merger is not a fixed or absolute state; it occurs to varying degrees. Pearlman (1989) describes three kinds of merger: (1) In some relationships, merger is transient and mainly present during times of sexual or emotional closeness; (2) in other relationships, merger is a normative preference for intense connection that can include some loss of individuality; (3) in a third kind of relationship, merger is more permanent and can reach a point of excessive dependency; there is acute tension or anxiety when physical or emotional distance occurs, an inability to function effectively without the presence of the other, and self–other confusions in terms of who is feeling what.

Pearlman (1989) builds on Chodorow's (1978) theory to describe how the ego boundary—the separation of self and other—is more fluid and less defined for women. Theoretically, female development is rooted in the early mother–daughter relationship of shared identity and sameness of biological sex. This results in the mother's expectations of sameness in her daughter, negative reactions to individuality and difference, and insistence on proximity, conformity, and prolonged dependency. Mothers can respond with emotional distancing if expectations for sameness are fixed and inflexible. Daughters change their different behaviors in order to retain their mother's closeness. Fathers tend to be exempt from these interactions, and society reinforces women's dependency and self-negation through sex-role socialization that requires women to put others first. Women learn to become acutely attuned to the needs and wishes of others, and they are especially vulnerable to emotional distancing and separateness in relationships.

Similar histories of relating to others, duplicated in relationships between women, shape lesbian couple dynamics (Pearlman, 1989). This contrasts with the difficulties heterosexual women report in trying to bridge the emotional differences between themselves and their male partners (Rubin, 1983); married women in Rubin's studies were painfully aware of the lack of merger in their relationships with husbands. Nevertheless, many long-term husband–wife relationships are characterized by intense merger. Additional research, from a feminist perspective, about how intense closeness gets played out in diverse relationships, regardless of gender, is needed to examine merger from women's perspectives.

In lesbian couple formation, merger is the intense bonding, romance, and discovery of mutuality of sexual passion and emotional connectedness (Pearlman, 1989). For many women, the bonding, interdependence, and intensity are unmatched and distinctly different from other types of coupling. There may be a loss of ego boundary and individuality as partners unite. The beginning of lesbian coupling can be labeled a "minor legend." Retelling their coming-together stories serves as "couple glue," helping to maintain their connection when they begin to recognize and deal with differences. Conflict characterizes the next phase of lesbian coupling, as partners reestablish individual boundaries and test couple solidarity. Some become uncomfortable with differences; they may stabilize around merger connectedness, producing boundary problems. If couples survive the conflict period and reorganize to accommodate their needs for individuality and separateness, they can move on to more permanent commitment.

Merger must be understood within a societal context. It is homophobia, the "irrational fear and hatred of those who love and sexually desire those of the same sex" (Pharr, 1988, p. 1), and legal sanctions (Harvard Law Review Association, 1990) that present problems for lesbian couples, not merger. Lesbian couples are expected to pass as heterosexuals. They are pressured to curtail affection and close interaction in public. This restraint can break couple connectedness, and partners may respond by isolating themselves. Pearlman (1989) notes, "The irony is that heterosexual women are more free to be publicly affectionate than lesbians are" (p. 84). Lesbian couples share these behavioral restraints with others, such as gay male couples, heterosexuals in a secret affair, and interracial couples. Distancing and invisibility are enforced through the potential of physical or verbal harassment and actual responses of attention and discomfort.

A lesbian–feminist perspective on merger redefines closeness between two women in a way that respects and validates lesbian couple dynamics. Rich (1980) challenges feminist object relations theories (Chodorow, 1978; Dinnerstein, 1976; Miller, 1986) for the implied assumption that mature adult women choose relationships with men only, whereas lesbians choose relationships that allow them to recreate mother–daughter emotions and connections. Certainly, fusion between women can create problems; lesbian couples must deal with overattunement to other women's needs, the hostilities of ex-lovers who remain in the lesbian community (Krieger, 1982, 1983), and internalized and projected homophobia (Pearlman, 1989). Thus, merger may be an adaptive and protective response to a society that oppresses women and denigrates their love and desire for each other. Couples need to work actively toward clear communication and ongoing discussion of feelings, reactions, and individual differences in order to maintain a positive partnership (Pearlman, 1989). Brown (1989a) suggests that merger in lesbian relationships is a model that may be helpful to heterosexual couples: "The merger that a healthy lesbian couple experiences is more normative and functional for intimate pairs than the illusion of autonomy and distance within a relationship that exists in heterosexual couples simply as an artifact of gender roles" (p. 454).

In many respects, lesbian couple formation and dynamics are similar to heterosexual relationship development. As they begin their relationship, all couples must make choices about how much time to spend with each other, how often to see each other, and whether to act on their sexual attraction. However, there are no courtship rituals, such as going steady, engagement, or legal marriage, for lesbian couples. Their relationships tend to progress more quickly as a result (Clunis & Green, 1988).

The contradiction between desires for individuality and connectedness is a familiar theme for women, but the lack of role models and rituals in lesbian relationships means that these women do not have the ready-made prescriptions to fall back on that, real or imagined, seem to help heterosexual couples through difficult passages. Thus, lesbian relationships are constrained by lack of institutional supports. Paradoxically, this may lead to more innovative patterns in negotiating the dynamics of the relationship.

NONMONOGAMOUS RELATIONSHIPS

Monogamy is legislated in the form of legal marriage. In spite of marital prescriptions and laws, about 50% of married men and 35% of married women have extramarital relationships (Atwater, 1982; Richardson, 1989). Lesbian couples confront the issue of monogamy and nonmonogamy, just as heterosexual couples do, but the dynamics may differ (Blumstein & Schwartz, 1983; Clunis & Green, 1988; Kassoff, 1989; Krieger, 1982). On the one hand, lesbians form relationships based on their own rules. On the other hand, they are not exempt from the pervasive influences of compulsory heterosexuality that require women to commit to only one partner (Rich, 1980).

The Politics of Lesbian Nonmonogamy

Without legal guidelines, lesbian couples have the freedom to negotiate their own boundaries around sexual exclusivity. Couples may choose to be monogamous as an expression of solidarity, or they may choose nonmonogamy for a variety of reasons (Clunis & Green, 1988). Lesbian nonmonogamy is defined as "a form of intimacy in which a woman concurrently engages in sexual and emotional relationships with more than one woman lover" (Kassoff, 1989, p. 167).

Kassoff (1989) identified five kinds of nonmonogamy in an in-depth, phenomenological study of lesbian–feminists. A total of 28 lesbians comprised the sample; they were predominantly white women, ranging in age from 21 to 39, and earned low to moderate income. First, "symbolic" nonmonogamy refers to lesbians who considered their relationships open, but were actually monogamous in their behavior. Second, "stable" nonmonogamy is based on an explicit choice for the couple to have other partners and for negotiations around multiple relationships to be openly discussed in an ongoing way. Third, "transitional" nonmonogamy is an unstable, nonconsensual relational system in which participants express conflict and dissatisfaction with their arrangements; it serves "as a transition into or out of a primary commitment to self or a lover" (Kassoff, 1989, p. 171). Fourth, "self-oriented" nonmonogamy is seen as an avenue for individual self-discovery and self-actualization. Commitments are made first to self needs; these women are reluctant to define themselves in a primary relationship. Finally, "couple-oriented" nonmonogamy occurs when primary partners are having interpersonal problems with merger or a strong political belief in liberating themselves from an exclusive, possessive, marriage type of partnership. They may wish to revitalize or differentiate their long-term primary relationship with a secondary partner who is "more transitional, more sexual, more emotional, less accountable and less of a responsibility than a primary partner" (Kassoff, 1989, p. 172).

Although these patterns appear remarkably similar to research conducted in the 1970s on heterosexual nonmonogamy (see Libby & Whitehurst, 1977), for lesbians monogamy may be more of a political issue. Lesbians' views about monogamy and nonmonogamy are related to their diversity. In Krieger's (1983) analysis of lesbian communities, women may couple more freely as a way to demonstrate loyalty to the community, rather than settling into pairs in a way that might reflect a traditional marriage. This type of partner exchange among lesbian communities consisting primarily of young, white, middle-class college students who are experimenting with sex, politics, and lesbianism does not seem to be shared by many third-world lesbian communities, where monogamy and long-term commitment are valued (Sandoval, 1984). The ideal of lesbian separatism can foster a community of like-minded women that exerts a subtle pressure on its members to conform (Sandoval, 1984). Zimmerman (1984) points out that women of color view lesbian separatism as a white woman's dream, where community becomes a "sameness that melts all women down into one mold" (p. 676).

The complex interplay among sexual orientation, age, race, class, religion, ethnicity, and gender is demonstrated in the writings of women of color. Moraga (1983) argues that the specificity of the oppression must continually be acknowledged; otherwise, there is a danger of homogenizing lesbian existence. In their analysis of homosexuality, homophobia, and revolution since 1959 in Cuba, Arguelles and Rich (1989) describe the extra discrimination Cuban lesbians faced before Castro's revolution. Whereas male homosexuals interacted with the upper-class Cuban tourist trade, lesbians were almost all closeted. Subservience to men was still required of women. Before the revolution, women suffered tremendous repression, and attitudes and behaviors toward lesbians changed slowly. When lesbian diversity is considered, changing opportunities for women's coupling can be understood as historically and culturally situated.

Women's Heterosexual Affairs

Extramarital sexual relationships are a normative part of American married life (Atwater, 1982; Bernard, 1977; Blumstein & Schwartz, 1983; Cuber & Harroff, 1965; Richardson, 1989). Although historically about half of husbands and one third of wives have affairs, rates of extramarital involvement are approaching the 50% mark for women. As more women enter the paid labor force, their opportunities to meet extramarital partners increase.

Richardson (1989) estimates that between 18% and 32% of single women become involved with married men. Secret relationships between married men and single women demonstrate how gender and power structure women's choices and chances for involvement in forbidden relationships. Cross-sex, secret, forbidden relationships offer men far more power than women because of men's gender, married status, superior socioeconomic position, and age. However, many of the women Richardson interviewed preferred such liasions because of the freedom from marital commitment they offered.

Richardson (1989) interviewed 65 single women who were or had been in intimate relationships with married men for over a year. Using a snowball sampling technique, the respondents were located from all regions of the country and ranged in age from 18 to 56, with a median age of 28. Women in both working-class and professional occupations were included. Their male lovers were all living with their wives at the time of the affair; none were in "open marriages." The extramarital relationships lasted from 1 to 25 years; none were one-night stands or short affairs.

Richardson (1989) identified two stages in the relationship development between forbidden partners. In the first stage, "becoming confidantes," a pattern of idealization of the male lover occurs in which "the man's marital status creates a context of privacy, time constraints, and expectations of temporariness that encourage revealing secrets about the self" (p. 111). The more the man reveals, the more the woman comes to trust and idealize him and their relationship, which then intensifies her commitment. In the second stage, "becoming a we," the couple do not have socially recognized events and transitions to aid in their relationship development, so they create their own meanings to overcome the sense of isolation they experience from being forbidden. This work is largely the hidden labor of the woman. They develop rites and rituals that are unique to the relationship as a way to "prove," if only to themselves, that the relationship exists. Enshrinement behavior also occurs, as demonstrated by bringing their scrapbook from its secret hiding place to show it to the researcher. Some women purposefully destroyed their "sacred objects" to mark the ending of the relationship:

> The same autonomy and freedom from social norms that affected the construction of the secret liaison affect its ending. Neither social interaction nor public rituals are available to signify to the self that the relationship no long exists. . . . The single woman has a paucity of forms through which to "deconstruct" her relationship. (Richardson, 1989, p. 116)

Atwater (1982) found that married women involved with single men have greater power in their relationships than do single women involved with married men. As Richardson (1989) points out, the status of being married enhances the gender status of being female.

Invisible Wives: Women Married to Gay or Bisexual Men

Researchers have neglected an experience that some women confront, the homosexual extramarital involvement of their husbands. Kinsey, Pomeroy and Martin (1948) concluded that the true incidence of homosexuality among married people is much higher than they were able to document. Far less is known about the wives of homosexual and bisexual men (Hays & Samuels, 1989). In an exploratory study of 21 heterosexual women who are or have been married to homosexual men and who have had children by them, Hays and Samuels (1989) recruited respondents through support groups of wives in major East Coast cities. These wives responded to a 27-page questionnaire on all aspects of their marital and personal histories. Their average age was 48 years, and the average length of marriage was 20 years. Eleven were still living with their husbands, but only three of these women felt that the marriages would last. The women were well-educated and predominantly middle class.

Eighteen of the women stated that they did not know their husbands were bisexual or homosexual when they married; the other three claimed they were naive about their husbands' sexual practices. The shame associated with "being blind to the facts" (Hays & Samuels, 1989, p. 98), as well as the social stigma still associated with homosexuality, left these women with very little support, apart from others in the same situation, for their experiences and feelings. There was no evidence from the early years of their courtship or marriage that their choice of a mate could have been prevented. Most women did not select their husbands for qualities different from those of heterosexual men, and they had experienced their marriages as generally satisfactory.

Realizing that their husbands were emotionally attached to other men caused far greater stress than the discovery of their husbands' homosexual activity. Preserving the continuity of the marriage was more important to them than their husband's extramarital behavior. The loss of trust when husbands had been deceitful was much more damaging than the fact of homosexuality. The women were also concerned about helping their children adjust to the discovery of their fathers' sexuality. Overall, the women described the shock of not being prepared for this experience and their need for support in integrating the experience themselves, with their children, and with those outside the family.

VIOLENCE AGAINST WOMEN
IN INTIMATE RELATIONSHIPS

The intimacy of close relationship also has a darker side. The violence that occurs in intimate relationships has been well documented and attests to the pervasiveness of power as a potent dimension of intimacy. Between 1979 and 1987, women reported being the victims of intimate violence three times as frequently as men; three fourths of these assaults were perpetrated by spouses (9%), ex-spouses (35%), and boyfriends or ex-boyfriends (32%) (Harlow, 1991). Separated or divorced women were 14 times more likely than women living with their husband to have been abused by a spouse or ex-spouse. These occurrences were not isolated; about 20% of these women had been assaulted by their partner at least three times in the 6 months before the survey. White women are more likely to be assaulted by their husbands or ex-husbands, and African-American women by their boyfriends or ex-boyfriends.

Harlow's (1991) analysis of data from the National Crime Survey indicated that about a quarter of these assaults involved the use of a weapon. It is not surprising that 28% of the murders of women in 1989 were believed to have been committed by husbands or boyfriends.

The question persists of why women who are battered do not leave the relationship. Research on this topic indicates that many women who are abused have low self-esteem and feel inadequate or helpless to leave the abusive partner (Gelles & Strauss, 1988). Women who experienced more violence as children are less likely to leave an abusive relationship, as are women who perceive themselves to be without educational and occupational skills necessary to support themselves and their children (Gelles & Cornell, 1985). Women also may stay with their abusers because they love them and believe the men will reform, because they believe their children need a father, or because their partners threaten to track them down if they do leave. The most reasonable explanation revolves around resources and vulnerability. If women do not have the economic or personal resources to make a satisfactory exit from the relationship, their alternatives are limited (see Yllo & Bograd, 1988). Family isolation and societal denial of the pervasiveness of violence are associated with woman battering. Women without peer and social supports are less likely to define brutality by their male partners as violence (Kelly, 1988).

Cultural constructions of traditional marriage indirectly support violence by depicting the male as the powerful and dominant partner. A man who feels inadequate and threatened in his own home often sees violence as a way to enforce his dominance and gain control of some aspect of his life (Gelles & Strauss, 1988). Couples who report the most sharing of decision making have the lowest level of violence; the highest reported level is in relationships where power is concentrated in the hands of one partner (Gelles & Strauss, 1988). Women who have personal resources and the potential for economic autonomy are in the best position to have relationships free of violence and to be able to leave if they feel at risk.

The repression that lesbians experience in mainstream society further silences lesbians who are victims of abuse and battering in their relationships (Evans & Bannister, 1990). Lesbians may have even less access to services such as battered women's shelters in light of pervasive homophobia. Funding agencies may threaten to close down shelters if there is a visible lesbian presence, thus leading to exclusion of women who do not fit the stereotype of a battered woman who deserves services (Hammond, 1989). Lesbians of color contend with racism, sexism, and homophobia, which may lead to further silencing in the very communities that "should be havens from the racist, sexist, classist institutions that comprise majority culture" (Kanuha, 1990, p. 176). Feminists have provided analyses documenting that battering can occur in any relationship. Given the pervasiveness of abuse, it is important to recognize that services are needed for all women, yet they are available for only a small minority. Feminists condemn all forms of physical, emotional, and sexual abuse, regardless of the type of relationship in which the abuse occurs.

THE ENDINGS OF RELATIONSHIPS

People and their relationships continue to develop and change over time. Some intimate relationships endure until the death of one partner, but, more frequently, contemporary relationships end in separation or divorce. Regardless of the sex of one's partner, the loss of a love relationship signals a major life transition and emotional suffering for at least one of the partners. For women who have been dependent economically on a partner, the end of the relationship can also be financially devastating.

Considerable research is available on the consequences of divorce, but little attention has been devoted to the disintegration of relationships. The process by which a couple disentangle their lives exhibits a fairly consistent pattern as the transition is made from a couple identity to individual identities that are defined by self and others as separate and distinct from the former partner (Vaughan, 1986). There is usually a period of conflict and discontent before one partner moves from deliberating about ending the relationship to actually taking steps to terminate it.

Although there is great variability in individual relationships, research on divorce reveals gender differences in experiences related to separation and divorce. Wives tend to evaluate their husbands much more severely and negatively than their husbands judge them (Spanier & Thompson, 1984). In Spanier and Thompson's study, women rated every item evaluating their marriage more negatively than men did and were particularly negative about the husbands' participation in household and parenting responsibilities. Men failed to meet women's expectations for sharing these demands. Men were twice as likely as women (35% vs. 18%) to report that they still loved their partners at the time of the final separation, whereas women were more likely to feel ambivalence (25%), mild affection (21%), or outright hate (19%).

One partner in a relationship usually becomes discontented or emotionally detached before the other. The initiator of the separation, having had time to consider and develop alternatives to the relationship, usually fares better emotionally. As one who is less invested in the continuation of the relationship, the initiator usually has more power and influence in the transition.

Vaughan (1986) found that resources are critical in understanding how people experience and survive the "uncoupling" process. She warns, however, that it is risky to predict how disruptive uncoupling will be by simply comparing partners' social and economic assets. Paramount is not the abundance of resources, but how connected the resources are to the partner's individual identity. She uses the example of a small bank account that is secret and separate as being a more firmly secured resource than a larger sum in an account that is jointly held by the couple.

Personal resources and perceived alternatives seem to be necessary, although perhaps not sufficient, to facilitate an adaptive recovery to the termination of an intimate relationship. The economic costs for women have been well documented. As the result of divorce, men's standard of living tends to improve while women's drops. The most often quoted statistics (Weitzman, 1988) claim that a woman's standard of living falls 73% in the first year and a man's rises 42%. Although Weitzman appears to have overstated the impact (Faludi, 1991), divorce carries greater economic risk for wives than for husbands because these women generally have lower incomes as well as physical custody of minor children. The most recent analysis (Bianchi & McArthur, 1991) indicates a 37% decrease in monthly family income when men leave the home. Only 15% of women who divorced in 1990 were awarded alimony, and only about half of the women who were awarded child support received it (Lester, 1991). Even when women received the total amount awarded, the mean amount of $3,268 is a relatively small contribution to the financial support of a family.

In the last decade, in-depth studies of women's experiences of divorce have revealed the difficulties that women face in ending their marriages, particularly if they have children. Arendell (1990) interviewed

60 women about their postdivorce situations. The significant drop in family income and the resulting economic uncertainty tended to shape most other aspects of these women's lives, aggravating emotional traumas and revealing the economic dependency that their marriages had obscured. All but three of the mothers were employed, but only two earned more than $1,500 a month. The women's low earnings were traced to limited job training and experience due to their commitment to marriage and childcare and to the continued discrimination against women in the workplace. More than a third of the women depended to some extent on their own parents for direct financial help because they could not support their children on their incomes alone.

Like most divorced mothers, these women continued to be the primary parent to their children even in the two cases in which the parents shared custody (Arendell, 1990). Women struggled with the conflicting demands of parenting and providing, but found their relationships with their children *better* after the divorce. They redefined relationships with their children and became more open and democratic mothers.

A persistent problem for women in this study was how to negotiate being a single mother and a single woman. Finding time and resources for a social life outside the family was difficult, as were the effects of altered friendships and the lack of guidelines regarding the changing social realities of adult sexual relationships. Ironically, the easiest and surest way women saw to resolve many of the issues facing them was to remarry (Arendell, 1990). However, most did not plan to do so and voiced a new appreciation of themselves as single individuals.

Much of the theory and research about divorce treats women as a homogeneous group and ignores the diversity of women's experiences by age, ethnicity, socioeconomic level, and whether they initiated the divorce. In a longitudinal study of the effects of divorce, Wallerstein and Blakeslee (1989) revealed the differences between the postdivorce lives of younger and older women. Women older than 40 were less likely to make social and psychological shifts and explore new opportunities. Many of these women, especially those who did not initiate the divorce, were described as intensely lonely and expressing a great sense of loss. More than half experienced a decline in their standard of living, and 80% were financially insecure. These older women faced different social, psychological, and economic barriers than the younger women, who were often able to improve their lives through remarriage and new careers.

Like other aspects of lesbian existence, the termination of committed lesbian relationships has been obscured. The process of uncoupling among lesbian couples is similar to that of other relationships (Vaughan, 1986). The ending of an intimate relationship means pain, sadness, and a sense of loss. However, there are differences between the situations of most heterosexual couples and lesbian couples that may mediate the way separation is experienced.

There may be less social pressure and support to maintain a lesbian relationship because of the lack of acknowledgment and support by family members and acquaintances. In heterosexual relationships, the legal process of separating and terminating a relationship provides some structural constraints that are not present in lesbian relationships. These legal activities provide for many heterosexual couples a rite of passage that marks the transition from their coupled state back to being single individuals. These institutionalized transitions are not part of the lesbian uncoupling process. In fact, any issue such as child custody or disputes over property that might draw a lesbian couple into the legal arena probably carries with it greater risks than similar issues do for heterosexual women.

However, lesbian women are probably in a better position to make a satisfactory transition from a deteriorating relationship than are many heterosexual women. Lesbians tend to have more egalitarian relationships in which both partners contribute to financial support and sharing responsibilities; thus, economic dependency tends to be less of an issue. Although one partner may decide to sacrifice her personal needs or interests to take primary responsibility for housework or childcare, unlike heterosexual couples there is no expectation about who this partner should be. Because there is less disparity between incomes in lesbian couples and both usually work, neither may be plunged into poverty as the result of the termination of the relationship.

Divorce does not have to be a kinship rupture. Examples from postmodern feminist families reveal that, despite the end of an economic and sexual partnership, the emotional component often continues. In her ethnography of working-class families, Stacey (1990) found that relationships with former partners continued, particularly when children were involved. Ex-spouses and their families became a kinship extension (Stacey, 1990). In lesbian communities as well, intimate partnerships ended, but women continued to be friends and political allies (Krieger, 1982).

A Feminist Vision for Enriching Women's Relationships

In this chapter, we have examined various perspectives on women's intimate relationships in adulthood. The ideas and experiences presented have been selective, not intended as an exhaustive survey of all that has been written about women and their partnerships. Instead, we have presented a way of looking at women's relationships that places the lifelong dialectic of gender on a critical plane. We focused on the dilemmas for adult relationships between an early socialization for homosociality and a later expectation for heterosociality, culminating in the major role of wife for women. We incorporated emotional and sexual relationships between women into the discussion as a central relational concern, first, because lesbians are literally ignored in treatments of women's family arrangements and, second, because of the possibilities for change and new ways of being that lesbian partnerships represent. And yet, we recognized the continued vitality that relationships with men hold for women.

Our point of view was motivated by the feminist project of deconstructing myths about a monolithic family experience for women and reconstructing a more comprehensive knowledge about women and their families. Uncovering diversity as we lift the veil from formerly invisible ways of living and being in the world is an exciting project, suggesting new ways in which women and those they love join and separate over the life course. We have found that relational commitment remains an organizing feature of women's lives. Indeed, women are innovators in attempting to generate and sustain relationships that are rooted not in hierarchy but in relational qualities such as empathy, responsibility, and cooperation.

Continued Vitality of Marriage

Stacey (1986) made the intriguing observation that feminism has yet to explain or appreciate the complexity and continued vitality of heterosexuality, even for women who are feminists. We extend Stacey's point to consider the continued vitality of marriage. In this chapter, we have examined the dialectic between autonomy and affiliation that is played out in women's lives and through their intimate relationships. Although we have examined numerous alternatives to compulsory marriage and heterosexuality, we cannot dismiss the pull of marriage or, in its less institutionalized version, the salience of lifelong commitment to a significant other. In some ways, feminist women and men are reclaiming marriage (Blaisure, 1992) as a potentially empowering option for all couples.

Thompson (1989) offers an insightful perspective on marital responsibility that is grounded in contextual and relational morality. This approach examines the dialectic between the critique of marriage as exchange and the simultaneous desire for a lifelong bond with an intimate partner. Thompson's argument, set within the context of heterosexual marriage, seems useful for other types of relationships as well.

We suggest a reconstruction of marriage, not as a legal arrangement between a man and his wife, but as a committed partnership based on economic cooperation, sexual expression, and emotional intimacy. In this conceptualization, diverse partnerships can be accommodated. Healthy lesbian relationships, for example, are characterized by the equality of best friendships (Peplau, 1982), rather than by the gender hierarchy found in traditional marriage (Glenn, 1987). Moreover, as Baruch et al. (1983) found, the most rewarding marital relationships were loving friendships characterized by caring and cooperation. Thus, we embrace Thompson's (1989) use of responsibility and equity as a new basis for multiple types of marriage relationships, including those that do not, as yet, have legal sanction.

Contextual morality deals with "the everyday experience of particular people in particular circumstances in a particular community and society at a particular historical moment" (Thompson, 1989, p. 3). Relational morality emerges out of the daily interactions of marital partners, "evident in how we treat each other day by day" (Thompson, 1989, p. 7). This framework liberates the discussion of moral responsibility in marriage from an absolutist, fixed stance. Thus, morality in marriage is an everyday construction, accomplished through words, actions, thoughts, and feelings, and set within a sociohistorical context that shifts according to hierarchies of age, race, gender, class, and sexual orientation. Marital responsibility has four processes: attribution, disclosure, empathy, and cooperation. These interactional processes seem to be a stronger basis for relationship growth and maintenance than the former view of marriage as role based. The commitment that emerges from two individuals acting in the best interests of self and partner offers possibilities for individuals to complete themselves in another, fulfilling the promise that legal marriage, which is rooted in hierarchy, has not been able to do.

Developing a Proactive Approach to Relationships

The development and maintenance of satisfying intimate relationships is not something that just happens *to* women. Rather, women can develop skills and make knowledgeable decisions that maximize the likelihood of mutually rewarding partnerships based on love, caring, and sustenance. Girls and young women can be socialized with the knowledge that they are valuable in and of themselves regardless of whether they are in a relationship. Attention can be devoted to helping young women develop decision-making and communication skills so that relationships are not initiated or continued through default.

Young women need to be raised with the understanding that it is no longer a viable option to expect that they can be economically or psychologically dependent upon a partner. They must grow up with the expectation that they will need to support themselves and their children. At some point in their lives they may choose to rely upon a partner's economic support for periods of time, but they must have the resources to be economically autonomous to protect themselves and their children from vulnerability.

Women who work and contribute to family income have a higher sense of control and self-esteem that allows them to have expectations of equality in their relationships (Vannoy-Hiller & Philliber, 1989). The potential to be financially autonomous provides women with more power, equality, and the resources needed to make a satisfactory exit from a relationship if necessary (Okin, 1989). The research findings on the postdivorce lives of women indicate the far-reaching effects of economic uncertainty for women who have sacrificed their own personal and career development to attend to being wives and mothers. Many of these effects are avoidable as women become more conscious in their decision making.

The lack of relationship permanence indicates that women and men need to make more careful choices before entering a committed relationship. Relationship development is romanticized in our society, perpetuating the notion that the heart is a better guide than the head when making decisions. Early and continuing relationship education would teach the basics of relationship skills and provide an understanding of how one identifies potentially healthy partners before making an emotional commitment. If both females and males learn a wide repertoire of skills that allow them to express and negotiate their needs, desires, and concerns in functional and caring ways, much of the miscommunication between women and men could be avoided.

Relationship contracts for marriage or cohabitation offer a useful tool for making decisions about partnerships. Even without using contracts as legal documents, they can be of value to women in assessing the benefits and risks of a particular relationship. Areas of potential difficulty can be identified and negotiated by working through aspects of the relationship, such as sharing household responsibilities, handling conflict, and deciding about childbearing, careers, money, and sexual fidelity.

The more experience and confidence a woman has, the more likely she will be to make decisions that are in her own best interests. The trend toward delaying first marriage means that women will be somewhat older, more mature, and probably more educated when they make long-term commitments. Women who make commitments later not only have more experience, but may also have more personal and economic resources, which maximize the likelihood of negotiating equal relationships with their partners.

Although individual women can take action to enhance the likelihood of having satisfying relationships, the social context is just as important. Relationships develop from, exist in, and are influenced by prevailing social norms and structures. The growing acceptance of relationship variations allows women to explore other opportunities for intimacy over the life course. The normalization of lesbian relationships and heterosexual cohabitation means that women are less likely to end up in a marriage by default. When information about the variety of relationship possibilities is presented to young people for consideration, they are more likely to make decisions that are consistent with their identity and interests than when marriage is presented as the only acceptable life choice.

CHAPTER THREE

Women's Sexualities

Although women are exploring, articulating, and (re)claiming their sexuality, female sexuality is virtually an uncharted landscape even in feminist discourse and analysis. There is no contemporary paradigm for understanding women as sexual beings, no clear strategy for replacing lingering myths with authentic sexual experiences.

The legends of Mary, the pure mother and wife, Eve, the insatiable temptress, and Mary Magdalene, the repentant prostitute, have pervaded Western cultural definitions of female sexuality, controlling and restricting women's experiences in an attempt to preserve social order and family relationships (Janeway, 1980). Revolutionary social changes demand a revision of thinking about women and sexuality. Half of all young women now experience sexual intercourse by age 16; virginity at marriage is the exception rather than the rule. Women seek out information about their own anatomy and physiology, as well as about how to enhance their sexual relationships. Women are becoming more assertive about their sexual desires and their expectation that there be sexual fulfillment for both partners in any sexual interaction.

Although norms have changed significantly regarding sexual behavior for women, existing ideas about female sexuality stress the victimization women experience and undermine the development of satisfying relationships. Fine (1988) identified four prevailing discourses of female sexuality that influence the way in which women and society construct sexual expectations and meanings: sexuality as violence, sexuality as victimization, sexuality as individual morality, and a discourse of desire. Our society suppresses a discourse of female desire, promotes a discourse of female victimization, and favors the married heterosexual state over other sexual options (Fine, 1988).

Little systematic research on women's sexuality exists. Kinsey made a pioneering effort in the 1950s, followed by Masters & Johnson's (1966) groundbreaking research. In the late 1970s and early 1980s there was a flurry of feminist work with the publication of Laws and Schwartz's (1977) *Sexual Scripts: The Social Construction of Female Sexuality*; Snitow, Stansell, and Thompson's *Powers of Desire: The Politics of Sexuality* (1983); Stimpson and Person's (1980) *Women: Sex and Sexuality*; and Vance's (1984) *Pleasure and Danger: Exploring Female Sexuality*. Differing opinions about the relationship between sexuality and pornography led to divisions among feminists in the 1980s (Leidholdt & Raymond, 1990). Reproductive rights issues overshadowed general female sexuality concerns in the late 1980s and early 1990s.

The lack of attention to women's sexuality is related to and compounded by the scarcity of research on human sexuality in general. Research on human sexuality is controversial, undervalued, and poorly funded. Theory development has been almost nonexistent. The research that has been done problemizes sex by focusing on topics like adolescent sexual activity, sexual abuse, and rape rather than on what might constitute normal sexual functioning. A decade review of marriage and family research in the 1980s shows only two articles related to sexual topics, and these addressed sexual abuse of children (Gelles & Conte, 1990) and teen pregnancy and childbearing (Miller & Moore, 1990).

Even feminist research has emphasized the victimization aspects of sexuality rather than exploring pleasure and empowerment. Nothing less than a "monumental overhaul" of the entire system of thought about sexuality is required (Schneider & Gould, 1987). A new paradigm is needed to guide exploration and understanding of sexuality in families in general. Maddock (1989) suggested criteria for judging the sexual health of families and an ecosystemic model that emphasizes dialectical balance among the various aspects of family sexuality. He identified gender as a key variable and acknowledged its influence on sexual thoughts, communications, perceptions, and behaviors. However, his use of "the family" as the unit of analysis obscures gender-related differences in sexuality. The family of which he speaks appears to be headed by married, heterosexual partners; the multiplicity of contemporary family configurations is ignored. A deconstruction of family sexuality would reveal the effects of gender, age, race, sexual orientation, and legal status on the meaning and experience of sexuality for the individuals involved.

An analysis of gender influences is critical. Historically, female sexuality has been repressed, distorted, and compared to male sexuality, which is used as the normative baseline for eroticism and sexual activity (Schneider & Gould, 1987). Most women form sexual partnerships with males and are affected by differential understandings, expectations, experiences, and attitudes. Female sexuality has not been controlled totally by external forces, however. Women are not merely victims of male sexual prerogative; they have made choices and taken actions to enhance their lives. Our goal in this chapter is to reveal women's sexual potential, examine their desires in sexual relationships, and clarify the meaning of these relationships to them.

Postmodern feminist theory deconstructs traditional understandings about women's sexual experiences and guides the construction of a discourse of empowerment and normalization regarding female sexualities. This approach rejects unitary notions of woman's experience and acknowledges the influences of class, religion, race, age, and sexual orientation (Fraser & Nicholson, 1990; Hawkesworth, 1989; Tong, 1989). Subsuming all women into a general category ignores differences in behavior, desire, and experience, thereby obscuring existing inequalities among women and emphasizing differences between women and men (Scott, 1990). The concept "sexualities" used in this chapter signifies the multiplicity of women's experiences.

A postmodern feminist perspective is inclusive enough to consider sexual diversity among women as well between men and women. There are differences among women in their sexual lives. There are those women who have different numbers of partners, different sexual values, and different degrees of interest in participating in a variety of sexual activities. One study of 868 nurses revealed a range of 1 to 75 sexual partners (Davidson & Darling, 1988). Black women appear to be more liberal in regard to sexuality, experience first intercourse at an earlier age, and have more frequent sexual activity than white women (Weinberg & Williams, 1988). Lesbians may define and experience sexual interactions differently than heterosexual women (Frye, 1990). Class, age, and religious orientation also influence sexual values and activities, but there has been no systematic research examining their effects (Francoeur, 1987; Fullilove, Fullilove, Haynes, & Gross, 1990).

A valid understanding of sexuality must acknowledge sociohistorical factors contributing to the diversity of women's sexual experiences in intimate and familial relationships. Part of the historical record is the sexual victimization of women by men through sexual assaults and rape, sexual harassment, prostitution, unplanned and unwanted pregnancies, and pornography, which degrades and objectifies women.

We deconstruct female sexualities and shift the focus from characterizing women as victims to affirming women as innovative agents in developing satisfying sexual relationships. The effects of power inequities on intimate relationships provide the context for this analysis. In this chapter, five dialectical themes provide a framework for exploring women's sexual experiences.

First, we consider some of the problems inherent in studying sexual topics. We look at interpretive issues such as the problem of how language and social control of ideas are used to limit the conceptualization and empirical investigation of sexuality.

Second, we consider the extent to which sexualities are biologically given or socially constructed. Are women's sexualities essentially different than men's, or have social forces and gender arrangements constrained female sexual expression, thereby distorting knowledge and understanding of their sexual potential? The concept of sexual scripts is used to explore the tension between the stability and variability of sexual identity over time and in different relationships.

Third, we consider the perception that women may be less interested and less sexually active than men. We examine the influences of gender differences, sexual orientation, and relationship duration on women's sexual interactions.

Fourth, we turn to the debate regarding the connection of reproduction and sexuality in women's lives. Although we address these aspects of women's experiences in separate chapters to differentiate the issues related to each, in this chapter we briefly consider their interconnections.

Fifth, we explore the relationship between sexuality and power. Power has been eroticized; symbolic resistance, submission, and conquest have been romanticized and internalized as normal aspects of sexuality. However, women have resisted male control and constructed their own personal and intimate identities, balancing between pleasure and danger in their sexual lives (Vance, 1984).

Last, we propose a feminist vision of women's sexualities. We offer proposals for sexual pluralism, education, and empowerment from a feminist perspective.

INTERPRETATION AND CONTROL IN SEXUALITY RESEARCH

The media saturate society with sexual messages. Paradoxically, there is resistance to dealing explicitly with sexuality through education and research. A nationwide survey of the health and sexual behavior of 20,000 people by the National Institute of Child Health and Human Development was planned to begin in 1989. The study was designed to gather information about people's sexual activity over the lifespan, how they choose partners, and their partners' characteristics. Data would have provided guidance in AIDS education and prevention programs. Health and Human Services Secretary Louis Sullivan, influenced by conservative members of the House of Representatives, blocked funding for the study (Reiss, 1990). In 1991, Sullivan also cancelled an $18 million 5-year survey of 24,000 adolescents in grades 7 to 11. The study was to gather information about sexual practices that place teens at risk for early pregnancy and sexually transmitted diseases (Gosselin, 1991).

Although government officials may stifle sexuality research, this action does not stop change. Social change often signals shifts in power that can threaten the control of dominant groups. This is true regarding female sexuality. Because women's sexualities have been simultaneously exploited and repressed, contemporary societal messages about women as sexual beings are conflicted and confusing to both women and men. Competing tensions and provocative themes threaten not only men's sexual control over women, but also women's sense of certainty about the determinants of their own sexuality.

Much of the early work on women's sexuality goes unmentioned in human sexuality texts. In a historical analysis of female sexuality in the United States, Lewis (1980) traced the ongoing attention to women's sexuality dating back to the colonial era. Although socialization, medical influences, and religion collaborated to promote belief in women as sexless and passive, Lewis (1980) revealed otherwise by documenting early research on female sexuality. A female physician, Clelia Mosher of Stanford University, conducted the first known sex survey between 1890 and 1920. By talking directly to women born around the time of the Civil War about their sexual feelings and responses, she found they were frank about their enjoyment of sexuality despite the prevailing societal view that sex was only for reproductive purposes. Mosher's work was followed in 1929 by Katherine Davis's *Factors in the Sex Life of Twenty-Five Hundred Women*. In the 1930s, Helena Wright (1959), a gynecologist, wrote a sex manual that gave women step-by-step instructions on how to masturbate and how to have orgasms through intercourse.

Recent feminist critiques continue to resist the notion of women as sexless. Feminists have examined common assumptions about women's sexuality and explored the ways in which women construct understandings of themselves as sexual beings (Golden, 1987; Hite, 1987; Rich, 1980; Sevely, 1987; Sherfey, 1973; Vance, 1984). Feminists disagree about some of the basic assumptions regarding sexuality, a tension discussed throughout this chapter. Some argue that sexuality is the arena in which male dominance and female subordination are produced and maintained (Jackson, 1987; MacKinnon, 1982). MacKinnon (1982) proposed that sexuality is to feminism what work is to Marxism. Society is organized hierarchically through male sexual dominance and the sexualization of inequality.

In contrast, Rubin (1984) argued that sex and gender are not simply interchangeable and that feminist theory is not powerful enough to totally explain the politics of sexuality. Sexual politics overlap gender politics; there are sexual hierarchies within and between genders. Because all sexuality issues are not based on gender inequality, Rubin (1984) claims that most contemporary feminist thought "lacks the angles of vision" to analyze comprehensively the social organization of sexuality.

A postmodern feminist perspective provides a corrective to the dialectic. Through attention to diversity and the tensions surrounding women's sexual lives, it offers a perspective for rethinking sexualities.

Deconstructing Sexualities

Explorations of women's sexualities take place in a terrain strewn with obstacles. The deconstructive function of a postmodern feminist perspective challenges and exposes beliefs and concepts that are taken for granted and used to legitimize apparently natural social arrangements. A major constraint in constructing an understanding of female sexualities and a discourse of desire is the lack of a nonpejorative vocabulary to capture and express women's sexual experiences, wishes, and feelings (Bernard, 1981; Schneider & Gould, 1987). Sexual language exhibits a male, heterosexist bias. Sexual activity is identified usually as premarital, marital, or extramarital. Some feminists have suggested renaming and reframing sexual terminology to address these biases. Penetration might be replaced with the concept of enclosure, foreplay transformed to heterosexual afterplay, and sexual activity released from its link to marriage (Schneider & Gould, 1987).

Renaming sexual terminology is important because it provides legitimacy. Legitimacy leads to integration into a society's way of thinking about the world. A valid vocabulary for naming their feelings and experiences allows women to reflect on their own sexuality and communicate their sexual interest and preferences. Because language frames thought and sets its limits, defining a clear conceptual basis for female sexualities can be a forerunner of internal change that allows women new ways of being in the world (Rubin, 1990). Opening up a feminist discourse with the goal of empowerment allows women to explore and define their sexualities by what they are or can be, not by what they are not or should not be (Newton & Walton, 1984).

Disentangling Dimensions of Sexualities

Deconstructing the concept of sexuality allows a clearer analysis of the factors that contribute to the creation of self as a sexual being. Sexuality is usually conceptualized as a unitary construct, but it is more useful to think of it as a complex blend of attitudes, feelings, behaviors, and responses. Newton and Walton's (1984) four-component model provides a blueprint for the deconstruction process. This model distinguishes sexual preference and desire among heterosexual and lesbian women, and sexual acts from culturally prescribed roles associated with masculinity and femininity. The four components in their model are erotic identity, erotic role, erotic acts, and sexual preference.

Erotic identity is one's "sexy persona" or how one imagines oneself as an erotic object (Newton & Walton, 1984). For each person, it is influenced uniquely by the interrelationship of personal history and culture such as gender, social class, and sexual orientation. The conventional gender categories of man or woman are assumed to be erotic identities in and of themselves for heterosexuals. The conflation of gender role and erotic identity is especially problematic for women, who are expected to conform to stereotypical ideals about how women should look in order to be attractive and desirable. Heterosexual women may have little opportunity to consider erotic identity apart from heterosexual roles that require them to be monogamous and to experience sexual desire within a long-term committed relationship to one man, presumably as a husband.

A second dimension, erotic role, is what one does in partnered sex (Newton & Walton, 1984). Whereas erotic identity is one's sexual self-image, erotic role refers to processes and interactions within relationships, such as initiating, responding, and resisting. The way one looks, one's gender category of male or female, and one's sexual orientation are not necessarily correlated with the role one plays during sexual interactions.

The third dimension, erotic acts, refers to the content of one's sexuality, the "particular acts that obsess, please, turn you on, either to do or have done, to watch or hear" (Newton & Walton, 1984, p. 246). Erotic acts involve body zones, objects, or specific scenes that provide the content and excitement for sexual expression.

Sexual preference and sexual orientation both refer to whether one's partners in sexual activity tend to be of the same or the other sex. Because sexual preference implies a sense of choice that most people do not experience regarding the sex of people to whom they are attracted, the term "sexual orientation" is a more precise term. In this book, sexual preference is reserved to designate situations where choice of partner by sex has been specifically considered and a decision made. A woman may be attracted to both males and females; clinically, she would be considered bisexual. However, for political reasons, she might choose female partners exclusively, thereby declaring her sexual preference.

The deconstruction of sexuality into these component parts leads to underlying questions about how, for each individual, these dimensions interrelate to present a sense of an integrated sexual being. By what process is the sense of sexual self developed? How and why do differences among people occur, and what are the implications of these differences?

SEXUALITY: BIOLOGICALLY DETERMINED OR SOCIALLY CONSTRUCTED?

The debate about the extent to which one's sexual identity is biologically determined or socially constructed is basic to critiques of sexuality. Disentangling the physiological and social contributions to sexuality is probably impossible. Human beings have certain inherent capacities to respond to stimulation of those parts of their bodies richly endowed with nerve endings. The basic physical response pattern of sexual arousal and orgasm is rather uniform across individuals. With adequate stimulation, regardless of the type of activity involved or the sex of the partner, males and females have the potential for similar response patterns (Masters & Johnson, 1966). The response cycle described by Masters and Johnson includes excitement, plateau , orgasm, and resolution phases. An alternative model proposed by Kaplan (1979) identified three stages—desire, excitement, and orgasm—characterizing human sexual response.

One of the few differences between males and females is the male refractory period. Following orgasm, men experience a period during which they cannot achieve a full erection or have another orgasm. Women do not require this recovery period; they are capable of having orgasms in quick succession. With self-controlled, mechanical manipulation such as with a vibrator, an average female may have 20 to 50 consecutive orgasms, stopping only because of exhaustion (Sherfey, 1973). In physiological terms, women potentially are more sexually responsive than are men. Despite this potential, there is great variety in women's response patterns. More than 50% of women in some studies report never having had any orgasms through penile–vaginal intercourse, much less experiencing multiple orgasms (Hite, 1976).

Physiological research indicates that it is not the lack of female orgasmic capacity that leaves them preorgasmic:

> The maximum physiologic intensity of orgasmic response subjectively reported or objectively recorded has been achieved by self-regulated mechanical or automanipulative techniques. The next highest level of erotic intensity has resulted from partner manipulation, again with established or self-regulated methods, and the lowest intensity of target-organ response was achieved during coition. (Masters & Johnson, 1966, p. 132)

Even though women are least likely to have an orgasm as the result of coitus, it is the normative activity among heterosexual couples. When most people talk about having "sex," it is assumed that they are referring to penile–vaginal intercourse. The lack of adequate stimulation that coitus provides and men's tendency to stop activity after their own orgasms contribute to women's orgasmic "difficulty" (Crooks & Baur, 1990).

The underlying uniformity in women's and men's physiological responsiveness tends to be obscured by the variety of ways in which sexuality is manifested in society. Social norms construct, define, promote, and proscribe certain acts and partners. Although there appear to be some physiological givens regarding sexual response, the evidence challenges the notion of sexuality as an unchanging or natural state. For most people, much of their sexual activity occurs with a partner. Sexual desire is produced in the context of a relationship; it is not a core component of the self that is fixed forever (Blumstein & Schwartz, 1989).

The Social Construction of Sexual Scripts

The view of the sexual self as socially constructed is supported by work as diverse in time and place as the Kinsey group's (1948, 1953) classic studies of men's and women's sexual behavior, Golden's (1987) contemporary investigation of women's sexual orientation, and the latest work from the Kinsey Institute (McWhirter, Sanders, & Reinisch, 1990). Clinicians and researchers have tended to see sexual behavior as flowing from sexual identity, but most women do not experience their sexuality with such congruence (Golden, 1987). Feminists (e.g., Aptheker, 1989; Blumstein & Schwartz, 1989; Golden, 1987; Kitzinger, 1987; Schneider & Gould, 1987; Smith, 1989; Vance, 1984) critique essentialism, which posits that sexual desire, identity, and behavior form an unchanging unified core of sexuality that is an inherent part of personality. Because they are socially constructed, women's sexualities offer, instead, the possibility for growth and change over the life course.

The concept of sexual scripts (Laws & Schwartz, 1977) is useful in understanding how social norms affect the construction of sexual identity, the integration of sexual roles, and the meaning attributed to sexual activity. Sexual scripts refer to a "repertoire of acts and statuses that are recognized by a social group, together with the rules, expectations, and sanctions governing these acts and sanctions" (Laws & Schwartz, 1977, p. 2). Through primary socialization, formal education, and personal experience, each individual constructs a sexual script for herself with rules about (1) with whom she has sex, (2) what sexual behaviors are acceptable, (3) when it is appropriate to have sex, (4) where it is acceptable to have sex, and (5) reasons for sexual activity. Sexual scripts include a subtext about the process of sexual activity and the enacting of erotic roles such as who should initiate, what is appropriate communication, and how power can be used. One's sexuality is a product of opportunity, socialization, and interpretation (Blumstein & Schwartz, 1990).

An individual's sexual script develops as the result of messages from parents, teachers, media, religion, peers, partners, and other social institutions. Although idiosyncrasies result from the ways individuals develop their sexual scripts, there are also shared cultural themes and symbols resulting from common childhood experiences and societal messages (Katchadourian, 1989). Because females and males are socialized and treated differently, it is not surprising that men's and women's sexual scripts provide different norms. Women learn to link love and sex; thus, eroticization tends to develop in the context of a relationship (Blumstein & Schwartz, 1990). For men, a relationship appears to be desirable but not necessary. Women who have many partners and a great deal of sexual activity are described as promiscuous, but men are likely to be described in terms acknowledging their prowess and expertise unless they are gay (Rubin, 1990).

Sexual scripts that reinforce and maintain existing social arrangements become institutionalized. Young women are still encouraged to "save themselves for marriage." If they cannot remain abstinent, they are urged to be selective sexually and very discreet so they do not "spoil" themselves for their future husbands.

Alternative scripts are denied and devalued in an attempt to keep them from being perceived as options (Laws & Schwartz, 1977). For example, cohabitation is seen as a poor substitute for marriage for women. Lesbian sexuality is rarely described or discussed. However, as sexual pluralism becomes more obvious through social activism, the media, and education, there is greater opportunity for women to perceive options and develop sexual scripts that deviate from prevailing notions of what is appropriate or acceptable.

The Development and Construction of Sexual Orientation

Sexual orientation is defined by the sex of the individuals to whom one is attracted, about whom one fantasizes, and with whom one falls in love. Money (1987) suggests that falling in love is the definitive criterion of heterosexual, homosexual, and bisexual orientation.

Little is known about how people develop a sexual orientation. No more is known about the development of heterosexuality than about homosexuality or bisexuality. Cross-cultural research on male homosexuality suggests some type of biological component contributes to sexual orientation. Homosexuals are found in all societies, regardless of the degree of acceptance or rejection of homosexuality (Katchadourian, 1989). About 10% of individuals in all societies are homosexually oriented, and this percentage tends to remain stable over time.

Money's (1987) theory about the development of sexual orientation proposes that prenatal hormonal influences on the brain interact with postnatal socialization to influence an individual's subsequent sexual orientation. As a result, there is a normal, natural variety of sexual orientations, which tend to be established in early childhood.

There has been a tendency to see heterosexuality and homosexuality as mutually exclusive, discrete categories, but research suggests otherwise (Katchadourian, 1989). Kinsey et al. (1953) originally proposed placing people on a scale with gradations of heterosexual and homosexual inclination. The scale was based on people's sexual feelings and experiences and represented a ratio of homosexuality to heterosexuality. A person's sexual orientation was identified on a seven-point continuum:

0 Exclusively heterosexual
1 Predominantly heterosexual, only incidentally homosexual
2 Predominantly heterosexual, but more than incidentally homosexual
3 Equally heterosexual and homosexual
4 Predominantly homosexual, but more than incidentally heterosexual
5 Predominantly homosexual, only incidentally heterosexual
6 Exclusively homosexual

In an extension of Kinsey's work, Klein (1990) proposed a more complex approach to thinking about sexual orientation. Rather than focusing only on sexual behaviors, Klein's model takes into consideration sexual attraction, sexual fantasies, emotional preference, social preference, self-identification, and lifestyle. For each dimension, one would be somewhere on a continuum from exclusively heterosexual (0) to exclusively homosexual (6). A bisexual person would be identified as equally heterosexually and homosexually oriented (3) regarding sexual fantasies, emotional preference, and so forth. Rather than dichotomously categorizing an individual as homosexual or heterosexual, this approach produces a rich montage of feelings, connections, and behaviors.

Most sex researchers and therapists tend to believe in a basic predisposition in sexual orientation, but this commonly held belief has not been challenged through systematic research (Blumstein & Schwartz, 1990). A critical feature of Klein's model is the temporal dimension. For example, change in the ratio of sexual fantasies about the same and other sex individuals from past to present can be captured. This dynamic perspective accommodates change over time and considers discontinuities in an individual's sexual orientation. Instead of a simple continuum,

Klein's (1990) Sexual Orientation Grid provides a complex model that includes seven variables and three time frames.

The Kinsey Institute recently convened a group of researchers to discuss sexual orientation and published the results in a book representing the state of the art at the end of the 1980s (McWhirter et al., 1990). The most compelling theme in this work is a new perspective that suggests developmental change and discontinuities in sexual behavior patterns and sexual orientation:

> The fact that sexual behavior patterns and sexual self-labelling can change dramatically and sometimes several times (e.g., from heterosexual to homosexual and back to heterosexual) within an individual over time challenges the view that sexual orientation is fixed or determined early in life and remains constant. (Sanders, Reinisch, & McWhirter, 1990, p. xxiv)

Sanders et al. note, however, that the existence of these transitions does not necessarily imply that individuals have conscious choice over their sexual orientation or that they can change it at will.

Feminists have contributed other perspectives regarding the social construction of sexual orientation that imply some sense of choice. Golden (1987) criticized the tendency among clinicians and scholars to categorize people into one of four rigid sexual groups: heterosexual, homosexual, bisexual, or asexual (celibate). Golden (1987) found that college-age women are able to handle the ambivalent feelings that may occur when sexual identities and sexual behaviors are independent of each other or incongruent.

Drawing upon Ponse's (1978) study of southern lesbians, Golden (1987) noted a distinction between whether a woman defines herself as primary (a born lesbian) or elective (a lesbian by choice). From an early age, primary lesbians had a conscious sense of being attracted sexually to females. Elective lesbians perceived their sexual identity as a conscious choice. They did not feel different from other girls, and no one had labeled their childhood behavior as deviant. As they aged, they usually had heterosexual identities and experiences. They came to label and identify themselves as lesbians during college.

The second distinction for elective lesbians was whether their lesbianism was seen as a central and enduring aspect of their self-concept or whether they perceived their sexuality as fluid and dynamic: "Then I was heterosexual, and now I'm a lesbian" (Golden, 1987, p. 26). Some women saw their past behavior and identity as inconsistent with their adult self-concept, whereas others did not view their current choice of lesbianism as dissonant or in need of reconstruction. Women's sense of the fluidity or essentiality of their sexuality was subject to change due to the process of self-definition, whereas the distinction between primary and elective lesbianism was more dichotomous over time.

The flexibility of sexual orientation is difficult to explore because of controversy and fear about homosexuality and bisexuality. Bisexuality is even more stigmatized than homosexuality (Klein, 1985, 1990; Shuster, 1987). In Golden's study (1987), elective lesbians were treated with much more suspicion by others than were primary lesbians, who felt their sexuality to be an enduring personality component. Given the combination of homophobia and sexuality, formerly heterosexual women who are now lesbian were less tolerated than women who experienced themselves as exclusively homosexual or heterosexual. The notion of change in sexual orientation could also be used as ammunition to push "to rehabilitate" both gays and lesbians as heterosexuals.

Many people who identify themselves as heterosexual have had same-sex partners, and many who identify themselves as homosexual had, and continue to have, sexual contact with other sex partners (Bell & Weinberg, 1978; Nichols, 1990). For women, it is not unusual for heterosexual marriage and motherhood to precede the coming out process. It is often unclear whether they are primary lesbians who have repressed or denied their homosexuality in order to conform to societal expectations, or whether they are elective lesbians who have chosen relationships with women after having lived heterosexually in the past.

Women's sexuality may be more fluid than men's because of contemporary childrearing arrangements, in which women raise children (Golden, 1987). For example, in interviews with 975 heterosexual men and women, Rubin (1990) found that about 10% of the sample had experimented with same-sex relationships, and that women were more likely than men to have done so. Object relations theories propose that during childhood the primary love object for females is likely to be of the same sex. Yet, Chodorow (1978) and Dinnerstein (1976) excluded lesbians from their theories of childrearing and gender socialization (Rich, 1980). This omission is critical because feminist theorists have not explained why more women seem to be exclusively heterosexual when they have been raised and loved primarily by women (Golden, 1987).

Claiming One's Sexual Orientation

Most American women are socialized with an assumption of heterosexual orientation. Therefore, even women who are primary lesbians, who grow up knowing that they are attracted to females, must come out. Coming out means that a lesbian must formally deny the expectations from family and society that she be heterosexual (Rothblum, 1989). Heterosexual women do not have a corresponding developmental task to accomplish; they are not expected to claim their sexual orientation.

Deciding how to come out can be difficult because some women engage in sexual activity with other women but do not have a lesbian consciousness; they may even be married to men (Aptheker, 1989; Green & Clunis, 1989). Other women may define themselves as lesbian but may not be sexually active (Golden, 1987). Historically, sexual behavior has not been important to the definition of lesbian, though in the late 20th century, sexuality is explicit and defining of lesbian existence (Aptheker, 1989).

Coleman (1981–82) suggests several steps in the coming out process for lesbians and gay men. Applied to lesbians, this clinical model proposes that a woman may feel different, alienated, and alone before coming out. Coming out involves facing one's own feelings toward other women, self-acceptance, and disclosure of one's lesbianism. Next, there is experimentation with one's new sexual identity. Finally, there is integration, involving the incorporation of both a private and public lesbian identity into one's self-image. Many individuals do not follow a predictable pattern.

Coming out is a process, and it may never be a completed act (Golden, 1987). Lesbians constantly come out to themselves, associates, acquaintances, and strangers. Daily challenges include the need to face internalized and externalized homophobia (Pharr, 1988). Women who identify themselves as bisexual reveal how sexuality is constructed in an ongoing way (Shuster, 1987). Their coming out process may be ongoing because of shifting identities and attractions to both women and men.

The Emotional–Sexual Continuum

Current constructions of women's sexualities are rooted in feminist revisions of Freudian and object relations theories. Heterosexuality is assumed to be normative; lesbian and bisexual experience is invisible or problemized. Radical feminists have challenged the presumed naturalness of heterosexuality and exposed the political implications underlying these theories. Rich (1980) proposed that women have been convinced, through the idealization of heterosexual romance and marriage, that sexual orientation to men is inevitable. This "compulsory heterosexuality" denies women the opportunity to determine the meaning and place of sexuality in their lives. Instead of a limited, clinical definition of lesbianism as a female version of male homosexuality, Rich (1980) suggested one based on the realities of women-identified existence.

Rich (1980) proposed the concept "lesbian continuum" to define the context of women's close associations with each other. Lesbian continuum should replace the narrower ideas of "lesbianism" or "heterosexuality" because almost all women are close to other women emotionally, yet only some women express their feelings sexually. To avoid the essentialist implications of "compulsory heterosexuality," women should be considered along a continuum from active sexual and emotional involvement with other women to emotional bonding only.

Rich's proposal expands the typical androcentric definition of women as sexual objects to a more inclusive, woman-centered view of women as emotional and sexual subjects. However, decentering male-defined notions of women's sexuality with female-defined notions may not be inclusive enough. Critics of Rich's lesbian continuum suggest that it, too, is essentialist (Weeks, 1987). If lesbian existence is posited as a profoundly female experience that promises a powerful female eroticism, then heterosexual women become newly marginalized as politically incorrect or unnatural. Defining lesbianism as the perfect vision of egalitarian sexuality suggests that women could "magically leap over our heterosexist conditioning into mutually orgasmic, struggle-free, trouble-free sex" (Hollibaugh & Moraga, 1983, p.395). Attributing women's oppression to compulsory heterosexuality implies that women are always controlled by men, and heterosexual women are perpetual victims (Weeks, 1987).

Thus, feminist ideas about the social construction of sexualities are by no means uniform or uncontested. Ideas about women's sexualities can devolve into opposing camps about what is natural versus what is chosen. Feminists continue to debate how to redistribute power, achieve equality, celebrate difference, and define gender. The social construction of women's sexualities is inextricably linked to power and perceived differences between women and men.

ARE WOMEN AND MEN THAT DIFFERENT?

For centuries, women have been characterized as less sexual than men. Male sexual arousal and behavior have been used as the standard to determine what is normal and natural (Schneider & Gould, 1987). The interrelationships among gender, sexual orientation, relationship duration, and sexual interactions reveal a more complex picture.

A major study of American couples examined the influences of gender, sexual orientation, and relationship status on sexuality. Blumstein and Schwartz (1983) explored sexuality issues in a sample of approximately 12,000 people, representing heterosexual, gay and lesbian, married, and cohabiting couples. Group comparisons revealed that gay men who had been together less than 10 years were the most sexually active; lesbians reported the lowest frequency of sexual activity of the four groups. Cohabiting heterosexual couples had sexual relations more often than did married couples, regardless of how long the cohabitants had been together. Of the couples who had been together for 2 years or less, 45% of the married couples, 61% of the cohabitants, 67% of the gay men, and 33% of lesbians reported sexual activity three times a week or more.

The lower frequency of sexual activity and fewer number of partners among lesbians (Bell & Weinberg, 1978; Blumstein & Schwartz, 1983) suggest that gender is a more important factor than sexual orientation in determining sexual interaction. The essence of the argument is that gay male relationships reveal male sexuality unfettered by the restraint of female sexuality; gay men have more frequent sexual encounters, more partners, and more variant forms of sexual activity, and display more potential for violence (Katchadourian, 1989). If gay relationships characterize "natural" male sexuality, the parallel to this argument would be that lesbian relationships demonstrate "natural" female sexuality. The behaviors of gay and lesbian couples would reflect extreme examples of the general approach that men and women take to sexuality and relationships (Nichols, 1990).

Is female sexuality inherently different from male sexuality, or is women's relatively low level of reported sexual activity due to socialization and societal repression of women as sexual beings? Cohabitants had sexual relations more frequently than married couples, suggesting that social norms may be influential in determining the pursuit of sexual satisfaction through interpersonal sexual activity. Women who cohabit may be less constrained personally by norms that dictate traditional behavior of any type and therefore feel freer to have sexual activity as desired. The fact that male and female cohabitants in Blumstein and Schwartz's (1983) study were more likely than other groups to report equal initiation of sexual activity supports this hypothesis. In married couples, both husbands and wives reported that men were usually the initiators. Messages that women may internalize about not initiating sexual activity may explain lower frequency in lesbian relationships (Blumstein & Schwartz, 1983). Nichols (1990) proposed fusing as another reason for the lower frequency of sexual activity among lesbian couples. If women are closely merged with little opportunity for autonomy and personal space, avoiding genital sexuality may be a way to achieve distance.

Evidence of lower frequency of sexual activity among lesbians is not conclusive, however. Some studies have found that lesbians have sex more frequently, are more sexually responsive, and are more sexually satisfied than heterosexual women. Coleman, Hoon, and Hoon (1983) compared sexual experiences of 407 lesbians and 370 heterosexuals, 17 to 68 years of age, with the goal of clarifying similarities and differences. Forty-two percent of the lesbians reported having sex two to four times per week, compared with 26% of the heterosexual women. Higher frequency may be correlated with experiences of orgasm; 89% of the lesbians reported having orgasms frequently or always compared with 66% of the heterosexual women. Sixty-nine percent of the lesbians were pleased or extremely happy with their sexual activity, compared with 53% of the heterosexual women. If the women who are usually pleased with their sexual experiences are included, the percentages increase to 85% and 78%, respectively.

The majority of the women in the Coleman et al. (1983) study, regardless of sexual orientation, found their sexual activity satisfying. These women generally had some college education and were comfortable enough about their sexuality to answer questions about it, so they may not be representative of women in general. However, the evidence indicates that both heterosexual and lesbian women have satisfying sexual lives.

Differences between the two groups of women may be explained in a variety of ways. Lesbians may be more skillful lovers because they know firsthand what may be arousing to female bodies and are more likely to prefer activities like cunnilingus or manual stimulation that are likely to lead to orgasm (Coleman et al., 1983). Penile–vaginal intercourse is less effective in arousing a woman to orgasm. If women are uncomfortable communicating what is most stimulating or their partners do not understand or do not want to provide more effective stimulation, orgasm may not occur. There is, then, less reinforcement for women to have intercourse more frequently.

Methodological factors must be considered, also. Coleman et al. (1983) found that lesbians had more partners than heterosexual women; 32% of the lesbians had had 15 or more partners compared to 4% of the heterosexuals. Half of the heterosexual women had had only one or two partners, compared to only 7% of the lesbians. Experience with a variety of partners provides opportunities for feedback about a woman's sexuality—what she does and does not enjoy and the potential of her own responsiveness (Laws & Schwartz, 1977).

Lesbian and heterosexual women may define "sex" and "sexual activity" differently, implicitly including and excluding various activities when they respond to questions about frequency. Heterosexual women might be more likely to report only penile–vaginal intercourse as occurrences of real sex, whereas lesbians may be more inclusive of the entire sexual and emotional experience of making love (see Frye, 1990).

Sexual activity in committed relationships, heterosexual or lesbian, decreases over time (Blumstein & Schwartz, 1983; Smith, 1991). Blumstein and Schwartz used statistical analyses to determine whether the effects of aging and a normal decline in sexual activity were most responsible for the decrease or whether it was the duration of the relationship. For married couples, the effects of age and duration of relationship seemed to be about equal; for cohabitants, gay men, and lesbians, duration was more significant.

Rubin's (1990) interviews with 300 adults about their sexual histories identified several reasons for decline in sexual activity over time. For one quarter of the couples, other conflicts in the relationship were manifested sexually in lack of interest, withholding of sex, or sexual dysfunction. More subtle reasons included decline in activity after the "chase and the conquest" of courtship. Familiarity and availability also affected frequency. One man in Rubin's (1990) study said:

> The problem is that there's no closed "paren"; nothing brackets the experience of marriage. The terrible thing about connubial life is that time is endless, and that gives you a whole different sense of time and possibilities. In a relationship that's not "til death do us part," you have to make each evening a good one, or else there won't be a next time. (p. 171)

Relationship duration does not just have a dampening impact on sexuality. As committed relationships evolve and become more complex, sexuality is only one of many options for sharing intimacy (Miller & Fowlkes, 1980). Sexual activity may also become more infused with eroticism as the result of the development of shared meaning and negotiation. A broader definition of intimacy would acknowledge the expanded repertoire of behaviors that couples construct over time.

Gender differences in sexual scripts can contribute to variations in reasons deemed appropriate for participating in sexual activity. Women report different reasons than do men for having sex. Leigh (1989) gathered information about why they do or do not have sex from 445 women and 477 men, 76% of whom were exclusively or primarily heterosexual and 24% of whom described themselves as bisexual or homosexual. Significant differences were found between males and females and between individuals of different sexual orientations, although the differences tended to be small. Women were more likely than men to say that they had sex to express emotional closeness. Men were more likely than women to say that the most important reasons for having sex were for pure pleasure, conquest, relief of tension, and pleasing one's partner. Heterosexuals said that reproduction, emotional closeness, and pleasing one's partner were more important reasons for sexual activity than did gay men and lesbians.

When asked why they might limit their sexual activity, men indicated that fear of AIDS and fear of rejection were the most important reasons; women rated more highly fear of pregnancy, lack of interest, and lack of enjoyment. Gay men were significantly more likely than the other groups to limit sexual activity because of fear of AIDS.

Leigh (1989) also looked at frequency of sexual activity for each of the groups to see whether there was a relationship between the importance of various reasons and actual behaviors. For women in a primary relationship, pleasure was the major predictor of frequency. For heterosexual women, it was the pleasure they derived from sexual activity; for lesbians, the most important predictor was the partner's pleasure. For women who were single, lack of opportunity was the major predictor of frequency. This may be a consequence of women's preference for sexuality to be linked to a relationship.

Leigh's (1989) results indicated that women and men had different reasons for sexual activity, but their reasons for being sexually inactive were similar. Women were more likely than men to express low interest in sex, conforming to the stereotype that women have less of a sex drive than men. Women may have less interest in sexual activity if they do not derive satisfaction from the experience. Socialized to satisfy their partner and to believe that their own satisfaction is optional, women may find sexual activity more frustrating than rewarding. Women who report greater frequency probably derive greater pleasure from their sexual activity.

Several findings from this study are provocative because they challenge existing stereotypes. Heterosexual men rated "because your partner wants to" and "to please your partner" higher than any of the other three groups as reasons for having sex. Although all groups rated "for conquest" among the least likely reasons for having sex, lesbian women were as likely as heterosexual men to give this reason, with both of these groups rating it slightly higher than did heterosexual women and slightly lower than gay men. For both women and men, regardless of sexual orientation, the most important reasons for having sex were pure pleasure and emotional closeness. These anomalous results may reflect women's increasing interest in experiencing and enjoying sexuality to the fullest and the pressure on men to help them do this (Leigh, 1989).

Elaborating Women's Sexual Scripts

The concept of sexual scripts is dynamic and consistent with the theme of growth and change over time. Through opportunity, experience, education, and introspection, scripts can be revised and reconstructed. Women can develop a more comprehensive understanding of themselves as sexual beings, modifying their sexual scripts to include and reflect new information that can result in greater pleasure. But how malleable are sexual scripts once they are constructed? Laws and Schwartz (1977) stress the potency of primary socialization, noting that it maintains much of its subjective reality even when later learning overlays and contradicts it. Although there may be considerable fluidity in women's thinking about where they participate in sexual activity, women may have more difficulty integrating activities like masturbation or oral–genital sexual stimulation into their sexual repertoire if early socialization has defined these activities as distasteful or wrong.

Taken together, studies on sexuality that include women suggest considerable change across cohorts of women in regard to sexual issues. Because there is no longitudinal research that follows the sexual development of individual women, we can only speculate about developmental changes in women's sexual lives during adulthood. By following different cohorts of women, it would be possible to identify changes that occur in their attitudes, partner choices, and sexual behaviors over time.

Women's sexual scripts are becoming more complex as they develop a wider range of sexual activities they find acceptable. In *Worlds of Pain*, Rubin (1976) noted that although 70% of working-class couples and 76% of the middle-class couples engaged in oral–genital stimulation, only about one fourth of the working-class and one third of the middle-class couples did so routinely. Few of the working-class women said they enjoyed it unreservedly or without guilt. In a later investigation, Rubin (1990) noted that 75% of the college students from whom she gathered data engaged in oral sex; most said it was a routine part of their repertoire. In the 1950s, Kinsey found that about 50% of women engaged in fellatio and cunnilingus. Of the more than 100,000 women responding to a sex survey in *Cosmopolitan* magazine in the early 1980s, 84% indicated that they regularly participated in oral sex (Wolfe, 1981). Blumstein and Schwartz (1983) found that only 10% of the heterosexual couples and 4% of the lesbian women in their study did not participate in oral–genital stimulation.

Traditional sexual scripts for women included only their husbands as appropriate sexual partners. If sexual intercourse occurred before marriage, it could be justified only if one was in love and planning to marry. Current sexual scripts for young women indicate a change in thinking about the essential link between sexuality and marriage. For many young women today, the belief that they are at the beginning of a relationship, without regard for relationship permanence, seems sufficient for them to feel comfortable with interpersonal sexual activity (Rubin, 1990). The increased visibility of gay and lesbian relationships and families provides other possibilities for thinking about appropriate partners as sexual scripts are constructed and reconstructed.

As women claim control in other areas of their lives, changes are likely in expectations regarding their sexual freedom and fulfillment. New sexual scripts will reflect women's increasing autonomy, posing new challenges for their partners. Perhaps the single most influential factor contributing to the emergence of more "agentic" (characterized by agency or the capacity to act in one's own interests) scripts for women has been the ability to separate sexuality and reproduction.

THE TENSION BETWEEN SEXUALITY AND REPRODUCTION

The linkages between sexual activity and pregnancy are undeniable; however, in this book sexuality and reproduction are discussed in separate chapters to stress that they are not synonymous. To merge the two obscures women's experiences of each and the intricate meanings associated with these central aspects of their lives (Schneider & Gould, 1987).

The interest and controversy generated by the appearance of actress Demi Moore, very pregnant and nude, on the cover of the August 1991 issue of *Vanity Fair* magazine revealed the powerful tensions surrounding pregnancy and sexuality. The cover presented an elegantly photographed Moore holding her belly with one hand and covering her breasts with the other. Public reaction was mixed: Some people decried such an "unspeakable mixture of sensuality and procreation," and others lauded it as "bold, taboo-breaking, and affirmative of the diversity of female experience" (Muro, 1991, p. 48). Although many raised questions about Moore's motivation for posing for the cover, it was clearly a marker event that disclosed a previously invisible aspect of women's lives in a way that challenged existing beliefs about pregnancy, sexuality, and beauty.

The process of conception generally involves sexual intercourse between a woman and a man. This understanding is integrated into most females' sexual scripts very early. Most young women learn that they should not be sexually active because they may become pregnant. Contraceptive education stresses the connection between sexuality and conception and urges women to prevent unwanted pregnancies. Even for women who are conscientious contraceptors, the possibility of method failure means that the dissociation of sexual activity and conception can never be accomplished totally by premenopausal women.

The association of sex and reproduction may be a problem for lesbian couples as well. Although they are free of the risk of pregnancy as a consequence of sexual behavior, they lack the opportunity to become pregnant as a result of their sexual union. Becoming pregnant involves a series of decisions about conception, donor choice, and legal arrangements (Harvard Law Review Association, 1990; Pies, 1988).

The tension between sexuality and motherhood may affect revisions of women's sexual scripts during their pregnancies. Many women abstain from intercourse during all or part of their pregnancies, even if they have not been medically advised to do so (Ussher, 1989). Despite great variability in women's interest and responsiveness during the first trimester, most women report an increase in responsiveness and desire during the second trimester. During the last trimester, there is generally a decrease in sexual activity (Katchadourian, 1989), probably because of physical discomfort, concern about body image, or worries about endangering the fetus.

Physicians often do not talk to women and their partners about sexual activity during pregnancy; thus, couples may have unfounded concerns and sacrifice sexual enjoyment needlessly. Unless women are at risk for bleeding or premature labor, they can continue sexual activity and have orgasms up to the onset of labor (Crooks & Baur, 1990). After childbirth, women's sexual interest and activity vary considerably. Although most can comfortably and safely resume sexual intercourse by about 3 weeks postpartum, psychological readiness and the impact of the baby on the couple may affect sexual interest (Crooks & Baur, 1990; Katchadourian, 1989).

Sexual arousal while breastfeeding is a common experience for many women and seems tied to degree of breast sensitivity (Ussher, 1989). There is no name for this experience, and such pleasurable feelings may be unspeakable or disturbing for some women . What should be a positive and unique aspect of mothering is distorted into something hidden and shameful.

Thus, the tension between sexuality and reproduction operates at many different levels. Ironically, prior to conception there is societal pressure to emphasize the linkage of sexuality and reproduction— particularly for young or unmarried women (e.g., Miller & Moore, 1990). This threat functions to a certain degree to control women's sexuality. Women are warned of the consequences of acting on their desires. After conception, there is a subtle societal expectation that women separate sexuality and the reproductive aspects of their lives. Underlying issues of control and power such as these pervade women's sexual experiences.

SEXUALITY AND POWER

The Eroticization of Power

Male privilege is embedded in the economic and social structure of society as a whole and played out personally in intimate and sexual relationships.

Although authentic love relationships between individual men and women exist, the societal foundation of such private relations is unbalanced; women are more likely to be at a disadvantage. For heterosexual women to maintain viable, intimate relationships with their male partners, they must "act within the cultural ground rules governing their relations with men" (Aptheker, 1989, p. 94). Women's sexual subordination has been institutionalized in the traditional marital relationship. Sexual scripts prescribe husbands as dominant and wives as submissive. Hierarchical role-playing becomes part of the script in the most private, intimate ways.

The analysis of the relation between sexuality and power in women's lives is compelling because females continue to be sexually victimized by men at an alarming rate. One percent of college women are survivors of incestuous relationships with their fathers (Finkelhor, 1979). In a probability sample of 930 women, Russell (1986) found that 4.5% had been sexually abused by their fathers by age 18. There is one forcible rape of a woman by a man every 6 minutes (Uniform Criminal Reports, 1987); one in every four adolescent females is likely to be raped. Among married couples, one in every ten wives are sexually assaulted at least once by their husbands (Finklehor & Yllo, 1985). In a national survey of 32 educational institutions, 28% of young women (mean age 21 years) reported that they had been subjected to sexual coercion since age 14 (Koss, Gidycz, & Wisniewski, 1987).

The general consensus is that male perpetrators are not pathological because they commit sexual violence against women, but rather that traditional sexual scripts legitimize male dominance and the linking of sexuality and aggression. Social constructions of relationships that give males approved power and control over women and children increase the likelihood of sexual assault and rape (Reiss, 1990). Sociocultural scripts enforce macho images of men as powerful, aggressive, and lusting after women who are vulnerable, coy, and needing to be convinced. Forced, coerced, or manipulated sexual encounters result from male perceptions that they have a right to control interactions with women, particularly if the other person—wife, partner, or child—"belongs" to them.

Sexual assault of women by their husbands provides the clearest example of how social institutions legitimize male sexual dominance. Wife rape has not been considered a crime because marriage is based on a contract that gives a man the right to "carnal knowledge" of his wife (Lott, 1987). Because marriage is presumed to imply a blanket consent to sexual intimacy, many states still have marital exclusions to rape laws on their books (Katchadourian, 1989).

Victims of sexual assaults suffer from emotional problems, self-destructive or suicidal behaviors, self-esteem problems, development of aversion to sexual activity, diminished interest in sex, embarrassment, and confusion about their responsibility (Burgess & Holmstrom, 1974; Butler & Burton, 1990; Gelles & Conte, 1990; Katchadourian, 1989; Lott, 1987). The perpetrator in cases of incest and partner rape is someone with whom a girl or woman has an intimate relationship and trust and with whom she is expected to continue to live.

The legacy that young females inherit as the result of pervasive sexual violence against women in our society is subtle intimidation against being truly autonomous and a sense of vulnerability to male dominance that is woven into women's sexual scripts. Although women understand that most men do not rape, women are continually reminded through media, education programs, and experience of the potential danger of a more powerful, and supposedly uncontrollable, male sexuality. This reinforces the existing power difference between men and women in their sexual lives.

The evidence from cross-cultural studies supports the position that contemporary sexual arrangements are socially constructed. Sanday's (1981) classic study of sexual assault compared rape-prone and rape-free societies and found certain shared characteristics in those that were rape prone. In these societies, male violence is glorified or at least tolerated, men and boys are encouraged to be aggressive and competitive, men demean women and rarely participate in family work, and women have less economic and political power. In rape-free societies, women and men share power and authority, and both sexes are raised to value nurturance and avoid aggression and violence.

The Ambiguities of Sexual Freedom

To act autonomously sexually, women must share the social, political, and economic power that men enjoy (Miller & Fowlkes, 1980). This position is supported by a study exploring the factors that contribute to fulfillment in women's lives (Baruch et al., 1983). Data from 300 women with various lifestyles and life circumstances revealed a positive relationship between occupational prestige and sexual satisfaction. Women who had better jobs and contributed more money to the family income had more satisfying sex lives. Women who felt better about themselves and had the power that came with income equal to their partners' felt less intimidated in their relationships.

Another analysis of 61 preindustrial societies found that greater economic equality between women and men was correlated with a lower degree of sexual double standards (Blumberg & Coleman, 1989). Husbands of wives with more economic power adopted behaviors—rationing sex or making excuses—that in industrial societies are associated stereo-typically with women who are economically dependent.

Economic power may be necessary but not sufficient to equalize females and males in sexual relationships. Several researchers (Fullilove et al., 1990; Weinberg & Williams, 1988) have discussed the seemingly paradoxical relationship between economic power and exploitation among black women and men. The shortage of eligible black men, particularly those who are stable economically, poses an additional problem for economically secure black women. Although these women are in a position to enjoy sexual interactions for their own sake, free of economic dependence on the men involved, there is greater competition for the men available (Weinberg & Williams, 1988). This gives men more leverage than they would otherwise have and discounts women's power in the relationship.

Without social, political, and economic equality, there is the risk that women merely become more available to men—increasing the likelihood of exploitation while limiting the protection and benefits women traditionally have derived by trading sexuality for marriage. Ironically, feminism's goal of sexual autonomy for women has the potential for "freeing men first" (English, 1983). By adopting male models of sexual freedom without corresponding changes in the social structure, women may be merely legitimizing and increasing men's access to them (Jackson, 1987). Rubin's (1990) interviews with women and men who were part of the sexual revolution of the 1960s captured this tension between sexual freedom and social inequality. Prevailing sexual scripts provided little guidance for dealing with women's new opportunities for sexual expression:

> So we had all this freedom and didn't know how to deal with it. And there were all these guys—just think what they were looking at; it was like a dream come true for them. All these women who suddenly weren't supposed to say no anymore. Well, the men didn't know what to do with it either, so it became a new version of the old male–female game. (Rubin, 1990, p. 94)

Neither women nor men have come to terms with the power that women acquire when they claim control of their own sexuality. In Hite's (1987) sample, 53% of the women fantasized about a very free sexual life, but also feared these thoughts and worried about becoming too sexual. Rubin (1990) found that among 600 students from whom she gathered data, 40% of the females said they understated their sexual experience because they believed others would not understand. She concluded that women hide their sexual behavior because men still hold the power to define what is acceptable.

Power issues are often played out in sexual relationships but can easily be obscured or misinterpreted. Initiation and refusal of sexual activity provide a window on power negotiations in intimate relationships. Blumstein and Schwartz (1983) found that among heterosexual couples, if there was not equal initiation, men were likely to be the initiators. Cohabitants were more likely than married couples or homosexual couples to share initiation and refusals, with 46% of the females and 42% of the males indicating that they and their partners shared the role. Among married couples, 33% of the men and 40% of the women perceived that they and their partners shared initiation. The discrepancy suggests that there may be different perceptions about what actions constitute the initiation of sexual activity. In cases where the initiator role was not shared, 51% of the husbands compared to 12% of the wives indicated that they were more likely to initiate sex. Being married—or being the type of person who marries rather than cohabits—appears to reinforce traditional sexual scripts regarding initiation.

Only 37% of the same-sex couples said that the initiator role was shared (Blumstein & Schwartz, 1983). Some lesbians apparently were not comfortable in initiating sex because they did not want to be seen as the aggressor. Among the lesbian couples who did not share initiation, it was likely to be the more emotionally expressive partner who initiated and maintained the couple's sexual life. The partner who exhibited the most typically female behaviors—encouraging discussion of problems, spontaneously kissing and hugging—was more likely to begin sexual activity.

Information on refusals of sexual activity indicated that the more powerful partner was more likely to refuse. Refusing involves controlling access to sexuality and increases power. Blumstein and Schwartz (1983) proposed that women's lesser interest in sexual activity may be the result of active suppression of their sexual desire, resulting in greater willingness to refuse. Paradoxically, they achieve more power in the relationship by withholding a valued resource, but do so at the cost of their own sexual interest and desire.

Another window on power negotiations in male–female relationships comes from media images. McMahon (1990) analyzed issues of *Cosmopolitan* magazine from 1976 to 1988 to see how sexuality represents power relations. Describing the magazine as an icon of feminine sexuality dating back to the mid-1960s, McMahon (1990) determined it to be a "dream book and strategy manual . . . that offers the fantasy of revenge for class and gender subordination through images of women's sexuality used to dominate and control men on their own turf" (p. 395). Her analysis revealed a model for heterosexual relationships based on a reversal of relations of domination and subordination rather than on mutual emotional safety and self-disclosure. The message projected by the magazine is that in order for women to be active agents, men must be objectified and subordinated.

A revenge scenario holds little promise for contemporary women. Women do resist male control over their sexuality, but role-reversal seems more of a media fantasy than a practical solution. Because sexual satisfaction is a powerful contributor to happiness and optimism in women's lives, greater long-term benefit will be derived from efforts to enhance the likelihood that women will have fulfilling and pleasurable sexual relationships.

The Tension between Pleasure and Danger

Women's growing sexual freedom has been a double-edged sword. The tension between pleasure and danger captures the dialectical aspects of sex in women's lives:

> To focus only on pleasure and gratification ignores the patriarchal structure in which women act, yet to speak only of sexual violence and oppression ignores women's experience with sexual agency and choice and unwittingly increases the sexual terror and despair in which women live. (Vance, 1984, p. 1)

Women's sexuality is complicated and difficult to grasp, and it may be unsettling to men. As more information becomes available on female sexuality, and it is legitimized as a vital topic in women's lives, acknowledging desire, investigating pleasure, and taking control of one's sexual activities become important.

The societal context of women's lives makes focusing on pleasure and gratification a risky undertaking. Most women are aware of the relative danger of fully experiencing their sexuality. Among the dangers are not only the very real threats of male violence perpetrated through rape, incest, and sexual harassment, but also the intrapsychic anxieties that sexuality engenders, the fear of competition for sexual partners, and the fear of pregnancy.

Sexual Initiation

Adolescent stories about sexual intitiation suggest varying themes of pleasure and danger in the development of erotic identity. Research exploring the early sexual experience of 300 teenage girls (Thompson, 1990) indicated that although some girls emphasized pleasure, curiosity, and desire, others spoke of pain and boredom with their first sexual encounters. The "pleasure narrators" were those who were more likely to initiate petting and intercourse and saw their early sexual experiences as "voyages of discovery." These young women had open discussions with their mothers, who often disclosed information about their own sexuality. The daughters learned about their own bodies and the potential pleasure of sexual relations. These young women looked forward to having sex with the knowledge that they could be subjects of their own sexual desire rather than merely the objects of others' desire. Most of these teens had had several sources of precoital sexual information.

The other group of sexually initiated teens provided narratives characterized by pain, boredom, and coercion, although they often failed to recognize or name it. Most denied any sexual volition and spoke as though they had had no sexual consciousness before first intercourse. Little understanding of sexuality contributed to the lack of desire and pleasure in these first experiences. In spite of their disappointment, many reported that "it was worth it" because they just liked being with their partner, it gave them status over other girls who were still virgins, or they saw it as a rite of passage that proved maturity and courage.

Sexual initiation is not always voluntary. Sexual assault and rape of girls and young women can have tragic consequences both immediately and long-term. Recent studies have identified a link between childhood sexual abuse and adolescent pregnancy. An exploratory study of 41 young, white, rural mothers who had been pregnant as teenagers found that 54% had experienced at least one unwanted sexual incident by age 18, a prevalence rate that is double the national estimates (Butler & Burton, 1990). The long-term consequences of the abuse depended on the type and duration of sexual abuse. Women who were forced to have sex, molested, or raped once had fewer lingering effects, such as anxiety, nightmares, and flashbacks, than those who had been raped or molested several times. Many of the abuse survivors said they did not know why they became pregnant. Butler and Burton (1990) suggested that for some girls sexual exploitation and the trauma of not being able to control their lives led to a resigned attitude in which life just happened to them: "They don't know why they become pregnant, they just are" (p. 78).

Another study (Boyer & Fine, 1992) found that of the 535 young women interviewed who became pregnant as adolescents, two thirds had been sexually abused, 55% had been molested, 42% were victims of attempted rape, and 44% had been raped. The age of first intercourse for these adolescents was 14, and only 26% used contraception at first intercourse. The rate of victimization varied by ethnic group. White adolescents had the highest rate (72%), followed by Native Americans (64%), blacks (50%), and Hispanics (46%). These results suggest that a large number of adolescents who become pregnant may have a history of sexual victimization that interferes with their development and undermines their self-esteem, confidence, and decision-making ability (Boyer & Fine, 1992).

The Risk of AIDS

The 1980s introduced a new danger in sexual activity. Since the identification of the virus that causes AIDS and the methods of its transmission in 1981, sexual behaviors have come under closer scrutiny. At first, it appeared that women, particularly those in monogamous relationships, were at relatively low risk. As the epidemic progressed, it became clear that not only are women at risk, but also they now make up the fastest-growing population of people with AIDS. In 1984, 6.4 % of those with AIDS were women; by July 1990 this figure had risen to 11% (Chu, Buehler, & Berkelman, 1990; Diaz, 1991; Minkoff & DeHovitz, 1991). Women of color comprise the greatest percentage of women diagnosed with AIDS, signaling a significant overlap between poverty and HIV infection among women. As of August 1990, 53% of women with AIDS were black and 21% were Hispanic (Diaz, 1991).

Women are at higher risk for being infected by their male partners than their partners are of being infected by them. A recent study (Holmes, Karon, & Kreiss, 1990) revealed that in 1988 the overall percentage of cases of AIDS attributed to heterosexual contact was 20 times higher for women than for men. Some women who contract AIDS through heterosexual means are workers in the sex industry, but many are infected by male partners who are IV drug users or who have been infected themselves through sexual intercourse with females or males. Married men's bisexual behavior has been identified as "the quietest of many silent factors" facilitating the spread of the virus (Osborn, 1990/91, p. 91). The source of heterosexually acquired AIDS differs by race. Black and Hispanic women are more likely to have been infected by an IV drug user; white women are more likely to have had bisexual men as their sexual partners than are black or Hispanic women (Holmes et al., 1990).

For women with AIDS, the proportion of cases attributable to heterosexual transmission rose from 13% in 1983 to 28% in 1988 (Holmes et al., 1990). Because the incubation period for AIDS is estimated to be 8–11 years, the increase in heterosexual cases actually reflects an increase in heterosexual transmission some years ago. Cole and Cooper (1990/91) point out that lesbians are also at risk because they can become HIV-infected in the way any woman can—by engaging in intercourse with men by choice, force, or necessity, using drugs and sharing needles, having blood transfusions, becoming inseminated, and exchanging blood and vaginal secretions during sexual contact with women.

Therefore, women may be even more at risk than current statistics indicate.

Rubin (1990) found that most of the men and women in her sample were not routine in their practice of safe sex. Because they saw themselves as heterosexuals, they did not think that they or their partners could get AIDS. Other research found evidence that women are changing their behaviors as the result of knowledge about HIV and AIDS (McNally & Mosher, 1991). Interviews with 8,450 women 15 to 44 years of age indicated that almost one third of single women surveyed had changed their behavior by reducing the number of sexual partners, reducing the frequency of intercourse, or stopping having intercourse entirely. Low-income women, black women, and women with more lifetime partners were the most likely to make behavioral changes.

The use of condoms and spermicides is the primary method available to prevent the spread of HIV through heterosexual intercourse. Male partners may resist the use of condoms, and women's attempts to protect themselves with condoms and other assertive behaviors in the sexual relationship may be met with violence (Osborn, 1990/91). If women do not have equal power in the relationship, they not only lose control over satisfaction and enjoyment in their sexuality, but also may be risking their health and ultimately their lives.

Feminist Tensions about Dominance and Equality

Although feminists agree that an analysis of power is central to an understanding of women's sexuality within a patriarchal society, opinions are divided about how to revolutionize traditional arrangements. What constitutes appropriate sexual expression in women's lives is hotly contested. Feminists disagree about the meaning of sexual equality for women. Does equality mean that women are free to adopt male-identified roles in sexual activities, that is, become dominant partners? Does it mean that women are to replace all role-playing with egalitarian sexuality? Can or should women enjoy dominance or submission as part of their sexual expression?

On the one hand, prosex feminists encourage diversity in women's sexuality (e.g., Snitow et al., 1983; Vance, 1984). They reject the notion that desire is unitary and are against censorship (Newton & Walton, 1984). Although recognizing the tension between pleasure and danger, they are critical of sexual prescriptions that would stamp out difference. On the other hand, feminists associated with the antipornography campaign provide an analysis that views all of women's sexuality as contaminated by patriarchy (Leidholdt & Raymond, 1990). They claim that women's subordination has been eroticized by the "prosex" group (Jeffreys, 1990). They call for a strict adherence to egalitarian relationships.

Prosex feminists take issue with the definition of sex in strictly egalitarian terms. They oppose the construction of women's sexuality as nonhierarchical, non-role-playing, with a de-emphasis on genital expression, penetration, and orgasm. They claim that this approach reflects Victorian ideals of "good girl" behavior and old class prejudices (Newton & Walton, 1984). In contrast, antipornography feminists argue that women's subordination is reflected in all sexual institutions and practices. They identify the interconnectedness of pornography (Dworkin, 1980; Lederer, 1980; MacKinnon, 1990), female sexual slavery (Barry, 1979), prostitution (Sheffield, 1987), and child sexual abuse (Russell, 1986) as related forms of the sexual victimization of women. In Russell's (1984) probability sample of 930 women, 24% reported being raped at least once. The figure rises to 44% if attempted rapes are included.

Antipornography feminists describe how the worldwide exploitation of women corrupts men as individuals as well as collectively and perpetuates sexual violence against women. They advocate a solution rooted in equality that condemns role-playing as based in male-originated dominance–submission rituals. The prosex group feels this view is "antisex" and intolerant of difference. At the core of this debate are class, gender, and sexual orientation issues. Late-20th-century feminism, like the suffrage and contraceptive movements of the 19th and early 20th centuries, is often criticized as a middle-class movement that has defined sexuality by the canon of equality (Newton & Walton, 1984; Smith, 1989). That is, women's sexual expression should not in any way mimic or support aspects of heterosexuality that have been used to limit women's control over their own experiences.

Newton and Walton (1984) criticized the canon of equality for feminist sexual practices, claiming that this ideology filters into the privacy of women's sexual choices. The emphasis on egalitarian sex "assumes functionally interchangeable partners and acts" (Newton & Walton, 1984, p. 243). According to this prescription, lesbians should not engage in any activity that seems like heterosexual sex. Lovers must be side by side, with no finger or object penetration. Orgasm should not be the end point or goal of sex. Fellatio, for heterosexual women, is seen as too submissive. The clitoris should be the only center of female sexual response, making male penetration a lesser activity (Newton & Walton, 1984).

Newton and Walton (1984) claim that the pressure for egalitarian sex reduces the power hierarchy between women and men to the simplistic notion that men have power and women do not; that is, heterosexuality involves "an oppressor and a victim. Masculinity equals sexual power, femininity equals sexual powerlessness" (p. 247). This notion is too simplistic because it suggests that the deeply entrenched ways in which power and desire are constructed can be interchanged with new, nonhierarchical ways of relating to self and others. Instead, Newton and Walton (1984) advocate that feminists should encourage open exploration of what sexuality and gender mean to women, rather than trying to stamp out difference.

The intensity of these debates has led to an unfortunate silencing of discussion about women-centered constructions of sexuality. Feminists on both sides have called for a new dialogue that recognizes women's oppression and exploitation but is not hopeless about their ability to control and empower their lives sexually (Jeffreys, 1990; Vance, 1984).

The Politics of a Woman-Centered Life

Lesbian identity is a 20th-century phenomenon, whereas female homosexual behavior is universal and has always been practiced (D'Emilio, 1989). As pointed out in Chapter 2, woman-centered bonds were strongly encouraged in the 19th century, as long as they did not threaten the power of the male head of household within the patriarchal family (Smith-Rosenberg, 1975). Not until the 20th century, when women began to claim their right to love each other, apart from men, did lesbian existence become defined in sexual terms (Faderman, 1981). The word "lesbian" as a sexual label did not appear until 1908, when it was first cited in The Shorter Oxford English Dictionary as "a female passion" (Stimpson, 1988, p. 98).

Women have always loved each other passionately, but the construction of lesbian identity as a sexual experience has emerged in recent history because women have found it possible to live openly with each other, economically independent of men (Aptheker, 1989). For educated, upper-middle-class working women of the late 19th and early 20th centuries, such as Jane Addams and Mary Rozet Smith, "Boston Marriage" was an alternative to the constrictions of Victorian heterosexual marriage. Addams and Smith lived together for 40 years in a union that was marked by social activism on behalf of the poor and a strong female support network (Cook, 1979). Regardless of their private activities, however, female couples were not considered sexual because women in general were not considered sexual (Aptheker, 1989).

One price lesbians have paid for their independence of men is the contemporary labeling of lesbian identity and behavior as deviant (Faderman, 1981). The association with deviance began with the medical establishment in the late 19th century and continues today in law and custom (Aptheker, 1989; Harvard Law Review Association, 1990; Robson & Valentine, 1990). However, laws and customs change. In 1973, homosexuality was removed as a mental disorder from the American Psychiatric Association's *Diagnostic and Statistical Manual* (Rothblum, 1989). Still, contemporary lesbians face censure and persecution for their resistance to male control, not the least of which is the threat of the loss of their children (Aptheker, 1989). Lesbianism is threatening because:

> Sexual access to women is a primary symbolic representation of manhood. Manhood and womanhood are encoded in relationship to each other. The lesbian, by stepping outside the code, cracks it. . . . A lesbian presence signals a potential for female independence that is as despised as it is feared. This potential is not only for an individual, personal escape from the conventional female subordination, but also for a far more general, structural challenge to the social relations between the sexes. (Aptheker, 1989, p. 90)

As a political movement, lesbian feminism has enhanced women's ability to create independent spaces for themselves and served as a corrective to the label of deviance (Aptheker, 1989; D'Emilio, 1989; Rich, 1980). Today, a lesbian is a woman "whose primary emotional, intellectual, and erotic relationships are with other women" (Aptheker, 1989, p. 87). Lesbians can choose to be with other women, in spite of structural limitations, not because it is an essential part of their nature or personality, but because they want to, and the opportunity exists.

Power, Class, and Butch–Femme Relations

Hierarchical role-playing characterizes many sexual encounters between women and men. How men act out a masculine script and how women act out a feminine script have become institutionalized as natural. Prescribed sexual roles constrain the range of possibilities for both sexes but have generally operated to the advantage of males.

Paradoxically, the vast majority of lesbians and gay men do not engage in gender role-playing. Indeed, lesbians and gays are "freed from the restrictions imposed by gender roles in traditional male–female relationships" (Peplau & Gordon, 1991, p. 483). Still, the stereotype persists that one partner adopts a masculine role of dominant, male breadwinner and the other acts the part of a submissive female. Scientific research and personal narratives of lesbians and gay men refute this stereotype as wrong. Lesbian and gay partnerships reject the husband–wife, role-playing script and tend to be modeled after friendships with an erotic and romantic component. These partnerships show that "successful love relationships can be built on models other than traditional marriage" (Peplau & Gordon, 1991, p. 486).

Although it is important to understand that role-playing is not prevalent among lesbians, a new feminist interpretation is available to examine the context of butch–femme relationships in mid-20th-century America. The comparison of these relations to the code of egalitarianism in late-20th-century lesbian feminism provides a sophisticated analysis of the intersections of historical context, gender relations, social class, and sexual orientation.

Butch–femme role-playing among lesbian partners reveals the dynamics of an intentional use of roles in women's attempts to construct nonexploitive sexual interactions. Class distinctions are important in how this role-playing was experienced and described, as well as in how it was treated historically by lesbian feminists, whose goal is personal and political change. Butch–femme refers not only to a type of sexual relationship between lesbians (Califia, 1988), but also to the pioneering ways working-class lesbians established an identity and created a culture during the pre-lesbian–feminist political climate of the 1940s to 1960s (Davis & Kennedy, 1986; D'Emilio, 1989; Smith, 1989).

Butch lesbians of the bar culture of mid-century America were not the first to explore sexual difference. In 1928, Radclyffe Hall published The Well of Loneliness, considered, until 1970, to be the lesbian novel (Newton, 1984). Newton's (1984) analysis of gender symbolization in the novel, as well as the cultural context in which lesbianism occurred, addressed the continued significance of a "mannish" look for lesbians in appearance and style. Hall chose a male appearance as a way to break out of the asexual mold of romantic female friendship that had characterized her Victorian sisters' experiences (Newton, 1984). The diversity among lesbians (Brown, 1989a) and the enduring significance of the "mannish" lesbian demand a social constructivist view of sexual preference but, paradoxically, do not solve the riddle of sexual orientation that continues to confound feminist psychology (Newton, 1984).

Considered in this analysis are the intersections of gender, sexual orientation, social class, and historical period, as well as the contributions of older lesbians and gay liberationists. Butch–femme remains prominent for some lesbians of color (Moraga, 1983) and lesbian fiction writers (Califia, 1988; Nestle, 1984). Butch–femme has been condemned as an antifeminist imitation of exploitive male–female relationships and outcast by lesbian feminists as embarrassing (Califia, 1988).

The new scholarship on butch–femme suggests a potential for sexual liberation in the playing out of difference. Butch–femme relations brought the exchange of power into the hands of women and "removed sexuality from the realm of the natural, challenging the notion that sexual performance is a function of biology and affirming the view that sexual gratification is socially constructed" (Davis & Kennedy, 1986, p. 15).

In contrast to its critics, butch–femme was not modeled on hetero-sexual interactions that are centered on male pleasure (Newton, 1984; Nestle, 1984; Smith, 1989). Lesbians have none of the social power that a man has. In fact, femmes, who looked and acted like heterosexual females, had more job opportunities than butch lesbians, and often were the main economic support within lesbian couples (Smith, 1989). Lesbian role-playing was not based on the heterosexual script of oppressor and oppressed that has come to characterize role-playing within the erotic masculine imagination of traditional gender roles (Schneider & Gould, 1987; Sheffield, 1987; Stimpson, 1988; Swedberg, 1989).

Instead, butch–femme relations reveal a class-based conflict between working-class lesbians in the 1940s–1960s and middle-class lesbian femin-ists. The former created an identity around role differentiation, and the latter developed an implicit creed of politically correct egalitarian sexual-ity (Smith, 1989) that falsely stereotyped the erotic relationships of butch–femme (Nestle, 1984).

Prior to the social and political movements of the 1960s and 1970s, lesbian existence was subject to more extreme censure and erasure than today (Aptheker, 1989). Working-class lesbians created social and politi-cal space by asserting their right to sexuality through a system of sexual communication carried out in dress, style, and behavior (Smith, 1989). In the 1950s, the street dyke emerged (Davis & Kennedy, 1986). A butch appearance, to the outsider, looked male: male clothing, short hair, tough appearance and demeanor. In their study of Buffalo, New York, lesbians, Davis and Kennedy (1986) found that the lesbians who fre-quented the bar culture held blue-collar occupations; they worked in factories, drove taxis, and tended bar.

The political climate of the time demanded an outward expression of sexuality because of the invisibility and repression to which lesbians were subjected. Other contextual factors affecting the choice of a lesbian appearance were the rigid sex roles within marriage and the political repression of the McCarthy era.

Bar culture, one of the few public spaces for working-class lesbians to mingle, was a way for lesbians to decode the meaning of others' behavior and identity (Smith, 1989). By asking, "Are you butch or femme?" lesbians were really saying, "Are you sexual?" and "How are you sexual?" (Nestle, 1984). The sexual role played by a butch lesbian, unlike a man in a heterosexual union, was to focus almost exclusively on her partner's pleasure. By satisfying her partner, she experienced and received sexual fulfillment (Davis & Kennedy, 1986). Unlike much of heterosexual coupling, giving pleasure was the role of the more masculinized partner, and receiving pleasure was part of the femme's role. Yet, it is important not to label simplistically the butch as the masculine partner or the femme her feminine counterpart, because butch–femme relationships "were complex erotic and social statements, not phony heterosexual replicas. They were filled with a deeply lesbian language of stance, dress, gesture, love, courage, and autonomy" (Nestle, 1984, p. 232). It is almost impossible to determine the extent to which the actual behavior of these lesbians conformed to stylized roles. Davis and Kennedy's (1986) respondents revealed a far greater range of sexual expression than the role-playing culture suggests. Thus, butch–femme relationships were not imitations of heterosexual sex; they were a sexual and political communication style that emerged from a resistance to a repressive dominant culture.

In contrast to working-class lesbians, middle-class lesbians belonged to the "gold earring set" (Smith, 1989, p. 400). By 1955, the Daughters of Bilitis (DOB) were founded, the only homophile organization open exclusively to women until the late 1960s, when lesbian feminist groups were formed. Class differences were evident between DOB and the working-class bar culture. Middle-class lesbians de-emphasized sexual difference and appealed to the normalcy and stability of relationships (Smith, 1989). DOB politics were assimilationist; they believed lesbians had to show they could fit in before public opinions changed (Davis & Kennedy, 1986; D'Emilio, 1989; Smith, 1989).

The DOB's criticism of butch lesbians was contradictory (Smith, 1989). Lesbian fiction published in the DOB's *The Ladder* emphasized sexual differentiation between two women, of which the more masculine-looking women were portrayed as highly desirable. Middle-class women in DOB feared the identification of lesbians as purely sexual beings or as preyers upon heterosexual women and girls (Smith, 1989). They downplayed sexuality, whereas working-class lesbians in the bar culture used butch–femme styles as a way to announce publicly that they were sexual.

The DOB was the forerunner of the lesbian feminist movement that emerged on college campuses in the late 1960s. Lesbian feminism resolved several problems faced by the 1950s DOB (Smith, 1989). It theorized a sisterhood for all women by providing an analysis of oppression that did not blame women, and by reconciling political activity with being out of the closet. However, lesbian feminism "embodied a fundamental rejection of butch–femme at its deepest level" (Smith, 1989, p. 409). The feminist critique of sexuality left lesbians and straight women with a code for what not to do, but it did not suggest an overtly feminist sexuality for women. Thus, middle-class values of repression and delayed gratification were as divisive and splintering as the whole issue of sexual orientation. Resistance to accepting sexual differences underlies threats to a unified feminist movement.

Conspicuous lesbians carried the brunt of institutionalized homophobia against lesbians (Smith, 1989). Being uncloseted to them meant sexual liberation. In contrast, to emerging lesbian feminists, being uncloseted meant political liberation. Using the overlay of radical feminist egalitarian politics as a lens to interpret earlier butch–femme working-class lesbianism is flawed because it is obscured by a middle-class bias. Postmodern feminism allows us to examine butch–femme relations as a class-based movement. Feminism is not just a middle-class, white women's movement, as evidenced by political, working-class lesbians of the 1940s to 1960s.

Building Coalitions between Lesbian and Heterosexual Feminists

Feminist constructions of women's sexualities have been inhibited by tensions about sexual orientation. A resurgence of this tension occurred in 1975, with the splitting or purging (depending on one's perspective) of lesbians from mainstream feminism (Zimmerman, 1984). Fueling the split were charges by radical feminists that lesbian sexuality is more "politically correct," and charges by psychodynamic theorists that the sexuality of heterosexual women is more mature (Aptheker, 1989).

Feminists face the challenge of acknowledging the contributions of lesbian feminists without undermining the contributions of heterosexual women as co-contributors of both radical and reformist change. Lesbians have taken the lead in initiating and staffing the feminist "movement's most immediate needs, like battered women's shelters, rape crisis and rape prevention centers, abortion clinics, and women's health centers" (Aptheker, 1989, p. 96). Until lesbian feminists began depathologizing lesbian sexuality, the medical establishment had convinced the public that women loving each other was aberrant. Part of the lesbian feminist movement has been to uncover and describe more affirmative stances toward lesbian existence (Smith, 1989) and female sexuality in general.

New questions, sensitive to heterosexual women's experiences, need to be asked as well. Most women's sexual partners are men, despite "the early psychic foundations of women's homoemotional needs and capacities" (Golden, 1987, p. 33). The problem with heterosexuality is that traditional sexual scripts subordinate women's interests and desires to those of their male partners and perpetuate the existing social power imbalance.

A critical challenge for women is to determine how heterosexuality can be constructed outside heterosexism. The very real feeling of attraction that women feel for men should not be denigrated. Rather, it can fuel a search for that which may be genuine between women and men but perverted by the compulsory nature of heterosexuality, traditional sexual scripts, and external forces that support inequality (Colker, 1991; Hollibaugh & Moraga, 1983).

Heterosexuality is not a unitary concept and is not experienced in the same way by all women. A deconstruction of heterosexuality could identify the variety of meanings it has for women and reveal how some women have reconstructed sexual relations with their male partners to be affirming, satisfying expressions of intimacy (Colker, 1991).

Compulsory heterosexuality has negative effects on both heterosexual women and lesbians. Heterosexual women are not encouraged to discuss their sexuality, to seriously question their sexual orientation, or to consider the implications of heterosexism (Newton & Walton, 1984). Lesbian women are ignored, silenced, and labeled as deviant. The result is that women's sexuality has been constructed in a reactive rather than proactive way. As a result, there is no coherent theory of female sexuality that encompasses the rich variety of experiences, attitudes, and desires.

Hollibaugh and Moraga (1983) proposed that women create sexual theory in the way that feminist theory was developed—by women getting together and suspending sexual values to talk about feelings, desires, and interests. Through an alliance between women with varied backgrounds and sexual orientations, a new synthesis could be constructed that originates in women's experiences and is for and about women.

A FEMINIST VISION OF FEMALE SEXUALITIES

The potential for pleasure and bonding through sexual relationships offers an opportunity for women to enrich their intimate relationships. The challenge is to transform existing social structures so that all sexual relationships can be rewarding and empowering to the partners involved. The vision of what egalitarian sexual relations could or should be like is in the process of being constructed.

A Commitment to Pluralism

Pluralism is at the heart of a feminist vision of sexualities (Laws & Schwartz, 1977). A pluralistic approach to sexuality means that a broad range of sexual choices are legitimate and asserts that honesty, equality, and responsibility are essential to any sexual relationship (Reiss, 1990, 1991). "All sexual encounters should be negotiated with an honest statement of your feelings, an equal treatment of the other person's feelings, and a responsibility for taking measures to avoid unwanted outcomes like pregnancy and disease" (Reiss, 1990, p. 219). Pluralism acknowledges the tension between pleasure and danger in sexuality and stresses the importance of making wise choices, which presupposes that one has accurate information and the power and willingness to use it to make sexual decisions.

Sexuality Education

Sexuality education is essential. For too long there has been a conspiracy of silence about sexuality that has been shattered only by the drastic threat of the HIV/AIDS epidemic. Today, talking about sexuality is a matter of life and death. The opportunity now exists to disseminate state-of-the-art information about sexual topics, to explore the meaning of people's sexual experiences, and to expand sexual scripts through awareness and understanding.

Access to information about their own bodies and those of their partners provides knowledge that women can use to make knowledgeable sexual decisions and to enhance their sexual enjoyment. Rather than remaining silent about their sexualities, women who share their experiences can rely on each other as sources of support and information. Research such as Thompson's (1990) work on teens' sexual initiation suggests mothers may be influential in the way daughters construct their own sexual scripts. Adolescents who had open discussions with their mothers and many sources of sexual information had more positive experiences.

Our goal is for people to have positive sexual experiences. Even in some of the more enlightened sexuality education programs, it is the negative aspects of sexuality that are stressed. Female adolescents, particularly, are socialized as "potential victims of sexual (male) desire" (Fine, 1988, p. 42). The role of pleasure in adolescents' sexual experiences is missing from education programs (Brick, 1989). The result is the perpetuation of sexual scripts within which pleasure is nonexistent, furtive, clandestine, and shameful. Only when people have the opportunity to explore their sexuality and determine what is pleasurable and positive will they gain control to say no to other sexual practices (Reiss, 1990).

Feminists need to advocate sexuality education that provides accurate and comprehensive information to both females and males. We need to begin and maintain conversations about the difficult choices involved in balancing pleasure and danger in sexual relationships. Each woman can contribute to a rethinking of existing sexual arrangements by being encouraged to question dominant sexual scripts and determine her own personal desires. Each woman also must assess the personal risks that she incurs in acting on her sexual choices. A postmodern feminist perspective encourages forming coalitions with others who support pluralism to neutralize the power of those who would silence public conversations about sexuality that do not reinforce traditional scripts.

The Need for Fresh Perspectives of Women's Sexualities

The concept of sexual scripts offers a vehicle for exploring sexual identity and behavioral change over time. By replacing a static, categorical model of sexuality with a dynamic, kinetic model, relational approaches to rethinking women's sexualities can be accommodated (Blumstein & Schwartz, 1990).

Alternative approaches to thinking about sexual identities stress the changing relationships through which sexuality is expressed over time (Blumstein & Schwartz, 1990; Klein, 1990; McWhirter et al., 1990; Newton & Walton, 1984; Weeks, 1987). The focus shifts away from categorizing people by actions or sex of partner and toward the quality of the involvement and the freedom to experience and enjoy relationships. This approach provides a new paradigm for considering sexuality and makes room for questions about diversity, power, and choice.

The idea that sexuality may be situational and contextual requires going beyond pluralism to challenge the naturalism of heterosexuality and the political correctness of lesbianism. How can we construct sexual relationships to allow women to define and control their sexualities without "flattening their sexual experiences in the name of equality" (Newton & Walton, 1984, p. 250)? While resisting essentialism and encouraging the deconstruction and reconstruction of traditional sexual scripts, it is important to maintain respect for the sexual choices that women make. Valuing these choices and acknowledging that they reflect the different social realities in which women live construct women as active agents rather than passive victims.

Women's sexualities are interwoven with other aspects of their lives and must be considered in context in order to be understood. To be sexually agentic, women must have equitable power and control in their other social roles. Only then can they comfortably communicate and negotiate effectively about their sexual desire and avoid sexual coercion.

Women's sexualities are significantly influenced by societal gender arrangements and power structures. Changes in women's roles have brought about analyses of the importance of sexuality in their lives. The debates among feminists regarding the politics of sexuality may be seen as bellwethers of change and empowerment. Although not the whole of feminist thinking about sexuality, these debates are exemplary because they provide a springboard for challenging old assumptions and a context for presenting ways in which women have become active constructors of their own sexualities. Feminists have placed women's lives and the social structures that affect them in the center of vision, revealing the constraints against which women struggle to define themselves sexually and the ways in which women are creating and exploring their sexual potential.

Women's Reproductive Lives

Women's unique ability to conceive and bear children is a fundamental difference between men and women. The capacity to give birth provides women with a potential source of great satisfaction and power. However, the responsibility of bearing and caring for children has limited women's autonomy and ability to participate in activities that enhance their personal development and their social and economic status. If women are unable to control the number and timing of their children, they are at risk for exclusion from many of the social, educational, and occupational opportunities that are open to men. Women's freedom to exercise reproductive control is essential to the goal of gender equality.

The current issue in the courts and before state legislatures is women's legal right to abortion. However, abortion is only the tip of the reproductive choice "iceberg." Equally important issues lying just under the surface include access to safe and effective contraceptives, explicit education about sexuality and reproduction, freedom to control one's own body and activities during pregnancy, and the availability and abuse of reproductive technologies. Reproductive freedom means more than the ability to choose whether, when, how, and with whom to have a child; it also means "having the economic means and social conditions that make it possible to effectuate one's choices" (Kolbert, 1988, p.8).

In this chapter, we explore the various reproductive issues that confront contemporary women and consider the meaning and consequences of these decisions for the women involved and their families. We focus on the choices women are making that challenge the norm of compulsory motherhood in which motherhood must occur "on time" and in the context of a heterosexual marriage. Because, to some extent, the concept of reproductive choice is more illusory than real, the personal and social contexts within which "choices" are made are also explored. Little research has been done on the reproductive choices and needs of women of color and disabled women, but the work that has been done suggests that women's reproductive experiences vary significantly, depending on their life circumstances. Sensitivity to these differences is critical in considering how to empower women with true reproductive freedom. What are the dilemmas that face women who choose to be child free, to delay motherhood, to have children in lesbian relationships, or to abort a pregnancy? We also examine potential costs and benefits for women of the new reproductive technologies, the tension associated with men's continued attempts to control reproductive decisions, and the implications for women of the fetal protection movement. We conclude the chapter with suggestions for ways in which women can empower themselves and each other to address the dialectics of reproduction.

THE POLITICS OF REPRODUCTIVE CONTROL

Women today have unprecedented power to make decisions about whether to have children, when to have them, and how many to have. The ability to control reproduction—and society's understanding that women have it—is a revolutionary change that O'Brien (1981b) has likened to the development of capitalism in its potential for changing the course of modern history. Because the care of young children has constrained women's educational and occupational opportunities, the availability of effective contraception and legal abortion has provided a material foundation for gender equality.

Women's changing consciousness regarding reproductive choice and the accompanying power to determine the course of their own lives necessitates a reciprocal transformation of social relations surrounding fertility decisions, childbirth, and child care. Sex and reproduction have never been linked inextricably for men. Now they no longer are for women. Ideally, with reproductive control women could have a new freedom to explore and enjoy their sexuality, to become mothers when they are ready and willing to do so, and to pursue a work life uninterrupted by unplanned and unwanted pregnancies. These possibilities can transform women's relationships with men, with their children, and with society in general.

Reproductive control will continue to be one of the major political themes in the late 20th century because of the potentially far-reaching consequences of women with the power to control their own fertility and expand their autonomy. Discussion and action regarding women's reproductive rights have generated a sociopolitical tension that is escalating in the 1990s. Although social thought and family policy have tended to see the rights and needs of women and children as synonymous, this is not the case in the area of reproductive decision making. Increasingly, the rights of the unborn child and the rights of the mother are being seen to conflict. For women, this conflict sets up a dialectical tension of the most basic type.

Reproductive control in the hands of women is a powerful social force, particularly if they choose not to have children. The current birthrate for American women is 2.0 children per woman (National Center for Health Statistics, 1991a). Since 1971 the total fertility rate has been below the 2.1 birthrate that is believed to be necessary to replace our population. Conservatives such as Ben Wattenberg of the American Enterprise Institute have written ominously about the consequences of the "shrinkage" of our population and the negative economic and political implications of this so-called birth dearth. In response to declining fertility rates, Wattenberg (1987) calls for measures that would be supportive of women trying to manage careers and motherhood simultaneously. Wattenberg proposes paid maternity leave, flextime, job sharing, day-care tax credit, and compensation to childbearing women at the rate of $2,000 per year per child age 16 or under. These funds, paid for from the Social Security Trust Fund, would encourage women to begin having children earlier and to have more of them.

Paradoxically, when women exercise fertility control and stop having children, support for programs and services that help women parent *and* pursue a job or career emerge. Women could gain political leverage by lowering their fertility rates.

Feminists have debated the consequences of refusing to conceive, bear children, and mother (Tong, 1989). On the one hand, the choice to remain child free has been described as women's unique opportunity for liberation (Firestone, 1970; Movius, 1976). By freeing themselves from the demands of caregiving, women would have the time and energy to commit to activities that would allow them to attain their own goals and achieve influential positions of power. If enough women chose this path, the result would be an opportunity to enhance the status of all women, which, in turn, would affect the balance of power in society.

By forgoing motherhood, however, women might relinquish experiences that are pleasurable and fulfilling. They also would give up the power associated with the ability to reproduce and the potentially close relationship to their own children when they chose not to mother. Rich (1986) has proposed that it is not the *experience* of motherhood from which women need to be liberated, but the *institution* of motherhood.

Although most women are probably not prepared collectively to use their fertility as a political tool, there is evidence that women are making more variant fertility decisions and becoming aware of their ability to control reproduction. More women are having only one child, postponing childbearing until later in their adult lives, or choosing to remain voluntarily child free. Each of these strategies allows women greater freedom in developing other aspects of their lives.

Not all women take advantage of the ability to control their fertility. A number of social factors have conspired to deter women from making fertility decisions in a conscious, deliberate manner. Chief among these is religion. Basic to many religions is the implicit belief that a woman's role is primarily procreative and that it is a sin to intervene in nature's course or God's plan. If women are to be devout and good conjugal partners, they risk spending most of their time and energy bearing and raising children, a role that keeps them dependent on and subservient to their husbands. To take control of their own fertility means challenging the most basic religious teachings and questioning traditional gender roles.

Another factor that interferes in women's reproductive control is lack of knowledge about effective contraceptive usage and the lack of availability of contraceptives that women are comfortable with and use consistently. This is particularly problematic for very young, less educated, and poor women. At a time when there is so much public controversy over abortion, several ironies are noteworthy: Contraceptive methods are disappearing from the market more quickly than new methods are being introduced; only one major pharmaceutical company is involved in contraceptive research; and the federal government has cut funding for contraceptive research.

An additional factor that influences women's fertility decisions is their partners' attitudes and preferences. Little research exists on the influence of a woman's partner in the childbearing decision, but a partner's influence may be extensive, particularly for women who are financially and emotionally dependent on male partners. As women gain greater reproductive control, urgent questions are raised regarding how these partners should be included in childbearing decisions. These questions are difficult and reflect the continuing tension that women face in integrating their partners' preferences with their own when the consequences of these decisions are manifested in the bodies of women.

Discussions of reproductive control tend to focus on abortion, but reproductive choice also includes the choice *to have* a child:

> We can no longer talk about reproductive choice in a vacuum. We must talk about the right to have as well as not to have children, the right to control the conditions under which we will have or not have them, and the right to a social system that allows a measure of real choice. (McDonnell, 1984, p. 80)

A narrow focus on abortion minimizes the importance of reproductive choice for all women and obscures the indirect factors that limit women's fertility choices.

The most consistent criticism of women's demands for reproductive control indicts women as selfish. Women's interest in self-fulfillment, according to conservatives, threatens the traditional family; abortion is the ultimate selfish act—pursuit of self-interest at the price of human life (Klatch, 1987). Opponents of women's reproductive freedom say that women will come to regard their obligations to children in the same way as men have over the years—that women will become "sociological fathers" (Hunt & Hunt, 1982).

The trend for women to make conscious decisions about reproductive issues is greeted with thinly veiled scorn. Nock (1987) labeled women "nontraditional" if they endorse male–female equality, calling these women "consumers" of children rather than "producers" of children. He suggested that such women "shop" for children by deciding rationally when conception will occur and consume children by carefully selecting the timing, number, and even the health of their children. Nock explained this transformation as the result of an emphasis on self and charged that women attempt to manage children to facilitate their own personal fulfillment, achievement, and success. Instead of scorn, women's concerns about reproductive control need to be treated with respect.

Compulsory Motherhood

Compulsory motherhood (Gordon, 1976) is part of the socialization process for women in our society. Most women think about whether or not to become a mother. If motherhood is normative in our society, choosing not to have children is seen as deviant or, at best, variant. Messages about the importance and appropriateness of motherhood as a prerequisite for full womanhood are so clear and pervasive that they are almost impossible to escape, regardless of sexual orientation. Infertility is seen as a tragedy, and couples may endure great financial and emotional expense to conceive.

Even feminist writers, with few exceptions, are pronatalist: "To the extent the movement does not subject the dominant pattern of universally prescribed parenthood to thorough analysis and criticism, it unwittingly contributes to the consolidation of one of the structural foundations of the situation it aims to change" (Gimenez, 1983, p. 289). The choice to remain child free should be one that is available to women as a socially accepted alternative. Yet, most females have grown up with the expectation that they, too, will one day become mothers. They have been encouraged to practice nurturing skills, first with dolls and later with younger children. Many theories have been used to explain the dynamics of sex role socialization and the reproduction of the desire to mother in generation after generation of women. The process by which one comes to integrate a vision of "self as mother" into one's sense of identity has eluded full understanding. Efforts to help women see motherhood as one of a number of options and opportunities, rather than a requirement for normal adult life, will result in more diversity in women's fertility decisions.

As women have gained autonomy and self-determination through increased educational and occupational opportunities, choices surrounding mothering have become problematic. Although children are an important source of joy, fulfillment, and power, children also have tied women to traditional roles and dependence on men. There are still strong pronatalist forces in our society, but a growing number of women are choosing, either actively or by default, to remain child free. Ironically, even decisions *not* to have children may actually be made in reaction to coercive pressures *to* be a mother and, therefore, are not freely made either (Johnson, 1989).

CHILD FREE BY CHOICE

Although most women become mothers, an increasing number of women complete their childbearing years without giving birth to a child. For some, childlessness is involuntary, but a significant portion of women without children are child free by choice. Regardless of women's reasons for not becoming mothers, they are still identified using terms that imply a deviation from the norm. A woman is childless, child free, or not a mother. For lack of a better term, in this book we use "child free" because it carries with it the sense of a choice having been made, although it suggests a negativity toward children that neither we, nor most women so identified, feel.

There has been a steep increase in the incidence of childlessness over the last two decades (National Center for Health Statistics, 1991a). In 1970, only 9% of women 35 years of age were childless; by 1989, 20% of women this age had no children. Some of these women will bear children in their late 30s or early 40s. Others will remain childless because of fertility problems. However, fertility impairment among couples with wives aged 35 to 44 declined from 48% in 1982 to 36% in 1988.

Although there have always been women who chose not to have children, only in the 1970s were this fertility choice and the resulting lifestyle given serious attention. Veevers's (1976, 1979, 1980) groundbreaking research on voluntary childlessness was one of the first systematic attempts to make visible and give voice to those choosing not to become mothers. This work explored various aspects of the decision not to have children, as well as the antecedents, correlates, and consequences of this choice.

Houseknecht's (1987) review on voluntary childlessness indicates that child-free women tend to be highly educated, employed in high-status jobs with above-average incomes, commonly claim no religious affiliation, and have nontraditional definitions of the female role. Most child-free women make the decision not to have children after being married rather than before and are more influential in the decision-making process if there is not consensus between partners. Of the studies reviewed regarding women's rationales for remaining child free, 79% found that "freedom from childcare responsibility/greater opportunity for self-fulfillment and spontaneous mobility" were given as primary reasons. "More satisfactory marital relationship" and "female career considerations" were the other most frequently mentioned rationales.

Women who choose to remain child free have been described as less traditional than other women (Bram, 1978; Greenglass & Borovilos, 1984; Houseknecht, 1987; Nock, 1987), even those who delay childbearing into their 30s (Baber & Dreyer, 1986). Nock (1987) analyzed data from the 1985 National Opinion Research Center (NORC) General Social Survey and reported that, although no women of reproductive age saw being child free as a "family ideal," nontraditional women (who supported male–female equality) were twice as likely to have no children. He argued that women remain child free or limit their fertility because of the symbolic significance of having a child. Motherhood is symbolic because "at a minimum it announces to the individual and others a decision about a woman's place in the world. Such a woman has chosen to be one of several types of American women, one who will not strive, primarily, for occupational success" (Nock, 1987, p. 382).

Decisions about motherhood reflect women's worldviews and their perceptions of women's role in society. Gerson (1985) suggests that women, even during childhood, differ in their expectations about adult roles and in their goals and aspirations regarding work and motherhood. These early orientations are shaped by life experiences and opportunities that support or interfere with their abilities to achieve their goals and aspirations. The development of these worldviews is a complex process about which there is little precise knowledge.

Nock's (1987) argument that fertility decisions are symbolic statements regarding women's beliefs about male–female equality and the relative importance of motherhood may be too simplistic because they mask the complexity and diversity of the decision process. His argument may be applicable only to women who actively choose to have no children rather than for women in general. Those who make an active, voluntary commitment to remain child free may be making a statement about their quest for worldly success and their preference for career involvement over motherhood (Nock, 1987). However, a feminist analysis provides alternative possibilities.

A radical feminist perspective on the "evacuation of motherhood" speaks of pregnancy and motherhood as a mark that signals male domination, making a connection between women's oppression and their role as "breeders." Allen (1983) suggests that if all women stopped having children for the next 20 years and focused on meeting women's needs worldwide for food, education, and energy resources, "the possibilities for developing new modes of thought and existence would be almost unimaginable" (p. 327). Turning from theory to praxis, Rich (1986) describes reports of slave women in Jamaica who "absolutely refused to reproduce—partly out of despair and outrage, as a gynecological revolt against the system" (p. xviii). Even though having and raising a certain number of children could get these women relieved from heavy field labor, they had few or no children. After emancipation, their birthrate increased. Similarly, some women in the United States, although in very different circumstances, may choose not to have children, at least in part because of a rejection of an environment that makes it physically, socially, or philosophically inhospitable, or even dangerous, for them to bear children.

Women who become mothers do so either as the result of an active decision process or by default. Merely becoming a mother may not be a symbol of a woman's thinking about the primacy of motherhood, as Nock (1987) suggests, but may reflect life circumstances that make fertility control difficult and motherhood the least undesirable of the perceived options. Another group of women become mothers because they see motherhood as one of women's most important rights and creative opportunities (see Ruddick, 1989). They do not see motherhood as sacrificing their occupational success, but attempt to integrate these two aspects of their lives. These women believe motherhood offers the potential for creating alternatives to oppressive societies through nurturant, maternal practices (Noddings, 1984; Ruddick, 1989).

The decision not to have a child and not to mother is a choice that can have a variety of implications for women. Not having the responsibility of dependent children means that women can pursue their own interests and goals and develop resources that allow them to be independent of a partner. Married, child-free women have marriages that are at least as happy and satisfying as women who are mothers, and they are no more likely to divorce (Bram, 1978; Houseknecht, 1979; Veevers, 1979).

Nevertheless, women who have no children forgo the uniquely female experiences of pregnancy, delivery, and breastfeeding and the joys that accompany the care and nurturing of young children. Child-free couples do not have the bond that joint childrearing can contribute to a loving, egalitarian relationship. Another consequence of choosing to remain child free is that a woman making this choice never has the opportunity to become part of the society of mothers. Even though being child free appears to be perceived as more variant than deviant today, there is little support for women who choose this fertility alternative. One reason why child-free women are seen as less deviant is because more educated, employed women are delaying their first birth until their 30s. It is no longer clear which women are choosing "no children" and which women are choosing "children later."

DELAYED CHILDBEARING

Since the early 1970s, there has been a trend for educated women to delay the birth of their first child until their 30s. Demographic data indicate that this trend is likely to continue and intensify. The recent increase in the first-birth rate for women in their 30s has occurred during a period of decline in the general fertility rate. From 1980 to 1985, the first-birth rate for women 20 to 24 declined 7% (National Center for Health Statistics, 1987). Rates for women aged 30 to 34 and 35 to 39 rose 32% and 69%, respectively, suggesting that women are waiting until their late 30s to have their first child. In 1976, births to women in their 30s comprised 19% of all first births (U.S. Bureau of the Census, 1989). By 1988, they accounted for 33%. The most recent data indicated that the increase in the first-birth rate for women aged 30 to 34 increased 4% in 1989, and the rate for women 35 to 39 and 40 to 44 increased by 9% and 13%, respectively (National Center for Health Statistics, 1991a).

Women who want to have children and to pursue their own education and career must balance conflicting demands. Rather than juggling the responsibilities of caring for young children and establishing a career simultaneously, many women are giving priority to their career during their 20s and delaying childbearing until later. Effective contraceptives and legal abortion allow women to control their fertility and defer motherhood until they are ready to become parents. By postponing their first births, women are free to pursue advanced degrees, to devote long hours to a career, and to amass economic and personal resources. These women are able to compete more equally with men in the labor market. They have higher incomes, providing financial security and independence. Because married career women who delay their first births have an income closer to that of their husbands, they may have more equal power in the marital relationship as well.

Women who delay childbearing are similar in many ways to those who choose to remain child free. Two thirds of the women in Veevers's (1980) sample of child-free women used a decision strategy of temporary postponement before making a commitment to have no children; only one third of the sample were "early articulators" who went into marriage planning to be child free. Even a decade ago, however, the choice to remain child free was less accepted, and a postponement process may have been necessary for many women to feel comfortable with their decisions.

Like child-free women, contemporary delayed childbearers are highly educated and tend to be employed in high-status professional positions (Baber & Dreyer, 1986; Wilkie, 1981). Most research on delayed childbearing has focused on white women, and vital statistics data indicate that black women are less likely to postpone their first births. However, Cohen (1985), drawing on data regarding Asian-American births, noted that first birthrates for women over 30 are higher for Japanese-American and Chinese-American women than for white women. In 1980, one third of all first births to Asian-American mothers were to women over 30, compared with only one fifth of white and one seventh of black women having their first child. Knowledge about delayed childbearing is clearly biased at this point because it has not included the experiences of women of color.

Education has been identified as a key factor in delayed childbearing (Bloom, 1984; Frankel & Wise, 1982). The more educated a woman is, the more likely she is to delay her first birth. The fact that more than one third of all Asian-American women in the United States complete college may help explain why so many delay their first birth (Cohen, 1985). Women who complete advanced degrees have more labor market opportunities, are more likely to have careers than jobs, and usually receive high salaries. The advantages of a high-status career may make it difficult, even for women who want children very much, to interrupt their work lives to become mothers. Marciano (1979) found that, even for women who married with the expectation of having a child, career advancement affected their willingness to give up their freedom and the rewards of working in order to become mothers. Education does not cause women to delay their first birth, but it makes options other than mothering possible. Once alternative choices are made, they become intrinsically important, and childbearing is postponed.

Wilkie (1981) presented a demographic analysis of delayed childbearing and concluded that for the educated group of career women who postponed their first birth, the delay was motivated by financial considerations, not career aspirations. Those who delayed differed little from early-childbearing women in regard to their attitudes and values about traditional roles and parenthood.

The results of subsequent research challenge these notions, however. Women who have a first child early in adult life and those who wait are different. Because no longitudinal study has explored women's childbearing decisions, it is not known whether women who postpone their first births are inherently different from women who have an early first birth or whether experiences during the postponement period contribute to the differences.

Daniels and Weingarten (1982) found a programmatic postponement to be the family timing scenario most characteristic of couples in their sample having their first child in their late 20s or early 30s. This programmatic postponement, which was characteristic of none of the early-timing parents, was based on participants' strategies for achieving a number of identity, intimacy, and career goals. Strategies included the achievement of a psychological readiness to commit to parenting, the selection of the right partner and creation of a strong marriage, and the accomplishment of career objectives.

The theme of personal goals and achievements was revealed in another study that compared late-timing mothers, aged 30 to 41, with mothers whose first births were at ages 19 to 25 (Walter, 1986). One of the most striking differences between the groups of mothers had to do with identity or sense of self. The delayed childbearers defined themselves both in terms of their roles as mothers and in terms of their own achievements and accomplishments. Women who had early first births were more likely to define themselves through their relationships with their children and husbands; their self-esteem and feelings of self-worth were dependent upon their involvement in caring for others. In ranking four factors that were most important in determining their sense of self (own achievements and activities, relationship with husband, relationship with child or children, or parental support), 67% of the delayed childbearers chose their own achievements and activities, compared with only 24% of the early childbearers. The early childbearers were most likely to say that their relationships with their husbands were most important in determining their sense of self. Fifty-seven percent of the early-timing women responded this way, compared with only 18% of the late-timing mothers.

Walter (1986) concluded that, although relationships are very important to older first-time mothers, they are comfortable and capable of depending upon themselves. These mothers were aware of their own emotional needs and willing and able to make demands on their environment to have these needs met. The early-timing mothers had had less time for personal development, were less comfortable with the prospect of having to depend upon themselves, and had more self-doubt. These findings suggest that delaying childbearing may allow women the time and experiences to develop a secure sense of self. Women who have established a firm identity, recognize the value of their own achievements, and feel confident of their own abilities are likely to approach mothering differently than other women (Walter, 1986).

Women who delay their first child are likely to have achieved other agendas in their lives, established their careers, and developed stable, intimate relationships (Baber, 1989). They express a readiness to mother and a deep sense of confidence in their ability to be a good mother, as two women noted:

> My life experiences were more varied because I waited. I feel that my children benefit from confidence derived from years of working. My own interests have broadened and I pass these interests on to my kids. Most importantly, my mature understanding of human nature helps me handle my children, their stages, moods, etc. with compassion. (Baber, 1989, p. 9)

> I am much more mature and happy. This made the birth of my son totally welcomed. I have more patience now. I have more confidence in myself enabling me to be a more confident parent. (Baber, 1989, p. 9)

Although the delayed childbearing trend has been well documented and the correlates of postponing the first birth established, little systematic research exists on the consequences of delayed childbearing for women and their families. It is not known whether delayed childbearing empowers women to take advantage of emerging opportunities without forgoing motherhood, or whether it is merely an adaptation to societal constraints that might, in itself, limit women's options in unsuspected ways.

It is difficult to determine the consequences of the trend toward delayed childbearing. A relatively long span of time is needed to determine the effects of postponing childbearing (Hofferth, 1984). Although some of the correlates or short-range effects of delayed childbearing, such as increased educational and occupational opportunities for women, may be easy to investigate, longer-term effects such as the consequences for children of having older parents may take many years to determine. Because variables such as educational level, career status, and income tend to be positively correlated with delayed childbearing, it is difficult to determine whether timing is the critical variable that explains the differences found (Walter, 1986).

Although there is little conclusive evidence regarding the costs and benefits of delayed childbearing, a growing body of information can be considered. Demographic studies indicate that a clear advantage of delayed childbearing is economic (Bloom, 1986; Hofferth, 1984). Analyzing data from the Panel Study of Income Dynamics for women aged 60 and older in 1976, Hofferth (1984) found that women who bore their first children at age 30 or older were better off economically than those who had their children at a more normative age or who were childless. Those who delayed their first birth had higher family incomes and living standards and had accumulated more assets than those who had children earlier.

Using data from more recent cohorts of women, Bloom (1986) found that women who delayed their first birth until 27 or older earned an average of 36% more per hour than women who have their first child before age 22 and 18% more than women having their first child between 22 and 26. Even controlling for education and work experience, Bloom (1986) found that delayers earned 10% more than the group having children before 22. Among professionals, those who delayed earned 22% more than the early-childbearing group.

In addition to allowing time for personal development, career establishment, and potential for financial security, delayed childbearing should be advantageous to the development of adult intimate relationships as well. Many couples who postpone their first births have had years to spend together and will have addressed the major adjustment issues during the early years of their relationships. Theoretically, having dealt with the identity and intimacy issues of early adulthood, they are prepared to approach parenting when they are less encumbered with individual concerns and with developing a satisfactory intimate relationship. An additional advantage for delayed childbearers is that the children are almost always planned and less likely to present a conflict between the demands of parenting and those of personal development.

Delaying childbearing also has disadvantages. Couples who have been child free for years have developed complex work and intimacy patterns and may be resentful of the interruptions generated by a baby who cannot always be scheduled and controlled. Women who have spent years preparing for and developing successful careers may have more difficulty than they anticipated with the competing demands of motherhood. The consequences of parenthood are more likely to be manifested in the worklives of women than in those of men, even among delayed-childbearing couples who are both equally career oriented. Conflict may result as work and parenting roles are negotiated and renegotiated.

Parents who are well educated and high achievers themselves may have higher than average expectations for their children. Delaying childbearing may mean less time available to have additional children. If a couple has only one child, they may have unusually high expectations of him or her because they will have only one opportunity to prove their parenting ability.

Women who delay having children may end up inadvertently childless. Women may delay marriage and childbearing until their 30s to devote their full energy to their careers and then may be unable to find a suitable partner. Although some women have chosen to have a child and parent alone, many others do not have children because they have not married or not married soon enough. Other women have married and delayed childbearing until their careers were established and then found themselves divorced, in a failing relationship, or married to a partner whose health problems preclude having a child.

There is considerable disagreement about the relationship between delayed childbearing and infertility. Couples who begin trying to conceive early in their adult life and have difficulty doing so may become delayed childbearers by default. However, infertility does not seem to be a significant contributor to the increase in first births to older women (Bianchi & Spain, 1986).

Difficulty conceiving, however, may result from delaying the birth of the first child. Postponing the first birth means more time at risk for sexually transmitted diseases that could result in damage to the reproductive tract. The more years that one is active sexually, particularly with multiple partners, the more years one is at risk for pelvic inflammatory disease (PID), a major contributor to infertility in women. However, without accurate data on the incidence of PID-related infertility, there is no reason to believe that delayed childbearers would be at any greater risk than the general population (Menken, 1985). The critical factor in determining risk appears to be the maintenance of a healthy reproductive tract. Because delayed childbearers are generally better educated and have access to medical care, they may be at lower risk than the general population in that they may be more likely to monitor their reproductive health. This, however, is speculative and needs to be studied systematically.

Although the general belief has been that fecundability (the probability of achieving a pregnancy in a month of unprotected intercourse) declines with age, the biological capacity to become pregnant does not vary much for women between the ages of 20 and 40 (James, 1979; Menken, 1985). However, there is a higher rate of unrecognized spontaneous abortions in older women. One study indicated that first-trimester, spontaneous abortions occurred 3.5 times more frequently in women 35 and older than in women aged 20 to 29 (Daniels & Weingarten, 1979). Reliable, systematic data are needed to allow women and their partners to judge the risks involved in delaying.

Fetal Abnormalities

The rate of fetal abnormalities rises exponentially with maternal age. The estimated risk for a chromosomal defect is 2.6 per 1,000 for children of women aged 30 and under; it is 5.6 if the woman is 35 years old, 15.8 at age 40, and 53.7 at age 45 (Hook, 1981). However, current screening technologies and legally accessible abortions allow considerable control over the likelihood of bearing a child with an abnormality.

Amniocentesis is the most frequently used test for fetal abnormalities. However, it cannot be done until the 14th week of gestation, and results may not be available for several additional weeks. If a serious defect is indicated and the decision is made to abort, a woman faces a second-trimester abortion. The decision to abort at this point may be more difficult psychologically, and the medical procedure itself may be riskier than that used in a first-trimester abortion.

A relatively new procedure, chorionic villi sampling, can be done as early as the eighth week of pregnancy, and the results are available in a matter of hours. Women who desire to terminate the pregnancy can make the decision during the first trimester. Although there were some early concerns about possible increased risk to the developing fetus with chorionic villi sampling, recent studies suggest that the risk is comparable to that of amniocentesis and that it is a safe and accurate prenatal diagnostic method when used by an experienced practitioner (Green, 1988). Unfortunately, this procedure is not yet generally available, and women may not be given information about it by their obstetricians.

A recent study of 3,917 women having a first child (Berkowitz, Skovron, Lapinski, & Berkowitz, 1990) compared the outcomes of pregnancy for women over 30 and those aged 20 to 29. Women who delayed childbearing were no more likely than the younger mothers to have preterm deliveries or babies who died, had low birth weight, or had low Apgar scores. The older mothers were more likely to experience pregnancy-induced hypertension, diabetes, and placental problems. They also were significantly more likely to deliver by cesarean section.

Maternal risks associated with later first pregnancies do not seem related to age per se, but to other variables that are confounded with maternal age (DeVore, 1983; Mansfield 1988). These include preexisting medical disorders, socioeconomic level, chronic diseases associated with aging, and the special medical management that older first-time mothers may receive because they are believed to be at high risk. The unexplainably high rate of cesarean sections for women over 30 may be due to the fact that these women are labeled high risk merely because of their age (Mansfield, 1988). Women's delivery outcomes may be dictated more by obstetricians' concerns than by actual birth complications.

Because more and more women are making the choice to postpone the birth of a first child until after age 30, accurate, valid information about the advantages and disadvantages of this timing strategy should be available. Only then can women and their partners make knowledgeable decisions. Delayed childbearing is advantageous to women. The disadvantages appear to be manageable if women are aware of the risks, have a long-term reproductive health plan that takes these risks into consideration, and have available health care.

ABORTION

Abortion is one of the most controversial social issues. The abortion debate has caused divisions between men and women, between feminists and antifeminists, and among feminists. In a comprehensive review of public policy issues affecting women, Gelb and Palley (1987) emphasized that abortion is an issue that appears to threaten traditional family values and signifies a fundamental change in women's role in society. Access to abortion means that women are no longer compelled to be mothers if they have an unplanned and unwanted pregnancy.

Prochoice advocates believe that reproductive freedom and women's control over their own bodies are a fundamental right. Antichoice activists see abortion as the ultimate act of callous indifference whereby women's fulfillment is achieved at the price of innocent human life, and women's reproductive capabilities are devalued (Klatch, 1987).

The abortion controversy is primarily about women's changing roles. Luker (1984) proposed that the debate about abortion is actually a "referendum on the place and meaning of motherhood" (p. 193). Her research on male and female activists in the abortion battle revealed that although male activists on both sides were similar in regard to social background variables, prochoice and prolife women (as they were identified in this study) differed on almost every variable considered.

Antiabortion, or prolife, women tended to have a bachelor's degree or some college and to be housewives or employed in traditional female occupations. They usually married early and had two or three children. Religion played a significant role in their lives; 80% were Catholics. They valued traditional gender roles highly and arranged their lives accordingly. Sex was valued for its procreative purpose, and unplanned pregnancies were often described as surprise pregnancies.

Prochoice women were more likely to have had postgraduate education and to be employed in professional occupations. Twenty-three percent had never married, and those who were married had an average of one or two children. Sixty-three percent indicated that they had no

religion, and none identified themselves as Catholics. They desired gender equality and saw the traditional division of labor in society as contrary
to their own best interests. Sex was valued as a means of developing
intimacy and mutual pleasure rather than as a reproductive activity. They
believed that pregnancies and children should be planned and wanted.

Luker (1984) concluded that the differences between the prolife and
prochoice women centered around their varying definitions of motherhood. Prolife women believed that motherhood was the most important
and satisfying role for women; prochoice women saw it only as one
possible role, not a primary or inevitable role for every woman. These two
groups of women had arranged their lives differently, consistent with their
beliefs about the appropriate role for women. Their everyday life experiences, in turn, tended to reinforce their values. Whatever choices a
woman has made, it is necessary for her to cling to the belief that the right
decisions were made. If prolife women, for example, do not maintain the
primacy of motherhood, they devalue their own life choices and the
meaning of their day-to-day existence.

Ginsburg (1989) collected life stories of 35 abortion activists from
Fargo, North Dakota. This study illustrates how different interpretations
of the meaning and value of motherhood in society contribute to the split
between even those who identify themselves as feminists. The life stories
of activists in Ginsburg's study revealed a tension between motherhood
and the workplace. Both prochoice and prolife activists saw themselves as
working to enhance women's position as they addressed the often contradictory demands of these two roles. Narratives of both groups stressed
the importance of nurturance and caretaking, but defined them differently. The prochoice activists viewed nurturance, or female cultural values,
as a goal for broad social change and in opposition to "a world that is
viewed as materialistic, male-defined, and lacking in compassion" (Ginsburg, 1989, p. 72).

Many of the prolife activists had left the work force to have children
and asserted the primacy of mothering and reproduction. Conversion to
the prolife cause often came after the birth of their first child and occurred
as the result of a reworking of their beliefs about women's place in our
culture and the possibilities of developing alternate models of motherhood.

If women are to relinquish paid work and choose mothering as the
primary role in their lives, it is necessary that they believe that they will
be well supported by their partners. A common theme that ran through
all of the prolife, antiabortion, right-to-life stories is the perception that
abortion weakens the social pressure on men to assume the consequences
of their sexual activity. Children and the moral and legal bonds of
traditional family life are seen to be the ties that bind a man to the woman

who has chosen domesticity over career. Whereas feminists encourage women to develop personal security by becoming independent through the ability to support themselves economically, the socially conservative, prolife women seek to develop and extend their security within the context of a traditional marriage (Klatch, 1987).

Even some of the prolife feminists support the idea that abortion offers men the opportunity for sex with no responsibility; Wiley (1989), a member of Feminists for Life, said:

> Sexual intercourse now implies for each of them—exactly nothing, no responsibility. So why should any man feel he's acquired an obligation if the woman decides to give birth? . . . Am I predicting that the elevation of sexual autonomy to the status of a "right," coupled with the availability of abortion, will cut men loose entirely? That paternal responsibility will sink to absolute zero? Hell, no. I'm not predicting that. I'm reporting it. (p. 76)

Because women have been socialized to be nurturant and to put others' needs before their own, the decision to abort a pregnancy causes great dissonance for many women. Studies involving women making abortion decisions (Gilligan, 1982) capture the dilemma of making a choice that calls into conflict responsibility for other and for self, "a dilemma in which there is no way of acting without consequences to other and self" (p. 108).

Reproductive choice is an essential tenet of feminism. However, even among those who identify themselves as feminists, there is dissension on the issue of abortion. This political ambivalence reflects women's personal struggles with decisions about voluntary termination of pregnancy. Recent court decisions and controversies regarding when life begins and the rights of biological fathers complicate the decision. Most feminists believe that the right to a safe, legal abortion is fundamental to women' s reproductive rights. Yet, there is dissonance between this stand on abortion and other core feminist issues (McDonnell, 1984), particularly if abortion is seen as a technique for screening out potentially "abnormal" individuals, doing violence against another in self-interest, or relieving men of their responsibility for the consequences of their sexual actions.

On July 3, 1989, in the case of *Webster v. Reproductive Health Services,* the Supreme Court rendered a decision that upheld a restrictive Missouri law that modified and narrowed women's rights to abortion as provided for by the *Roe v. Wade* decision in 1973. Based on the *Webster* case, individual states were given the right to enact laws that limit women's rights to abortion. Many state legislatures moved immediately to introduce legislation that limits who can seek legal abortions, sets time limits on abortion, and/or requires permission from parents or husbands. Most disturbing was the fact that the Supreme Court upheld as a permissible state value judgment the Missouri law's statement in its preamble that life begins at conception. This finding may be used by opponents of reproductive choice not only to make abortion illegal, but also to limit further contraceptive choices such as the intrauterine device (IUD) and open up the possibility of charging women with fetal neglect and abuse.

A 1991 Supreme Court decision further eroded women's rights to make informed reproductive decisions. Regulatory changes to Title X, the only federal program that specifically targets domestic family planning services, were developed by the Reagan administration in 1988. These regulations prohibited any family planning programs receiving Title X funds from providing counseling or referral for abortion (*Federal Register*, 1988).

Federal courts temporarily stopped the implementation of the new regulations. In May 1991, the Supreme Court decided in *Rust v. Sullivan* that the regulations were constitutional. Health care providers at family planning clinics were effectively barred from mentioning abortion, even if the pregnancy threatened a woman's health.

In 1992, the Bush administration loosened the regulations to exclude physicians from the ban. This step will have minimal impact because most family planning clinics are not staffed by physicians. These regulations victimize poor women who are the primary clients of government-funded health care programs. More affluent women who can afford private health care will be the only ones able to make informed decisions based on knowledge of all legally available options.

The growing body of Supreme Court decisions and government regulations have the effect of pitting the rights of the developing fetus against those of the pregnant woman. Abortion institutionalizes the dilemma of the conflicting rights of self and other. If a woman seeks an abortion for an unplanned, unwanted pregnancy, she is seen as putting her own needs and desires selfishly before those of the fetus and the biological father if he opposes the abortion. However, if a woman continues a pregnancy against her will because of coercion from others or self-abnegation, she is not only resigning and surrendering her body to the will of others, but also she is often faced with sole responsibility for the child's care after its birth.

Although abortion is one of the most frequently performed medical procedures in the United States, there has been little research done on the topic, primarily because of political pressures. In order for women to make knowledgeable decisions, valid, reliable information must be available to everyone. Systematically gathered data are also crucial for policy development.

In July 1987, President Reagan directed Surgeon General Koop to prepare a comprehensive report on the health effects of abortion on women. The contents of the report were not released, but Koop sent a letter to Reagan stating that "the scientific studies do not provide conclusive data about the health effects of abortion on women" (Measured Response, 1989). A House of Representatives subcommittee later conducted hearings into apparent discrepancies between the report and the information that had been made public (More on Koop's, 1990). Although the report and Koop's letter both concluded that the psychological effects of abortion are unclear, the report stated that abortion does not pose a physical risk to women. Data in the report indicated that "the risk of death from abortion . . . is less than the risk of death from an injection of penicillin" (p. 36) and that "infertility, miscarriage, low birth weight and other reproductive problems are no more frequent among women who experienced abortion than they are among the general population of women" (Measured Response, 1989, p. 37).

There is little evidence of psychological problems for women as the result of abortion. A panel convened by the American Psychological Association reviewed research on the psychological consequences of abortion. The panel's analysis indicated that women most frequently report feeling relief and happiness after first-trimester abortions (Adler et al., 1990). Women showed few signs of psychopathology after their abortions; the time of greatest distress was before the abortion.

Those who did experience negative responses after abortion tended to be women who wanted a pregnancy and were ambivalent about terminating it and women who were undergoing second-trimester abortions. Women who had negative feelings toward their partners, were making the decision alone, or whose parents opposed the abortion were more likely to experience greater distress. The degree of social support is the deciding factor in making a positive adjustment to an abortion (Zimmerman, 1989).

Some women may indeed experience guilt, regret, and other negative feelings, particularly if the abortion was not their choice, or if they are ambivalent about the decision. In discussing their reasons for having an abortion, 23% of the 1,900 women in one study on abortion indicated that their husbands or partners wanted them to have an abortion; 7% said that their parents wanted them to have an abortion (Torres & Forrest, 1988). Women may experience considerable pressure from parents or partners to seek an abortion that they themselves may not want to have.

Zabin, Hirsch, and Emerson (1989) investigated the effects of abortion on adolescents in one of the few studies that compared the effects of having an abortion with other fertility decisions. Zabin and her colleagues interviewed 360 young black women who came to a Maryland clinic for a pregnancy test. Baseline psychological data, as well as demographic and behavioral information, were collected during interviews with the young women before the results of the pregnancy tests were known. The study followed 334 teenagers—141 who terminated their pregnancies, 93 who carried them to term, and 92 who had negative pregnancy tests—for 2 years. The adolescents who chose abortion experienced no more stress or anxiety than did the teens in the other two groups and were no more likely to have psychological problems 2 years later. They were, however, subsequently more likely to use contraceptives and less likely to become pregnant again or drop out of school.

Who Has Abortions?

Information about who has abortions comes from the National Center for Health Statistics (Kochanek, 1991) and from the Alan Guttmacher Institute (Henshaw, Koonin, & Smith, 1991). The national abortion ratio in 1987 was 29 abortions per 100 pregnancies ending in birth or abortion; the ratio was highest for adolescents (42 per 100) and for women over age 40 (44 per 100) and lowest for women 30 to 34 (Henshaw et al., 1991).

One fourth of the abortions in 1988 were to women under age 20 and one third to those 20 to 24. Median age at abortion was about 24 years; the highest abortion rates were for the youngest and oldest women, with married women reporting lower rates than unmarried (Kochanek, 1991). In 1988, 21% of reported abortions were for currently married women. The mean age of these women was 28.1 years, about 5 years older than unmarried women having abortions.

The abortion rate tends to decrease with more years of schooling, but there tends to be a different pattern for women of different races. For white women, the highest abortion rate was for women with 12 years of education; the highest for black women was for those with 16 years of education (Kochanek, 1991). White teens experienced a slight reduction in abortion rates in 1987, but there was an increase in the abortion rate for black adolescents (Henshaw et al., 1991).

Women who report no religious preference have a higher abortion rate that those who have a religious affiliation (Henshaw & Silverman, 1988). Among women in Henshaw and Silverman's nationally representative sample of women having abortions in 1987, Catholic women were more likely than Protestant or Jewish women to terminate a pregnancy. Even though similar proportions of Protestants (88%) and Catholics (89%) report using a contraceptive method, Protestants use more effective methods, such as oral contraceptives and sterilization (Bachrach,

1984), and therefore are probably less likely to experience unplanned, unwanted pregnancies.

Most pregnancies are aborted during the first trimester. The median duration of pregnancy before abortion in 1988 was 9.3 weeks; only 11% of pregnancies terminated lasted longer than 12 weeks (Kochanek, 1991). Delayed terminations were more likely for younger, less educated, and black women. These women may have more difficulty finding the money to pay for an abortion and making arrangements to secure the abortion.

Why Women Have Abortions

Women seek abortions for a variety of reasons. A sample of 1,900 women gave an average of four factors that contributed to their decision to have an abortion (Torres & Forrest, 1988). More than three quarters of the women indicated that they were concerned about how a baby would change their life by interfering with their job, schooling, or responsibilities in caring for others. Sixty-eight percent said that they could not afford a baby at that time, and 51% were having problems with a relationship or were single.

When women indicated the most important reason why they had abortions, it was because they could not afford a child or because they were not ready for the responsibility. Other reasons that contributed to women's decisions to have abortions included being too young, not wanting others to know they were pregnant, having all the children desired, maternal or fetal health problems, parents or spouse wanting the abortion, and being the victim of rape or incest.

These data are important in contextualizing the results of public opinion polls since the *Webster* decision and many of the state laws that have been proposed to restrict women's access to abortion. In both cases, the tendency is to allow abortions in the event of fetal abnormalities, maternal health problems, rape, or incest. These were the primary reasons for abortion for only 7% of the women in Torres and Forrest's (1988) study. Under the more restrictive laws being proposed in many states, 93% of these women would be unable to secure a legal abortion.

Limiting women's access to abortion, or even making abortion illegal, will not stop women from terminating unwanted pregnancies. It will only make abortion less available and more dangerous, particularly for poor women who can least afford additional children. Before 1973 and the enactment of *Roe v. Wade*, there were probably 1 million abortions performed each year. If *Roe v. Wade* is overturned, the number of abortions will decrease, but they will not be eliminated, even in states that make abortion again illegal.

Even before the 1989 *Webster* decision, activists in the women's health movement began making plans for a nationwide underground network that would provide abortions to women in states where they may be limited or illegal. A spokeswoman for one feminist health center suggested, "This might be the time for women to reclaim this procedure and stop begging for abortion rights and just learn to do it ourselves" (McNamara, 1989a, p. 30).

There is precedent for women taking action when abortions are not available to those who need them. In 1969 a group of women in Chicago, collectively known as Jane, began making abortion referrals. In time they learned how to do abortions themselves and performed some 11,000 abortions over a 4-year period. According to an interview with a member of Jane, the group's goal was to make the alternative of terminating a pregnancy available to all women, not just the affluent (Addelson, 1986). The service operated on a sliding scale, and women who paid more helped to cover the cost for poorer women.

In addition to providing an important service to many women when abortion was illegal, Jane provided a model for women working together to empower themselves and other women. The member interviewed said that what Jane did was to try to show women that "they have the power to counsel and give a shot" and "have the power to change things and build alternatives" (Addelson, 1986, p. 303).

Although our position is that it will always be necessary to have safe, legal abortions available to women who experience unwanted pregnancies, lower abortion rates can be accomplished by ways other than outlawing abortions and making women and children suffer the consequences. Clearly, contraception is preferable to abortion. However, a recent survey of more than 10,000 women having abortions indicated that over half of the women were using a contraceptive at the time they conceived, 91% had practiced contraception at some time, and 70% had used a contraceptive method within the last 3 months (Henshaw & Silverman, 1988). Information is needed about why women who do not want to become pregnant stop using contraceptives. Effective contraceptive methods that women feel comfortable using and can integrate into their sexual lifestyle should be available.

Given the intense controversy surrounding abortion, it is reasonable to expect a significant push to develop new and safer contraceptive methods, but just the opposite is happening. Only one major pharmaceutical company in the United States is doing contraceptive research, and funding for the development of new contraceptive technology has not been a governmental priority. Low existing birthrates in the United States, the abortion controversy itself, and the costs and liabilities of contraceptive development and production have been cited as other reasons for the decreasing availability of contraceptive choices (Lincoln & Kaeser, 1988). Ironically, feminist opposition has also been given as a reason for contraceptive unavailability. Because women protested the use of potentially dangerous contraceptive methods and brought suit, for example, in the case of the Dalkon shield, pharmaceutical companies decided the liability involved with contraceptives was not worth the costs.

A new drug developed in France could radically change the abortion debate and give women even greater control over fertility decisions. RU-486, a drug that can be prescribed by a physician and taken in a woman's own home, can be more than 95% effective in inducing an abortion when taken within 49 days of a woman's last menstrual period and followed with a prostaglandin (Rosenfield, 1989). Abortion opponents have lobbied successfully to date to keep RU-486 from being introduced for review by the Food and Drug Administration. There is increasing interest and activity around bringing this drug to the United States. In July 1990, the American Medical Association took the position that testing of RU-486 should begin. On the grassroots level, the RU-486 Task Force has been formed in Santa Cruz, California, to educate people and generate support for the introduction of the drug into the United States.

Abortion Rights in 1992

The *Webster* decision freed states to introduce laws regulating the provision of abortion. By early 1992, more than half of all states had passed laws limiting women's access to abortion (NARAL, 1992). Louisiana, Utah, and the territory of Guam passed laws prohibiting virtually all abortions, but these laws were challenged and found unenforceable as long as *Roe v. Wade* prevails. Ten states require spousal consent or notice before a married woman can have an abortion. Twenty-five states have informed-consent laws requiring that women be given material that might dissuade them from abortion. Thirty-three states passed laws that prevent minors from obtaining an abortion without parental consent or notice.

In 1992, the Supreme Court further extended the right of states to restrict abortion. On June 29, 1992, the Supreme Court decided the Pennsylvania case *Planned Parenthood v. Casey* by voting 5 to 4 to maintain a woman's constitutional right to terminate a pregnancy prior to viability, but gave states broad new powers to impose restrictions. The Court decided that the states could pass restrictions as long as they did not impose "undue burden" on women seeking abortion.

The ruling in the Pennsylvania case upheld the provisions of the law that required (1) doctors to keep records on the abortions that they perform, (2) counseling for women on alternatives to abortion, (3) a 24-hour waiting period after counseling before abortion, and (4) parental or judicial consent for unmarried women under age 18 to have an abortion. The only provision of the law that was not upheld was a requirement that a woman inform her husband before having an abortion. This was defined as an undue burden on a woman.

Both the U.S. Senate and the House of Representatives began formulating versions of a Freedom of Choice Act that would codify the provisions of *Roe v. Wade* and prevent states from restricting abortions until fetal viability. The version of the act prepared by the Senate after the *Casey* decision, however, did not prohibit states passing laws (1) requiring parental involvement in a minor's decision, (2) banning public funding for abortion, or (3) protecting doctors from being forced to perform abortions (Neuffer, 1992).

SEXUAL ORIENTATION AND REPRODUCTIVE DECISIONS

Lesbians face additional obstacles in exercising their right to reproductive control. Lesbians and their families can be caught between two worlds: the lesbian community of which they are a part, and the predominantly heterosexual world that they will contact in raising children (Crawford, 1987; Hall, 1978). Lesbians must deal with internal and external homophobic reactions to their desire to parent. Lesbian parents of color must deal with racism as well (Hill, 1987; Morales, 1990).

Conceptualizations about ethnic and racial diversity within families include the culturally deviant, equivalent, and variant (Allen, 1978). Allen's scheme is applicable to cultural views about lesbian parenting. In comparison to parenting within a heterosexual context, views about lesbian parenting range from deviant to equivalent to variant.

The deviant approach is in direct contradiction to the ideology of compulsive motherhood. Lesbians are subjected to the contradictory expectation of compulsory childlessness (Crawford, 1987). Even if being a lesbian is tolerated, a new set of issues arises if a woman wants to have children. A deviant view suggests that what is considered natural for women who are heterosexual is considered unnatural for lesbians.

Lesbians must deal with the beliefs of some members of society that lesbian families are not a real family, and that children must be protected from this lifestyle (Crawford, 1987). Lesbians are expected to answer questions about why they want to parent and how they will do it, questions that are rarely, if ever, asked of heterosexual women and their male partners who choose to become parents (Pies, 1990).

Another problematic conceptualization is the culturally equivalent approach, which suggests that lesbians and their families are no different than any other type of family. Although well-meaning, the equivalent approach ignores and fails to understand the unique stresses, problems, and strengths with which lesbians cope in a homophobic world (Crawford, 1987). The equivalent approach asks lesbians to pretend that they are not lesbian. Certainly, lesbians share some realities with all other women, yet homophobia is a unique experience for them:

> Sameness offers one invisibility, it is true. It levels out differences and denies who one really is. It would deny the stigma and the history of oppression against gays. Likewise, it would deny consideration of lesbians as a discrete population. Different, they are, and precisely because of that stigma and minority status. To deny stigma is to close one's eyes to the lack of rights accorded lesbians, foremost among which is the right to be different. Those who say, "It makes no difference who you sleep with" trivialize lesbianism, reducing it to mere sexuality. (Maggiore, 1988, p. 45)

A third perspective on lesbian parenting is the culturally variant approach. This point of view suggests that in many ways lesbians are like other women and parents, yet, in other important ways, they differ. The dilemma posed by the contradictory messages of compulsory motherhood and compulsory childlessness is a case in point. The variant approach makes understandable this dialectic between two contradictory norms for lesbians who wish to be mothers.

Legal Issues Facing Lesbian Mothers

The Harvard Law Review Association (1990) reported that about "three million gay men and lesbians in the United States are parents, and between eight and ten million children are raised in gay or lesbian households" (p. 119). One fifth of lesbians have children (Bell & Weinberg, 1978). New means to becoming a parent as well as the desire and choice to do so are increasingly available to lesbians (Money, 1988) yet, lesbians and gay men are inhibited in their desire to procreate by legal barriers:

> First, lesbians and gay men may be denied access to necessary reproductive techniques such as artificial insemination, in vitro fertilization, or surrogate motherhood. Second, once they have children, gay and lesbian parents face further problems in defining the legal relationships both between the child and the second biological parent, and between the child and the "co-parent"—the nonbiological parent in a same-sex couple. (Harvard Law Review Association, 1990, p. 139)

Most lesbians can become pregnant at home through sexual intercourse or alternative insemination, a process where "semen is introduced into a woman's uterus or vagina by means other than sexual intercourse" (Harvard Law Review Association, 1990, p. 139). Insemination can be done by a woman herself with a needleless syringe or eyedropper. Some states have statutes that can be interpreted as prohibiting the alternative insemination of unmarried women, but these techniques are not easily prevented. By contrast, physician-performed alternative insemination is more problematic legally because of the parental rights of the donor.

The editors of the *Harvard Law Review* (1990) strongly recommend that "statutes that prohibit the artificial insemination of or fornication by unmarried women should be invalidated as an unconstitutional restriction of the right to procreate" (p. 140). These prohibitive laws are based on the belief that children fare better in "traditional" two-parent households, thereby discouraging single-parent families and encouraging marriage. Current realities, however, belie the belief reflected in antifornication and insemination statutes: "It is overinclusive in that many children conceived by unmarried women will be raised by two adults; it is underinclusive since many children born to married women are raised by only one parent" (p. 141). As Blumstein and Schwartz (1983) found, about 50% of first marriages between heterosexuals are likely to end in divorce, and the more children a woman has, the less likely she is to remarry.

The second legal issue affecting lesbian parenting choices regards the rights of the donor and the rights of the nonbiological coparent. The natural mother of a child is a legal parent, unless the child is adopted. Beyond this relationship, legal parenthood depends on a variety of circumstances. If the mother is unmarried and the child has been conceived through sexual intercourse, the natural father is considered the child's other legal parent. However, if the child is conceived through alternative insemination, paternity depends on whether the state has a law regulating insemination of unmarried women:

> Of the twenty-eight states with artificial insemination statutes, only seven have statutes that facially apply to the paternity of an unmarried woman's child. In five [California, Colorado, New Jersey, Washington, Wyoming] of these states, a donor of semen for physician-performed insemination will not be the legal father, but these statutes do not cover at-home inseminations. The other two states [Oregon, Texas] eliminate donor paternity regardless of a physician's participation. (Harvard Law Review Association, 1990, pp. 142–143)

The nonbiological coparent in a same-sex couple does not have legal protection. If the biological parent dies, the surviving coparent could "lose custody to either the child's other biological parent or other relatives of the child" (Harvard Law Review Association, 1990, p. 145). Several avenues have been used to avoid loss of custody. First, in three states (California, Alaska, North Dakota), coparent adoptions have been permitted by the courts. Like a stepparent adoption, coparent adoption allows the same-sex partner to adopt the child without affecting the other parent's rights. Although at this time a rare occurrence in most states, the editors of the *Harvard Law Review* argue that it is in the best interests of children raised in lesbian or gay households to be adopted by the coparent. Adoption gives children the additional security of having two legal parents who are willing to assume responsibility for them.

A strategy available when coadoption is not permitted is for the biological parent to nominate the coparent in his or her will "to be the testamentary guardian of the child" (Harvard Law Review Association, 1990, p. 148). A third strategy is for the coparent to argue that he or she is a psychological parent of the child and thus entitled to custody or visitation rights if the legal parent dies or the couple separates. The psychological parent theory has held in cases involving heterosexual parents; although not yet tried for homosexual parents, it is equally applicable.

A significant number of children are raised in lesbian households, yet laws do not formally or automatically establish their ties to the parents who care for them. Sexual orientation alone is irrelevant to parenting ability, and states should ensure continuity of care for all children rather than "promoting prejudice by basing decisions on false stereotypes or perceived community intolerance" (Harvard Law Review Association, 1990, p. 150).

Drawing up a legal document that spells out the exact nature of the parenting relationships and agreements for the biological mother, coparent, and donor is imperative (Pies, 1990). The best defense against going to court is to deal with these issues among partners and parents outside the courtroom. Most of the cases that go to court usually involve situations in which no contract existed beforehand (Pies, 1990). Bias against lesbian parenting and the cultural tradition that a child has only one mother are likely to affect judges and lawyers; a contract offers a safety net for these uncharted waters.

Pathways to Lesbian Parenting

There are many ways lesbians become parents. Lesbian motherhood may result from a previous heterosexual relationship or marriage (DiLapi, 1989). Many women do not realize they are lesbians until after they have children. Their unions with other women usually involve a stepparenting or coparenting arrangement.

Other lesbians have children in less traditional ways. Becoming a parent after a woman has acknowledged she is a lesbian involves much preparation and forethought. Unlike heterosexual couples, lesbian couples rarely find themselves pregnant and then have to decide what to do next (Pies, 1990).

Having a child requires that lesbians deal with a number of practical, financial, emotional, and ethical issues (Pies, 1990; Wismont & Reame, 1989). Decisions include whether to get pregnant deliberately with a male friend or to use alternative insemination (Hill, 1987; Pies, 1990). If alternative insemination is used, choices must be made about "whether to have a known or an unknown donor, whether to have the donor involved in the parenting, whether to use fresh or frozen semen" (Pies, 1990, p. 147).

On the one hand, choosing an unknown donor has several benefits. Legal battles with a child's father can be avoided, and parenting will be shared only by the lesbian couple. On the other hand, the costs of using an unknown donor include possible illnesses inherited from the donor and a child's strong desire to know about his or her paternity. If a sperm bank or private clinician is used, some background information about the donor may be known (Pies, 1990). However, many health care providers will not inseminate unmarried women, much less lesbians (Hanscombe & Forster, 1982, p. 17). Therefore, many lesbians have turned to men they know.

Choosing a known donor is a practice that has increased in recent years (Pies, 1990). Options include using the semen of a brother of the woman who is not going to be pregnant; then, both women in a lesbian relationship have a biological tie to their child. Close male friends who plan to participate in the life of the child are also involved as donors. Before the AIDS epidemic, Pies (1990) found that lesbians preferred gay men as their donors. Now that AIDS is so prevalent within the gay male community, decisions about donors must be considered carefully to prevent the risk of HIV disease (Hanscombe & Forster, 1982; Pies, 1990). Clearly, not all gay men are infected with HIV, but "this epidemic has had a profound effect on the course of the lesbian and gay parenting movement" (Pies, 1990, p. 149).

Not all pathways to lesbian parenting involve conception. Although adoption is less preferred to becoming pregnant as a pathway to parenthood (Hill, 1987), many lesbians do adopt children or become foster parents. Adoption may be chosen because a lesbian herself was adopted and wants to give in kind to another child. Some lesbian couples cannot conceive, so adoption is an alternative for them. Still others prefer adoption to having a biological child who might bring an imbalance to a couple relationship. Adopting a child may ensure a more equal relationship for the comothers with their child (Pies, 1990).

Lesbians considering adoption must decide how much of their intimate lives to disclose to agencies. Should both partners in a lesbian couple apply, or should they attempt to adopt a child through one woman only, as a single-parent adoption (Pies, 1990)? Given the volatile nature of the issue of homosexuality and children and the widespread homophobia in the child-welfare system, it is difficult for openly gay or lesbian parents to get fair treatment (Ricketts & Achtenberg, 1990). Yet, it is important for gay and lesbian parents to be open about their orientation if only to counter the myths and harmful stereotypes about them.

Foster care provides a temporary home for a child until the child can be adopted or returned to biological parents (Harvard Law Review Association, 1990). Foster parenting has always been an invisible way in which lesbians have raised children (Ricketts & Achtenberg, 1990, p. 84). Restrictions on placing children in foster care with lesbians have not occurred typically, unless the homosexuality of the parents is known. Only New Hampshire and Massachusetts have statutes prohibiting the placement of foster children in the homes of homosexuals (Harvard Law Review Association, 1990). Sexual orientation is irrelevant to provision of child care; it runs counter to children's welfare to deny them access to an acceptable, stable home (Harvard Law Review Association, 1990).

One way in which states and child-welfare agencies are including gay and lesbian parents in foster care and adoption is with hard-to-place children, those who are older, nonwhite, disabled, or emotionally disturbed (Harvard Law Review Association, 1990). There is a shortage of heterosexual couples willing to care for or adopt these children, and a permanent home is critical for their development.

Another situation involves foster care of gay and lesbian youth. Courts and agencies now recognize the benefits to the children, to the parents, and to society of placing children where they will be loved and understood. Gay and lesbian youth are frequently victims of physical and emotional violence in their own families when they reveal their sexual orientation (Ricketts & Achtenberg, 1990). Often they are turned out of their homes with no place to go. Ricketts and Achtenberg (1990) report estimates from the child-welfare system that between 30 and 70% of the juvenile prostitute, street, and runaway population are lesbian or gay adolescents. They are also prevalent within the suicide-prevention network. The effects of trauma they experience in homophobic, heterosexist homes is incalculable (Ricketts & Achtenberg, 1990). Still, some homophobia continues to underlie agencies' willingness to place these adolescents with gay and lesbian parents. Such parents may be considered a last resort, only for older and "confirmed" lesbian and gay adolescents (Ricketts & Achtenberg, 1990). Institutionalized homophobia is the problem, not the suitability of lesbians and gay men as parents.

Finally, there are special problems and potentials faced by a lesbian who becomes the nonbiological coparent of her partner's biological child. Couples must make decisions about who will carry the child they plan to raise together. They must find creative solutions to the nonbiological coparent's lack of legal protection, as well as the child's lack of protection in that he or she probably cannot be adopted by the other mother. Lesbian couples must consider a host of other issues that are romanticized for heterosexual mothers and even biological lesbian mothers. Nevertheless, the lack of societal rewards and the need to carve a meaningful role and a connection with a child attest to the resilience and the intense connection that some lesbians establish with children they parent but have not borne. The prototype of the chosen family of lesbians is the coparent–child relationship.

THE NEW REPRODUCTIVE TECHNOLOGIES

The incidence of infertility among young women is increasing. Because the ability to conceive and bear a child is closely tied to societal perceptions of full womanhood and most women desire to have children, infertility is defined as a problem. A variety of factors, some treatable and some not, may cause infertility in women. Among these are failure to ovulate, blockage of the fallopian tubes, defects in reproductive organs, hormonal imbalances, diseases, or malnutrition. Male factors such as sperm number and motility are implicated in 40–50% of fertility cases in heterosexual couples (Crooks & Baur, 1990).

In response to the problem of infertility, reproductive technologies continue to be developed to assist conception. The growth of reproductive technologies presents a dilemma for society in general and for feminists in particular. The development and use of reproductive technologies, although they may help those who are infertile to conceive and have a child of "their own," have raised unprecedented social, legal, and ethical issues. Processes such as in vitro fertilization, the freezing of embryos, and surrogate mothering are techniques that are revolutionizing the reproductive process, but minimizing women's roles in, and control over, the act of conception and the process of pregnancy.

Women are at risk for exploitation as the result of these technological innovations. Although it is men who control the technology and contract for the surrogates, it is women whose bodies are manipulated, monitored, and experimented upon. The concern is that

through these technologies men will intensify and consolidate their control over the reproductive process, and that women will become reduced
to their reproductive functions as egg providers and gestation vessels
(Corea, 1985; Rothman, 1989; Tong, 1989).

In Vitro Fertilization

One of the more frequently used reproductive technologies is in vitro
fertilization (IVF). In this procedure, a woman's ovaries are hyperstimu-
lated with fertility drugs to produce a number of ova. The ova are
retrieved surgically, fertilized in a petri dish, and the resulting embryos are
placed in the woman's uterus. In a slight variation on the procedure,
called "gamete intrafallopian transfer" (GIFT), the ova are mixed with
sperm and placed in the fallopian tubes.

Although it is possible that women will conceive through one of
these procedures, many risks are involved, and clinics have resisted
providing the information women need to make informed decisions. As a
result of growing concern about exploitation of infertile couples, the U.S.
House of Representatives Committee on Small Business held hearings
and gathered data on consumer protection issues in the IVF industry. The
data released indicated that 2,463 live births had occurred as the result of
26,332 IVF attempts—a success rate of about 9% per stimulation cycle
(Committee on Small Business, 1989). The success rate for the GIFT
procedure may be higher, about 20%, probably because it is used with less
severe infertility problems (Diamant, 1989).

This low success rate is costly to women and their partners. The
financial cost of the procedures usually ranges from $4,000 to $7,000 per
attempt. Women are at physical risk for complications and side effects
from taking fertility drugs and the procedures related to IVF. There are
also high emotional costs as women become invested in the procedure.
Many women have to take off work for hospital visits; some put their
careers on hold or quit work (Diamant, 1989).

One dilemma associated with IVF is that because several embryos are
usually transferred to the woman's uterus to enhance the likelihood of
implantation, multiple pregnancies are frequent. The woman and her
partner either must be willing to rear twins, triplets, or quadruplets or
make the decision to use a selective abortion procedure that is done in
utero, usually prior to the third month of pregnancy (Sher, Marriage, &
Stoess, 1988).

Access to reproductive technologies such as in vitro fertilization may
be limited in a number of ways. The financial costs are often prohibitive,
although several states require insurance companies to cover the expense
of infertility treatment. In addition, most programs do IVF only with

married couples, thereby limiting access for single women or lesbian couples (Rowland, 1987).

Surrogacy

There are several variations of surrogate mothering. A woman may be inseminated with the sperm of a man who will be the biological and legal father of the resulting child. In another situation, a woman may have implanted in her uterus an embryo conceived through in vitro fertilization using the sperm and ovum of another couple who are contracting with her for the resulting child. In either case, the surrogate carries the child to term and surrenders it in return for a certain sum of money.

The most immediate concerns in surrogacy situations involve the often conflicting rights of the individuals involved. Most feminists believe that surrogacy promotes the exploitation of women—physically, emotionally, and economically (Corea, 1985; Rothman, 1989; Rowland, 1987). Surrogacy has generated some of the most controversial and publicized ethical dilemmas associated with reproductive technologies. The outcomes of the Whitehead–Stern case involving "Baby M" in 1988 and the more recent Johnson–Calvert case in 1990 exemplify the problems associated with surrogacy and the ease with which women can become mere vessels for the gestation of children for others.

In the Baby M case, Mary Beth Whitehead was paid $10,000 to be inseminated with the sperm of William Stern. She carried the child to term and then changed her mind about relinquishing the child after it was born. After an extended custody battle, the surrogacy contract was ruled invalid, the child was placed in Stern's legal custody, and Whitehead was awarded visitation rights. The New Jersey Supreme Court ruled that paying a woman to have a baby amounted to baby selling and outlawed such contracts. In its ruling, the court found the payment of money to a surrogate mother illegal, perhaps criminal, and potentially degrading to women (Associated Press, 1988). Paradoxically, the child was removed from its birth mother and placed with the biological father.

Although many states rushed to introduce legislation to control surrogacy after the Whitehead–Stern case, the business of surrogacy contracting continues. In October 1990, a California judge issued a ruling in a surrogacy case involving Anna Johnson and Mark and Crispina Calvert. The Calverts had donated the sperm and ovum that resulted in the embryo that was implanted in Johnson. In return for $10,000, Johnson carried the pregnancy to term and was to relinquish the baby to the Calverts. After the birth, Johnson changed her mind and a custody battle ensued. The judge hearing the case ruled that Johnson had no parental rights to the child and that the Calverts would have permanent

custody of the child unless the decision is overturned by a higher court
(Peterson & Kelleher, 1990). This was the first court ruling in a surrogacy
case in which the birth mother was not the genetic mother. This decision
sends the message that women's bodies *can* be used in the service of those
more affluent.

Issues evolving from reproductive technologies, particularly surrogacy, have divided feminists. Although some maintain a woman's right
to control her body, even to the extent of serving as a contracted
surrogate, most feminists are strongly opposed to reproductive technologies because of the great potential for the exploitation of women, for the
commodification of women and children, for the increasing medicaliza-
tion of birth, and men's domination of the processes involved (Corea,
1985; Rothman, 1989; Rowland, 1987; Spallone & Steinberg, 1987).

For some feminists, the dilemma in not completely opposing reproductive technologies is that one of the touchstones of feminism is the
belief that women should have complete control over their own bodies.
Women should have the right to use their bodies in the way they choose,
including making money with them and their products, if they so desire.
This position acknowledges women's right to enter into surrogacy contracts, to consent to any medical procedures, and to sell their eggs or
embryos as men have sold their sperm in the past. Prohibiting women
from participating in reproductive technologies "for their own good"
demeans women and treats them as less than rational adults.

Rothman (1989) counters this argument, however, noting that defending women's rights to be exploited and demeaned is like defending
blacks' rights to sell themselves back into slavery if they want. Taking a
more sociocultural approach to the issue, she asks what kinds of alternatives people face that make such choices seem rational. Would reproductive technologies that require manipulation of women's hormonal
systems, voluntary surgical procedures, great financial expense, and often
psychological and relationship distress be seen as rational choices in a
society in which motherhood was an option for women rather than the
marker of full womanhood? Would the donation of eggs or embryos for
$250 or the voluntary release at birth of a child in return for $10,000 be
seen as rational choices in a society in which women did not live in
poverty with unequal access to the resources that would allow them to
have and support the number of children they wanted to mother?

MEN'S ROLES IN REPRODUCTIVE DECISIONS

Risking alpha bias (the exaggeration of difference), we take the position
that sociohistorical forces in the United States, as well as biological

necessity, have resulted in gendered reproductive consciousness. Men and women think about and experience reproduction in different ways. Women's reproductive consciousness is continuous and integrative (O'Brien, 1981b). As the result of the experience of pregnancy and the labor of delivery, women have a clearer understanding of their relationship to their children and a consciousness of species continuity that men will never experience. O'Brien characterizes the male reproductive consciousness as splintered and discontinuous because men are "separated" from all parts of the reproductive process except copulation. Paternity is based on a proprietary right to a child rather than on a natural relationship. It is only through a relationship of trust with the mother of the child and/or by an exclusion of all other possible fathers that a man can claim the right to a particular child.

Traditionally, men have enjoyed the rights of parenthood without assuming many of the responsibilities. Men have chosen the extent to which they actively parent. The concept "fathering a child" still is more likely to bring to mind procreative rather than nurturant aspects of parenting. There is a growing expectation that men take equal contraceptive responsibility in heterosexual relationships; that fathers be involved, active, loving parents; and, in the event of divorce or separation, that men maintain financial, emotional, and physical coresponsibility for their children. This expectation raises the dialectical tension between rights and responsibility regarding children.

Women, increasingly, are taking the position that men who want to have the rights to their children also need to take responsibility. A number of feminists have called for men to "prove their paternity" by becoming actively involved in coparenting, coming together with women in an experience that is freely chosen by both partners (O'Brien, 1981a; Rothman, 1989).

However, many women have a thinly veiled concern that, until there is gender equality on a societal basis, there may be significant risk in relinquishing any reproductive control to men or giving men more power by increasing their parenting roles. Among these concerns is the fear that if men get involved, they will take over, and that men may use these roles to further their own interests and manipulate mothers (Rowland, 1987).

As they assume responsibility, men expect to increase their rights regarding reproductive decisions and childbearing experiences. Should men have the right to veto a woman's abortion, have parental rights in artificial insemination cases, or control women's reproductive choices in other ways? To date, women have maintained the right to make the final choice, but is this position maintainable in light of a conservative Supreme Court and a growing contingent of men calling for equal rights to their children? What price might women be required to pay in terms of control over reproductive choice in return for men's acceptance of equal responsibility for children and child care?

How do we determine a man's right to a particular child? Under existing laws, a man is the father if he contributes the sperm from which the child was conceived, unless, by virtue of marriage, the child's mother "belongs" to another man. The child then also "belongs" to that legal husband. If a child belongs to a man in this sense, does that imply that the man has a right, from conception, to participate in decisions about that child?

Among the most controversial examples of conflicting rights to a particular child are those in which a woman wants to have an abortion and her partner, the biological father, wants the fetus to be carried to term. Several highly publicized cases have reached the highest courts in the United States and Canada. In each case, lower courts had issued injunctions to keep women from having abortions after their partners had petitioned the court. In a 1988 Michigan case, Shawn Lewis was barred from having an abortion by a judge who ruled that because she was in the midst of a divorce, she no longer had the right to seek an abortion (Smith, 1988). The judge indicated that the fetus needed to be protected like any child involved in a custody battle. This perspective elevates the rights of the fetus and the father above the rights of the mother to have control over her own body. Lewis was told that if she had an abortion anyway, she could be fined, jailed, and possibly lose custody of her son. The decision was overturned by an appeals court. The U.S. Supreme Court, after hearing the case, decided without comment that Lewis could not stop his estranged wife from exercising her constitutional right to terminate her pregnancy.

In another case, a Quebec court ordered Chantal Daigle not to seek an abortion after a petition by Jean-Guy Tremblay, the man with whom she had been living and decided not to marry. Ironically, Tremblay indicated through his attorney that he had planned to "allow" Daigle to raise the child, but had changed his mind and would take care of the baby himself (Palmer, 1989). The indication was not that Tremblay wanted to parent the child, but rather that he wanted to control Daigle's reproductive decisions.

Antiabortion groups have taken an interest in cases dealing with the rights of prospective fathers and supported the men financially and politically in an attempt to further the cause of outlawing abortion (McDonnell, 1984). The involvement of antiabortion groups confuses the issue, making it unclear in which cases the fathers are expressing serious desire to have and care for the children, in which cases they merely seek revenge against the women, and in which cases the men themselves are being exploited by those using the situation to further their own political agenda.

McDonnell (1984) asks, "How can we create a greater space, a more substantive role in abortion decisions for men without surrendering our legitimate right to control our own bodies?" (p. 64). She suggests that women allow the expression of men's feelings about the abortion. Services should be made available to address men's needs regarding the abortion, and men should be involved as much as possible during the abortion process. In this way, men are more likely to be a source of emotional support for women as they make the often agonizing decision to terminate the pregnancy. This approach assumes that the men involved are sensitive to the needs of the women and are willing to accede to the women's decision. If men take seriously their participation in the decision-making process, it is difficult to believe that they would be satisfied playing a role with no power to determine the final outcome.

There can be no single prescription for involving men in fertility decisions. If men have participated in the process by talking about fertility preferences before having sexual intercourse, have shared responsibility for contraception, and have communicated their position in the case of unplanned pregnancy, women may feel more comfortable in expanding the role men may play in other reproductive decisions. Our position is that men should be women's allies in the project of ensuring that their sexuality can be experienced and fully enjoyed without the risk of unplanned and unwanted pregancy. Every child should be a wanted child.

FETAL PROTECTION POLICIES

Another contemporary reproductive issue for women is the growing interest in monitoring their reproductive health and behavior during pregnancy. Women are being charged with child abuse and neglect and losing custody of their newborns if they participate in activities that endanger the fetus during pregnancy. Nineteen states now have laws making it possible to charge with child abuse any woman who gives birth to a child with illegal drugs in her or his bloodstream (Willwerth, 1991). The National Organization of Women's Legal Defense and Education Fund (NOW LDEF, 1990) completed a state-by-state summary of criminal prosecutions against pregnant women. At least 17 states have brought charges against pregnant women, usually for drug or alcohol use during pregnancy. The first woman to be charged under these laws, Jennifer Johnson from Florida, was sentenced to mandatory drug treatment and 15 years of probation (Willwerth, 1991). Other approaches to controlling addicted women's fertility have been suggested. A representative in the Kansas legislature introduced a bill that would give convicted female addicts the option of having a Norplant implant or going to jail. The Norplant implant is a recently approved contraceptive device that is implanted in the upper arm and is effective for 5 years or until removal. Paradoxically, there has been no action to increase the availability of drug treatment programs.

Economic deprivation and racial discrimination provide the context for maternal and infant addiction problems (Berrien, 1990). The impact of fetal protection policies falls most heavily upon poor women and women of color, who are disproportionately dependent on government-financed health care. More affluent women under the care of private physicians are less likely to be monitored or tested.

There are well-documented risks to the developing fetus if the mother ingests alcohol or other drugs during the pregnancy. However, the appropriate response to such a situation is not as clear because in order to protect the fetus, the activities of the mother must be constrained in some way. Again, the rights of the fetus are pitted against the rights of the woman carrying the fetus. There is growing concern about the "slippery slope" phenomenon. Now the attention of those policing pregnancies are focusing on drug and alcohol use. In the future, criminal charges may be brought against any woman who disobeys her doctor's orders by drinking, smoking, getting too much or too little exercise, not having prescribed tests done, and so on (NOW LDEF, 1990).

The dilemma is to ensure the health of newborns without treating women as though they are only the vessels within which fetuses gestate. The concept of fetal protection extends the antiabortion agenda to elevate the status of the fetus and to treat the woman as having only contingent value (Pollitt, 1990). Women are viewed with suspicion and portrayed as selfish, potentially violent, and incapable of making responsible choices.

Policing and criminalizing women's behavior during pregnancy has paradoxical effects. Monitoring women's pregnancies in this way undermines their relationships to care providers and destroys confidentiality (Berrien, 1990). Punitive tactics discourage women from getting prenatal care and increase the likelihood that women will seek late abortions rather than face criminal charges (McNamara, 1989b; Pollitt, 1990; Willwerth, 1991).

Punishing pregnant women by sending them to jail where prenatal care is inadequate or placing their children in foster homes is likely to have equally negative effects on the children. The most successful programs for addicted mothers provide comprehensive services that begin with detoxification and include pediatric services, psychological and job counseling for the mother, and parenting classes (Willwerth, 1991). The surest way to help a developing fetus is to help the woman carrying the fetus. By providing access to supportive prenatal care and drug treatment programs, the risk to a fetus can be reduced without invading a woman's right to privacy and control over her own body. However, the average waiting period for most drug treatment programs is 6 months to a year, and most do not accept pregnant women (NOW LDEF, 1990). A recent survey in New York City revealed that of the 78 treatment programs, 54% did not treat pregnant women, and 87% did not accept pregnant women on Medicaid who were addicted to crack cocaine (McNamara, 1989b).

Monitoring pregnant women for drug and alcohol use easily could be extended to include women who are HIV positive. Laws and pending bills in 14 states that criminalize the willful transmission of HIV could provide a vehicle for charging infected women with intentional homicide or child abuse if the virus was transmitted to their fetuses (Amaro, 1990). Routine counseling and testing of pregnant women may be important strategies for preventing pediatric AIDS, but they also invade women's privacy and put them at risk for biased treatment.

Infected women face a dilemma regarding abortion. Some women may be coerced into having an abortion to prevent the possibility of bearing an infected child. Restrictions on discussing abortion as an option have not been placed on federally funded AIDS projects as they have been on family planning programs (Amaro, 1990). However, if an HIV-positive woman *did* want to get an abortion, she might have great difficulty finding a provider; more than one fourth of abortion providers in the United States will not serve women who test positive for HIV (Henshaw, 1991).

A FEMINIST VISION OF WOMEN'S REPRODUCTIVE FREEDOM

Reproductive decisions are central to the lives of all women. Reproductive control is essential to women's ability to pursue educational and occupational opportunities that will make gender equality possible. The right to safe, legal abortions is only one aspect of a comprehensive approach to ensuring reproductive control. Women also need to have access to information and resources that will allow them to make knowledgeable reproductive decisions and to act confidently on those decisions. Thus, education about reproductive issues, a range of effective contraceptive techniques, and high-quality health care should be available to all women.

Required, comprehensive sexuality education in the public schools would provide an informational foundation for both females and males. By high school, every individual could be encouraged to formulate an individual reproductive health plan. Such a plan would be a heuristic device to guide an explicit, proactive consideration of the various reproductive decisions one might face. In addition to providing accurate information about reproductive anatomy and physiology, sexuality education and related courses could provide knowledge about preventing sexually transmitted diseases, choosing and effectively using contraceptives, and understanding pregnancy and childbirth. Opportunities also could be provided to explore decisions about having or not having children and the costs and benefits of various timing options.

Because there will always be unplanned, unwanted pregnancies, the availability of legal abortion is necessary. The number of abortions in the United States could be reduced, however, if adequate funds and research attention were devoted to developing new contraceptives for both women and men. Tax incentives could be provided to pharmaceutical companies to do this work.

Whenever private enterprise becomes involved with reproductive issues, there is the potential for exploitation of women. The commercial developers of reproductive technologies taught us this lesson. To prevent exploitation, women must be involved in planning, developing, testing, and overseeing reproductive technologies of all kinds. Women will be unable to control their reproduction unless they participate in the means of controlling reproduction: the research, the medical and contraceptive industries, education, and the law (Moen, 1979).

We believe that every woman should have the right to make the decision about having or not having a child. We are reluctant, therefore, to advocate banning reproductive techniques such as in vitro fertilization, GIFT, or surrogacy. Given women's active involvement in all aspects of reproductive technologies, including ethical and legal decisions, such techniques offer new options for women and their partners who may otherwise be unable to have children.

In this chapter, we have explored some of the contemporary issues relevant to women's childbearing experiences. Our goal has been to deconstruct compulsory motherhood as a monolithic concept and to begin the reconstruction of mothering as one choice of the many available. We have attempted to reveal some of the invisible aspects of reproductive decisions and provide information that allows a more comprehensive understanding of the dialectical nature of motherhood.

Each day women make complicated reproductive decisions—
sometimes with the support of a partner, sometimes in opposition to a
partner, and sometimes alone. Our feminist agenda strives to help women
become proactive regarding reproductive issues. Although we must continue to advocate for societal support, we cannot wait to act. Women can
take action to limit the likelihood that their ability to control their
reproductive lives are jeopardized. If women are to have the benefit of
separating the sexual and reproductive aspects of their lives, they must
make active decisions, rather than having outcomes determined by default. Therefore, each woman needs to have a working knowledge of the
reproductive process, understand the relative effectiveness of different
contraceptive methods, have confidence in her own fertility values and
preferences, and have the skills necessary to clearly communicate her
position to her partner(s) and negotiate effectively.

All of this sounds very idealistic in an era when most people have
not had any formal sexuality education, explicit discussion of sexual issues
is considered controversial, and discussing intercourse before participating in it is viewed as unromantic. Women can take the initiative to
empower themselves, other women, and their children to be more assertive regarding their reproductive lives. One of the most effective ways of
doing this is by breaking the silence about sexuality and conception that
isolates women from others and their experiences.

Women and Caregiving

Caregiving is an activity that is both tension filled and pleasure giving for most women. A postmodern feminist analysis of caregiving as a gendered activity deconstructs this aspect of women's experience as a "natural" manifestation of being female. A dialectical perspective invites examination of the contradictions within women's "labours of love" (Finch & Groves, 1983). In this chapter, we consider essentialist and socially constructed arguments surrounding the culture and the conduct of caregiving (Dressel & Clark, 1990).

The everyday usage of the concept "caregiving" implies the work involved in meeting the physical and emotional needs of others and being responsible for nurturing their growth and development. According to Noddings (1984), caring presupposes maintenance of the self and clear self-knowledge. Reflective caring involves perceiving the needs of another and using one's energy to meet those needs, just as one would if acting on one's own behalf. Caring is a social relationship that must be considered in the context of the political realities, material conditions, and social structures of the world (Hoaglund, 1991).

Some accounts of women's relationship to caregiving are prone to alpha bias, in which differences between men and women are exaggerated and commonalities ignored (Hare-Mustin & Marecek, 1990). These approaches begin with a maximalist, or "difference," position, proposing that women do the bulk of caregiving because it is their nature to do so. Women's responsibility for the overt and hidden caregiving activities in society, such as housework, teaching, nursing, childcare, and parent care, are attributed to the perception that they are more nurturant than men. The difference perspective emphasizes that women are more invested in their relationships because they have a greater need for connectedness.

Conversely, other perspectives of caregiving are characterized by beta bias, in which important differences in the experiences of women

and men are minimized (Hare-Mustin & Marecek, 1990). Consistent
with the minimalist position is the idea that caregiving is gendered only
in terms of socialized behaviors. Risman (1989) found, for example, that
when men are responsible for children, they function just like mothers by
providing the same kinds of instrumental (e.g., housekeeping) and expressive (e.g., sharing feelings) tasks of childrearing. When professionally
employed mothers leave their children with paid caregivers, they are just
as likely as men to undervalue the work of the women they employ to care
for their children and to perceive them as mere substitutes for their own
more important role as parent (Enarson, 1990; Nelson, 1990).

A postmodern feminist perspective holds in tension both maximalist
and minimalist aspects of feminist discussions of caregiving. Defining the
tensions allows examination of the ways that real and illusory differences
associated with gender, race, age, class, and sexual orientation are constructed and distorted. In this chapter, we review these tensions and
propose other ways of conceptualizing caregiving in women's lives.
Bridenthal's (1982) questions, What does the family do *for* women? and
What does the family do *to* women? lead us to ask, What does caregiving
do for women, and What does it do to women? Most important, what is
the relationship between power and caregiving? Whose interests are
served by women's nearly exclusive responsibility for caregiving? What
are the societal implications if women, as they gain economic power, "buy
out" of caregiving? What are the implications for women when they do
not provide care in ways that are expected of them? How might an ethic
of care be structured in an egalitarian society? What kinds of caregiving
behaviors do not depend on the oppression of a subordinate group?

This examination of caregiving is organized around several paradoxical debates about women and caring labor. First, we consider motherhood, which is the cornerstone of women's caring labor (Ruddick, 1989).
The deconstruction of ideas about motherhood reveals contradictions
that all women face, regardless of their maternal status. Whether a
woman becomes a mother or not, she confronts societal expectations that
a female is not yet an adult until she has a child.

Yet, motherhood is not the whole of care (Ruddick, 1989). Contemporary adult women are likely to spend more years caring for elderly
parents or ill spouses than for small children (Abel & Nelson, 1990). In a
recent survey of 7,000 federal workers, nearly half said that they cared for
dependent adults (Beck et al., 1990). Women also provide care for their
partners and their friends. Being a "second mother" to another woman's
children is likely to be a part of women's life course experience, particularly for African-American women (Stack, 1974), working-class women
(Rapp, 1982; Stacey, 1990), lifelong single women (Allen, 1989), and
lesbian comothers (Crawford, 1987; Falk, 1989), all of whom participate

in female-centered kin and friendship networks of mutual support. Thus, the first set of tensions we address is: In what ways is motherhood glorified and pathologized? How do women benefit or lose from the mystification of motherhood as their proper sphere?

Second, we turn to tensions in the conduct of caregiving. Are women the primary caregivers because it is natural to them or because of their subordination in a male-centered society? At issue is whether caregiving is a chosen, rewarding, and valuable activity—a labor of love—or whether caregiving is work that only women will do because they are more oppressed as a group than men. Are women subordinated to men because they engage in a devalued activity like caregiving or do they engage in this activity because they are subordinated? As subordinates, is caregiving the only way in which women are allowed access to power and rewards? If so, in what ways do women rationalize their subordination by claiming to find it rewarding?

Third, we examine ways in which the recipients of care are valued or problemized as burdens. Care receivers are often children, husbands, partners, and the elderly. How are care recipients treated as commodities whose value is determined by their extrinsic usefulness or their intrinsic worth?

Finally, we propose a feminist vision of caregiving. We consider implications for women, men, and children. We look for practical applications that arise from feminist principles to structure an agenda for nonoppressive caregiving.

THE MYSTIFICATION OF MOTHERHOOD

The first set of questions on caregiving concerns the ways in which women experience, contribute to, and resist the mystification of motherhood. Motherhood is sanctified when the experience of mothering is romanticized as a natural, primary, and inherently rewarding part of being female, yet the reality of child care and the lack of institutional supports for mothers are ignored (Rich, 1986).

A constructivist perspective is needed to consider the actual experiences and behaviors of caregiving because caregiving is a deeply personal and practical type of work. Every person receives some kind of care when young and continues to receive and give care throughout life. The feminist view that the personal is political suggests that ideologies about caregiving are mediated by personal experiences of being cared for and providing care to others.

The idealization of motherhood is a relatively recent phenomenon, initiated about two centuries ago with the rise of the middle class during the industrial revolution (Ehrenreich, 1989; Stacey, 1990). As the new merchant class family became more child centered and the spheres of women and men became more separate, white middle- and upper-middle-class women's lives became influenced by a "cult of true womanhood" (Welter, 1966). Their experience and influence became limited to love, marriage, motherhood, and the home (Smith-Rosenberg, 1975).

Thus, the mystification of motherhood is a legacy that is carried into the late 20th century. When the diversity of women's experiences is considered, the inaccuracy of the myths about motherhood are even more pronounced. The portrayal of women's lives as focused only on expressive functions excludes racial and ethnic women who labored first for others and then for their own families in order to survive economically and physically (Collins, 1989, 1990; Dill, 1988). The cruel irony of the mystification of motherhood is that only certain women were ever included in the few tenuous protections offered. Stacey (1990) documents that even as working-class wives began to achieve these kinds of protections, the postindustrial economic system unraveled whatever gains they had made toward the middle class ideal. The publication of Friedan's (1963) book, The Feminine Mystique, a cultural marker ushering in the second wave of the women's movement, helped to expose the myth of motherhood as a lifelong fulfilling vocation for women who had followed its pathway.

High divorce rates and no-fault laws have made a life devoted to caregiving a risky undertaking for contemporary women. Child support awards rarely are adequate to meet the costs of raising children and often are not paid regularly. Fewer than 15% of women receive alimony (Lester, 1991). If women have devoted themselves to homemaking and caregiving while forgoing their own careers and personal development, they and their children are likely to find themselves living in poverty in the event of divorce (Weitzman, 1988). Traditional motherhood is not a rational life choice unless a woman has a contingency plan for supporting herself and her children.

Contradictions in the Experiences of Motherhood

Motherhood, the cornerstone of caring labor, is shrouded in romantic language that obscures its practical nature. Being a mother is filled with contradictions in a patriarchal society (Ferree, 1990; Rich, 1986; Ruddick, 1989; Thompson & Walker, 1989; Trebilcot, 1983). Women are defined by their ability to fulfill the reproductive role; those who do not become mothers face social sanctions for their child-free lifestyle.

Complicating the experience and practice of motherhood is the fact that being a mother, knowing how to mother, and the actual work of mothering are three different processes. Being a mother is idealized as an important, natural, and fulfilling lifelong activity. However, the only training most young women get for this critical role is through indirect socialization, modeling their own and other mothers, and, perhaps, brief courses before their babies are born.

Mothers have been responsible traditionally for the way their children turn out. Yet, mothers are allowed less control over their children's lives than the ideology presumes (Rich, 1986). By the time a child enters a school system, peers, teachers, media, and community influences exert pressures on shaping the child's behaviors and identities. Preschoolers who stay at home during the day may watch hours of television and view explicitly violent and sexual content at a very young age. Mothers rear children in an environment that is often hostile to their aims of preserving the lives and nurturing the growth of their children (Ruddick, 1989). Mothers in inner cities are in constant competition with drugs, crime, and an environment of poverty that pose numerous threats to the lives and health of their children (Katz, 1989; Sidel, 1992; Wilson, 1987).

Parents are given few guidelines for raising children, and the script directing much of maternal practice contradicts human needs for bonding and attachment. Psychodynamic theories of development suggest that for a boy to become a man, he must break free from his mother emotionally and develop an autonomous self (Chodorow, 1978). Daughters are under pressure to formulate their own identities, but not until they marry or become mothers themselves (Fischer, 1981). A mother's work is to help her child form boundaries and develop autonomy, but this script is mediated by covert beliefs about proper gender-related identities and behaviors. The anxiety built into mothering is expressed in the contradictory sentiment: Grow up to be an independent person, but not too independent from me.

Blaming Mothers

Maternal caregiving is defined as necessary for a child's healthy growth and development, but, paradoxically, mothers are offered few clear guideposts and little support for the work they are expected to do. On the one hand, Belsky (1990) argues that the best situation for optimal child development is for mothers to stay home with their children for at least the first year of a child's life. Negative outcomes, he claims, are associated with maternal employment and nonmaternal child care if it is low-quality child care, such as high child–caregiver ratios and space limitations. One outcome is poor school performance for elementary schoolchildren whose mothers returned to full-time work within their first year of life (Belsky, 1990). Conversely, Demo (1992) argues that employed mothers are singled out unfairly for blame as the cause of a variety of child problems. He concludes that the problems allegedly encountered by children of employed mothers are vastly overstated. Paternal abandonment and neglect are far more likely to be at the root of the problems that are blamed on single or employed mothers.

Yet, mothers are held accountable for child outcomes. Great attention has been given in the popular press to the phenomenon of adult children of dysfunctional families blaming their parents for the anger, disappointment, and pain from their childhoods (Adult Children of Alcoholics, 1990; Brown, 1990). Even when the alcoholic or abusive father is implicated, the "codependent" mother is more often the one who is blamed (Gavey, Florence, Pezaro, & Tan, 1990; Holten, 1990). Mothers, rather than patriarchal society, are usually cited as responsible for the problems of postmodern families (Stacey, 1990).

The ideology of motherhood stands in sharp contrast to the reality of child caregiving. Perhaps it is not motherhood per se that is valued, but particular types of motherhood—motherhood within the context of a male–female relationship. Proponents of the maximalist argument would emphasize the importance of what mothers do to and for their children, but ignore how women's lives are regulated by social institutions. Within the traditional family, the father is theorized as a distant figure in child development. His status as breadwinner and ultimate authority is taken for granted. The contradiction of the maximalist position is that it presumes the need for a traditional marriage in which to rear children; yet, in a traditional marriage, the mother is overburdened with responsibility and blame, and the father is undervalued in meeting the child's immediate needs (cf. Dressel & Clark, 1990; Ferree, 1990; Thompson & Walker, 1989).

A minimalist position, by denying gender differences and suggesting that anyone can mother, is unsatisfactory from a postmodern feminist perspective, as well. If fathers are just as good as mothers, then why are men so negligent or absent in their child care responsibilities (see Demo, 1992; Ferree, 1990; LaRossa, 1988; Thompson & Walker, 1989 for recent reviews)? Ferree (1990) and Thompson (1991) concluded that unless women expect and negotiate changes in their relationships with husbands, changes will not occur. One reason men resist taking on more responsibility is that they are excused by the women with whom they live (Goode, 1982). It may be that women relieve men of the responsibility because they are reluctant to entrust men with the care of their children (Gerson, 1985; LaRossa & LaRossa, 1989; Rubin, 1983; Stacey, 1990).

Women may act as gatekeepers to their children for personal reasons, as well. As the one who carried and gave birth to the child, a woman may feel she has a different investment in the child than her partner and wants to know that the child is cared for in the way she thinks best. Other women may want to retain primary responsibility for children as a means of justifying the choice of a traditional homemaking role (Grossman, Pollack, & Golding, 1988). Caregiving and kinkeeping provide women with a type of power within the family that they may be reluctant to give up or share (Kranichfeld, 1988). Mothers have some sense of control and authority over their children's growth and development and receive credit if they are good mothers (Ehrensaft, 1983). The relationships that women cultivate with those for whom they care provide an unduplicated opportunity for influence, particularly if there are no alternatives that give them the same sense of accomplishment.

The Motherhood Hierarchy

Rearing a child is complicated by characterizing motherhood as the natural province of women. DiLapi (1989) proposed a conceptual framework to understand the social context of motherhood and the sanctions women confront if they mother outside the context of legal marriage. The framework is conceptualized as a three-tiered triangle. At the apex of the triangle are "appropriate mothers," who are married, heterosexual, and thus the most acceptable women for raising children. In the middle are "marginal mothers," including single mothers, teenage mothers, disabled mothers, and foster mothers. They differ from appropriate mothers in terms of family form. At the bottom of the hierarchy are lesbian mothers, who differ from marginal mothers in terms of sexual orientation.

Drawing on Rubin's (1984) ideas about the sex gender system, DiLapi (1989) chose a hierarchical model to describe the "system of unequal distribution of power and resources supporting motherhood" (p. 108). Married heterosexual women have the most access to motherhood services and support and are rewarded for being mothers. Marginal mothers have more tenuous relationships with institutional support systems. Lesbian mothers, through invisibility and denial of their existence, have limited access to external resources and options for parenthood.

Motherhood outside the context of the traditional family is poorly tolerated in a patriarchal society. All mothers face oppressive situations in which their childrearing goals can become compromised (Ruddick, 1989), but intense pressure is reserved for women who reproduce and parent apart from male control (DiLapi, 1989).

Other examples of invisible and marginalized motherhood are women who are unable to care for their children because of sickness or drug and alcohol addiction, women who neglect and abuse their children, and women who give up custody of their children. Rarely has research been conducted to understand mothering within these contexts from the point of view of the mothers themselves. Research specifically geared toward these mothers is needed to understand their circumstances and choices in terms other than deviance.

The Contradictions of Lesbian Mothering

In a postmodern feminist world, contradictory combinations of rela-tionships, previously invisible, demand consideration. Relationships once construed as implausible challenge us to reexamine definitions of love, marriage, and parenthood (Stacey, 1990). In Chapter 2, we considered the tensions involved in being a feminist and being married to a man. In the present chapter, we consider the tensions in caregiving when one departs from the traditional script of mothering.

If mothering is so important and if child care is best done by women, then why are lesbian mothers so criticized in society (Falk, 1989)? If having one mother is so important, then would not having two mothers be even better? The response to this question, from a patriarchal point of view, is a resounding no. Women raising children without a male partner violate the context in which women are allowed to be mothers in our society (DiLapi, 1989). Mothering is good only as long as a man or the patriarchal state supervises it.

Tensions about motherhood as an institution rooted in patriarchy and heterosexism get played out in the pluralistic lesbian community, as well. Personal narratives of male children of lesbians document the occasional, yet unique, experience of not being as welcomed as female children (Lorde, 1984; Rafkin, 1990). The intersections of gender, generation, and sexual orientation produce a script for parenting that offers unique challenges, dilemmas, and possibilities. Lesbians raising sons do so under unique constraints and opportunities, as Lorde (1984) depicts in her description of an interracial lesbian family in which her 14-year-old son, Jonathan, has lived since he was 3 years old. She describes the advantage for her son of growing up within a nonsexist household and the valuable contribution his family circumstances made to his human sensitivity:

> These assumptions of power relationships are being questioned because Frances and I, often painfully and with varying degrees of success, attempt to evaluate and measure over and over again our feelings concerning power, our own and others. And we explore with care those areas concerning how it is used and expressed between us and between us and the children, openly and otherwise. (Lorde, 1984, p. 79)

This passage reveals the deliberate, conscious choices involved in lesbian mothering. Lesbian mothers must overcome enormous constraints in order to have and to retain custody of their children (Falk, 1989; Pies, 1988).

The positive side of such oppression is that parenting in this context often becomes a shared, negotiated, and purposeful process. Koepke, Hare, and Moran (1992) compared lesbian couples with children and lesbian couples without children. Although they saw all relationships as solid and happy, those relationships with children were characterized by greater relationship satisfaction and sexual intimacy. This finding is contrary to the research on heterosexual relationships and children. Koepke et al. (1992) speculate that reasons for this discrepancy include the possible inflation of satisfaction scores for lesbians who were formerly married. In comparing their current lives to their past relationships with husbands, they may have been unaware of their sexual orientation. Now, being in a relationship with a woman may be a better fit for them. Second, perhaps lesbian couples with children may represent lesbian families that are exceptions; these women were willing to risk negative consequences, such as loss of custody of their children or the child's rejection of the mother, in order to be together. Perhaps only highly satisfied and solidly committed couples would risk such consequences (Koepke et al., 1992).

Resistance

Women both resist and collude with the motherhood hierarchy and the social control of their reproduction and parenting decisions. A sizable portion of the female population chooses to limit childbearing, and millions of women have children or raise them without male partners. More than 1 million babies were born to single women in 1988, 51% more than in 1980 (National Center for Health Statistics, 1990). Single women accounted for 18% of all white births and 64% of all black births in 1988. There has been a rapid increase in births by older single women in recent years, suggesting that some single women who had delayed childbearing and marriage decided to have a child without marrying.

Women have been innovative by creating their own means of support in response to the motherhood hierarchy. Lesbian mothers receive more support from their cohabiting partners in child care and household duties than do mothers who live with male partners (McGuire & Alexander, 1985). Having two adult women in the household in a supportive living arrangement alleviates the burden that married women and single mothers feel in attempting to "do it all," or at least most of it

(Ferree, 1990). Among middle-class married couples, shared parenting is possible when fathers define their involvement in parenting as a choice (Ehrensaft, 1987).

Motherhood is not just the domain of "appropriate mothers" who are heterosexual and married. Historically, unmarried women, whether heterosexual or lesbian, have relied on partners, relatives, and friends to pool resources and to share child care. Recent research indicates that fathers or father figures are more present in children's lives than is indicated by the social address "single-mother home." Mott (1990) used longitudinal and cross-sectional data from the National Longitudinal Survey of Youth to examine family transitions in terms of paternal presence or absence in homes lacking a biological father. The data, drawn from female respondents aged 14 to 21, indicated that in general, and for all races, 60% of children of unmarried mothers are likely to have at least weekly contact with their nonresident fathers or other father figures, such as their mother's new partner. Although the nature of father presence or absence is highly complex, these data indicate a way other than the traditional nuclear family that women conduct their motherhood careers.

Other types of mothers about whom there is little research are single mothers by choice (Merritt & Steiner, 1984) and lesbians choosing parenthood (Pies, 1988, 1990). In increasing numbers, women are becoming single parents by choice and not through divorce or desertion, or they are becoming parents in partnerships without husbands. By describing the experiences of marginalized mothers, we can examine the social regulation of motherhood that limits women's choices to live independent lives. By examining the constraints under which women and men rear children, we can deconstruct the "blame the mother" ideology that accompanies a society in which childrearing is individually, rather than communally, oriented (see Ehrensaft, 1987; Ruddick, 1989; Trebilcot, 1983).

WOMEN AS NATURAL CAREGIVERS OR SUBORDINATES?

Women are expected to be nurturant toward others and to put their own needs aside. Because women and caregiving are seen as synonymous in our society, women who fail to live up to these expectations are denigrated for not fulfilling their adult developmental tasks. Women who do not participate in maternal or caregiving activities are subject to psychological and social sanctions including charges of selfishness and lack of femininity.

Feminist theories of caregiving reflect traditional disciplines, such as psychology and sociology, yet also critique, contradict, and transcend such traditional views (see Walker, 1992). As feminists deconstruct the extent to which women perform the "expressive" role in families and society, new visions of agentic caregiving become possible (e.g., Jordan, Kaplan, Miller, Stiver, & Surrey, 1991).

Contested Issues Regarding the Ethic of Care

Is women's caregiving a natural part of being female or a consequence of subordination? Once again, gender differences in biological and psychological predispositions come into question. This issue has been framed dichotomously. Are gender differences responsible for women's greater involvement in caregiving, or does caregiving encompass certain behaviors that anyone, regardless of gender, can express?

As suggested previously, theories of caregiving range from a maximalist (men and women are opposites) perspective to a minimalist (men and women are alike) perspective (Kaufman, 1985; Risman & Schwartz, 1989). Maximalists argue for a more inherent or essentialist basis of women's greater involvement in nurturant activities; allegedly, it is women's nature to be more concerned with care and peace (for a critique of these theorists, see Echols, 1989). Men, in contrast, are theorized to possess a more destructive, warriorlike nature, rendering them incapable of providing the life-sustaining care that women provide (Echols, 1989). Minimalists posit a microsociological explanation for differences in caregiving. If placed in the role of caregiver, men, too, can provide the same kind of caregiving to children as do mothers (Risman, 1989). When men and women are in similar circumstances, gender differences are less obvious.

A related issue is whether caregiving derives from an ethic of care based on a particular type of moral thinking or whether it is merely a manifestation of women's oppression as subordinates in the social hierarchy. Do women provide the bulk of caring work in society because of a sense of responsibility to care for those who are dependent or do they do it because men with more power do not want to do it?

Psychological explanations support the ethic of care perspective; sociological explanations provide evidence for the subordination argument. Gilligan (1982) proposed a developmental explanation for women's moral orientation toward relationships and care that contrasts with Kohlberg's (1976) view of moral development as culminating in an ethic of justice. Tronto (1987) challenged this psychological explanation and suggested a sociopolitical explanation.

Tronto (1987) is one of a growing number of feminists (see also Dressel & Clark, 1990; Hare-Mustin, 1989) who critique theories of care that are based on the concept of psychological gender difference. Hare-

Mustin and Marecek (1990) suggested that differences between men and women are socially constructed, not rooted in biology or psychology; it is in the interest of the political structure to polarize men and women and to allocate social roles according to gender. Tronto (1987) and Dressel and Clark (1990) argued that social and political subordination, rather than psychological gender difference, is a better explanation for why women are the primary caregivers in our society. By taking a feminist view of the social construction of gender differences, women's propensity to care is seen as rooted in power dynamics and hierarchies (Ferree, 1990). Women's greater involvement in caregiving is perpetuated by socialization practices that stress the virtues of nurturant behaviors for young females while encouraging autonomous development for males.

The job of caregiving, with no salary, low status, long hours, and domestic isolation, interferes with the ability to accumulate resources that translate into power (Polatnick, 1983). Women who are primary caregivers become locked in a vicious cycle. Caregiving responsibilities limit the time and energy that they can commit to paid work. Without the status and earning power that accompany breadwinning, women continue to have less influence in renegotiating family responsibilities in order to redistribute caregiving responsibilities. Women assume or get assigned caring labor because someone has to do it and, since they generally have less earning power, it "makes more sense" for them rather than their male partners to make the occupational sacrifice. There is little incentive for men to assume caregiving responsibilities and little evidence that they want the job (Polatnick, 1983).

Certainly, both arguments about the ethic and practice of care have merit. The caring labor of women requires both critical deconstruction as well as celebration and honor. Caring labor is essential to human life both at the micro (family) level and the macro (societal) level. Women may be more oriented toward and attuned to providing attentive, reflective care because of socialization practices. Reproductive experiences sensitize women further to issues of care. Ehrensaft (1987) suggested that biological aspects of pregnancy and childbearing may prime parents for a different experience in gender-specific ways. The mother's "perception of the child as her product, and her experience of the child as an extension of herself all grow out of mothering's being deeply embedded within her as a core part of who she is and a prime determinant of her worth in the world" (Ehrensaft, 1987, p. 627).

Caregiving is socially constructed with different scripts for males and females. Women bear children, so it is easy to argue that they should have primary responsibility for them. After carrying a baby for 9 months, it is not surprising that a woman would have a significant investment in the care and nurturance of that infant, even if she had not been socialized to believe that it was her specific responsibility. The experience of caring for a vulnerable and dependent other is likely to result in the development of a certain degree of skill and knowledge about caregiving that is generalizable to other contexts (Noddings, 1984; Ruddick, 1989). Knowing *how* to care, women are identified as the logical choice for continued caregiving, particularly if individuals in positions of higher power have little interest in providing this service to others.

Although scholars and practitioners argue about women's proper place, caregiving is a very real, practical, and pervasive part of women's lives. Women juggle a variety of caregiving acts and the feelings associated with them in the course of any day. They rely on their own labor or the work of other women, such as secretaries and child care workers, to tend to personal and professional lives, for example, prepare dinner, type a manuscript, or pick up a child at school. Yet, it is usually men with few caregiving responsibilities in supervisory positions who preside over decisions about professional development and success. Although more women are moving into elite positions in society and sharing positions of dominance in the social structure with men, the old reality remains that it is nearly always women who provide care for themselves and others. Furthermore, as some women move into positions of power, they conform to the traditional male model that tends to devalue caregiving. By remaining child free and avoiding committed relationships, they limit the demands that caregiving might place upon them.

If caregiving responsibilities cannot be avoided, they can be minimized by hiring others, often women in a more subordinate position, to do them. The relationship between affluent mothers and the subordinates they hire is similar to that between fathers and mothers. Women in elite positions can hire others to relieve them of caregiving responsibilities so that they can pursue more economically and socially rewarding activities (Polatnick, 1983). Poor pay for licensed child care workers and the unregulated cottage industry that has evolved around the care of other people's children are examples of the gross devaluation of caregiving, affecting the women who provide the care, the children who receive the care (Nelson, 1990), and, ultimately, the women who use the care because all caregiving is devalued or undervalued.

By deconstructing women's nearly exclusive involvement in caregiving, we attempt to go beyond the dialectic of alpha and beta bias (Hare-Mustin & Marecek, 1990). A postmodern feminist perspective allows a reconstruction of caring labor that acknowledges differences, affirms the value of nurturance, and sets women's caregiving as a standard against which all other forms of caring labor can be evaluated.

Are Women Natural Caregivers?

The Reproduction of Gender Differences

Chodorow (1978) proposed a revision of psychoanalytic theory to explain how women become society's caregivers. She argued that women's mothering is one of the few universals in the sexual division of labor and is reproduced in women generation after generation. In the early psychodynamic environment, infants come to internalize the social structure of the sexual division of labor. Fathers are relatively absent, and mothers provide their care. Boys are raised to separate from their mothers, and girls are raised to identify and merge with their mothers:

> The sexual and familial division of labor in which women mother and are more involved in interpersonal, affective relationships than men produces in daughters and sons a division of psychological capacities which leads them to reproduce this sexual and familial divison of labor. (Chodorow, 1978, p. 7)

As a result, females experience themselves as more continuous with others and come to value close personal connectedness, thereby perpetuating a relational basis for mothering. Because male children learn to repress their attachment to their mothers, the relational basis for mothering is inhibited. Males do not tend to define themselves in terms of their relationships or try to relocate themselves in a primary parent–child relationship.

Chodorow (1978) provides a feminist explanation for the work that women do in maintaining and sustaining families. Her theory has influenced explanations about the relational difficulties of adult men and women. Rubin (1983) extended Chodorow's theory about the construction of gender differences through early socialization to explain the lack of intimacy between husbands and wives. Rubin argued that these early dynamics relate to the fact that women are the primary caregivers in our society. Differences between males and females in regard to attachment and autonomy are reinforced within families and through broader social structures as children grow to be adults. Rubin conducted in-depth interviews with a diverse group of 150 couples between the ages of 25 and 55. Data revealed how most couples were virtual strangers to each other as the result of being socialized in very different ways. At the core of these differences was the fact that females were raised primarily by a same-sex parent who encouraged connection and attachment and males by an opposite sex parent from whom they had to separate in order to develop an appropriate masculinity. As adults, women and men struggled in their relationships with conflicting tendencies regarding the reciprocal disclosure of feeling and thought necessary for deep and sustained intimacy (Rubin, 1983).

Rooting the reproduction of mothering in the normative nuclear family is problematic, however (Jackson, 1989). Chodorow's (1978) psychological theory assumes that the social context in which childrearing occurs includes only one mother and one father who live together with their child. Many children do not live within this type of family environment.

To some extent, Chodorow's theory suggests that because it is women who mother, women are responsible for the reproduction of gendered personalities and the resulting problems. The dynamics that create affiliative, nurturant females and individualistic, autonomous males are time and culture bound. Children's personality and developmental outcomes are influenced by changes in social structures as well. Less polarization in gender socialization may be evident in family and community structures where diversity is more normative. More examination is needed of males and females raised in family circumstances other than traditional two-parent, heterosexual, nuclear arrangements, such as in lesbian and gay male families, single-mother and single-father families, and stepfamilies.

The danger of emphasizing gender differences is that it becomes a justification of the status quo. Change becomes less likely, and women are blamed for their own subordination. If mothering is considered natural to women, then it is assumed that they choose to provide care or that they just cannot help taking care of others. If it is normal and natural for women to provide care, changing social arrangements will have little effect, and intervention stategies will be of little use.

The underlying assumptions of gender differences are unsupported and untested (Hare-Mustin & Marecek, 1990). Summarizing the qualities of males as "essentially autonomous" and the qualities of females as "essentially affiliative" is both a simplification and a caricature that obscures the real differences and similarities of men and women. It sets up a false dualism of gender opposites:

> The symmetrical pseudomutuality of male and female can be challenged. Not-"a" is not necessarily the opposite of "a." What do we observe in opposition to man? Man or mouse? Man or beast? Man or superman? Man or child? Man or mountain? Man or machine? Man or woman? Which is the opposite? (Hare-Mustin, 1989, p. 69)

Equating autonomy with masculinity and relatedness with femininity implies mutual exclusivity. Men and women are not seen as whole persons without the other. A false dependence of the sexes is proposed, although, paradoxically, men are seen as more "whole" than women (Bem, 1987). The dependence of men on women becomes masked (Rubin, 1983).

Theories explaining gender differences have been widely embraced because they are simplistic and appealing intuitively. Perceiving females and males as different reinforces the belief that they are so inherently. In constructing an understanding of the world, people try to make sense of and explain differences. Yet, the belief in gender differences reinforces the status quo (Hare-Mustin & Marecek, 1990). A belief in the inevitability of inherent differences between women and men leaves unrecognized the costs of social and political inequities that accrue to women and to minority group members. Society or privileged individuals do not have to change or even feel responsible if the ethic of care is prescribed only for those in a subordinate position. The focus on gender differences does not resolve the contradictions faced by women who do not want to be caregivers, whether they are in elite positions or not.

Women and Relational Morality

Chodorow's (1978) pioneering work on the early childrearing environment sparked numerous theories about the nature of women's caring labor. Gilligan's (1982) theory of relational morality draws on the differences Chodorow (1978) posits between females and males. Gilligan argues that women's concern with relationships is more pronounced than men's, and it is rooted in the nearly exclusive female role of childrearing, at least in infancy and early childhood.

Gilligan's view of women's difference from men is based on two assertions. First, there is a unique feminine orientation toward relationships that differs from a masculine orientation of individual achievement. Female children come to know themselves through the similarity between themselves and their mothers. They experience an enduring connection between themselves and others, whereas male children develop their identity through the contrast between self and mother (Colby & Damon, 1987).

Second, most developmental psychological theories are derived from research using male samples. Male development is seen as normative, and women's development is evaluated as deficient (Colby & Damon, 1987). Masculinity and male anatomy become the human standard, and femininity and female anatomy are seen as deviations from that standard (Hare-Mustin & Marecek, 1990). From a developmental perspective, adult thinking proceeds from adolescence to redefine moral judgments from context specific to ultimately reconciling the tension *between* self and other. Women's thinking is contextualized by perceptions of self more embedded in relationships *with* others. Their reasoning and judgments are more grounded in real life, and, therefore, according to male theorists such as Kohlberg, Erikson, and Freud, reflect a lower level of development (Gilligan, 1982). Gilligan takes issue with Kohlberg's view that women get stuck in his third of six possible stages of development. This third level, which is relationally oriented, is a form of conventional morality. Adult males are more likely to develop a more principled, postconventional moral logic according to Kohlberg's model.

Gilligan's original research contrasted with Kohlberg's by using a real-life dilemma, rather than a hypothetical one, to test moral reasoning. The women in her sample were referred to her by pregnancy and abortion services and were actually facing an abortion. The sample consisted of 29 women, diverse in age, race, and social class. Four decided to have the baby, 1 miscarried, 21 chose abortion, and 3 were still in doubt about the decision. The important part of the research, however, was not what decision the women made, but rather how they reasoned about a situation that involved conflicting claims.

The theory of relational morality was developed inductively. The first part of the interview asked women questions about their reasons for or against their choices, the conflicts they experienced, and their decision-making processes. The second part of the interview assessed their moral judgment in the hypothetical mode by presenting for resolution three of Kohlberg's standard research dilemmas. Then, how each woman constructed the abortion dilemma was analyzed. The following tentative developmental sequence was proposed.

The first level of judgment is an orientation to individual survival. There is an initial focus on the self as the locus of the decision. Then, there is a transition from selfishness to responsibility. In the transition to the second level, one discovers the concept of responsibility as the basis for a new equilibrium between self and others.

The second level is termed "goodness as self-sacrifice." The concept of responsibility is elaborated and fused with a maternal concept of morality, which seeks to ensure protection for those who are dependent. Good is equated with caring for others. The second transition is from goodness to truth. It is initiated when the conventions of feminine goodness legitimize only others as the recipients of moral care. The inequality between self and other creates psychological violence and thus disequilibrium. Now the relationship between self and others is reconsidered in an effort to sort out the confusion between conformity and care in the conventional definition of feminine goodness and to establish a new equilibrium, which dissipates the tension between selfishness and responsibility.

The third level is the morality of nonviolence. The self becomes the arbiter of an independent judgment that now subsumes both conventions and individual needs under the moral principle of nonviolence. What is universal now is the condemnation of exploitation and hurt. Violence against the self is included in moral judgments on par with violence against others (Gilligan, 1982).

Gilligan's work, whether she intended it or not, has been used to support the notion that women prefer to be caregivers. A number of debates have surfaced about the implications of her work (Colby & Damon, 1987; Kerber et al., 1986). A major criticism is that women's connection to care appears to be rooted in the assumption of their moral superiority. Although Gilligan (1982) states clearly that moral development is linked to theme, not gender, conclusions drawn from her empirical studies allow for the interpretation that men express a proclivity toward an individual rights or justice orientation and women toward a relational or care orientation.

Does Caregiving Reflect Women's Subordination?

Tronto (1987) argued that the ethic of care needs to be separated from gender so that a much broader range of options for all women and men emerges. The ethic of care is linked more to the intersections of class, race, gender and other statuses in life than strictly to gender. In contemporary American society, women and minority men are concentrated in service and caretaking occupations, often receiving substandard wages or doing unpaid labor at home. Through their service and work in taking care of others, caregivers develop a concern for the objects of their care and construct an understanding of them.

Tronto (1987) argued against Kohlberg's theory that an individualistic perspective, achieved by higher levels of abstract thinking, leads to the morally superior justice orientation over the lesser relational–contextual orientation. By Kohlberg's criteria, the people most likely to achieve a justice orientation of abstract, individualistic thought are males. The most moral figures he cites are religious and political leaders such as Jesus, Martin Luther King, Jr., and Gandhi. These men are idealized for their bravery, but on a more practical level, people who are most likely to develop a highly abstract, individualistic orientation in contemporary society are white men who occupy privileged positions in the social structure. It may be that privileged white males, who have the opportunity to develop a justice orientation, actually become morally impoverished:

> In order for an ethic of care to develop, individuals need to experience caring for others and being cared for by others. . . . The dearth of caretaking

experiences makes privileged males morally deprived. Their experiences mislead them to think that moral beliefs can be expressed in abstract, univeralistic terms as if they were purely cognitive questions, like mathematical formulae. (Tronto, 1987, p. 652)

In contrast, black culture "emphasizes basic respect for others, a commitment to honesty, generosity motivated by the knowledge that you might need help someday, and respect for the choices of others" (Tronto, 1987, p. 650). Stack's (1974) ethnography of a black community revealed ways in which resource pooling and kin arrangements were used to support individual, family, and community survival. Collins (1990) cites the motto Lifting as We Climb that was adopted by educated black women who founded the National Association of Colored Women's Clubs as characteristic of upwardly mobile black women's ethic of care. Historically, black women adopted an Afrocentric family orientation toward racial uplift for the black community, one that balances the needs of individuals and the group to move forward collectively. Black women's contributions to black churches has been a primary arena for this work (see Collins, 1990; Gilkes, 1985; Grant, 1982). Africanity (traditional African family/community culture) involves ties toward the kin group, a clear value on children's lives, and sharing resources (Kilbride & Kilbride, 1990). Women are at the center of this kin group, just as women are central in maintaining kin networks in working class family life (Rapp, 1982; Stacey, 1990). Thus, gender intersects with class and race in important ways. What Gilligan and associates linked to psychological differences between women and men may be based in power differences across social groups in terms of gender, race, and class.

Care may be an ethic created in industrial society by the condition of subordination. Tronto (1987) argued that the expansion of the ethic of care beyond an exclusive focus on gender is consistent with Gilligan's theory because Gilligan found that women are capable of using both the ethic of justice and the ethic of care more often than men. Privilege associated with gender, race, and class, therefore, lessens a person's ability to be more flexible in moral reasoning because those with greater privilege are not required to do much perspective taking.

The ability to use both orientations is a valuable asset in contemporary society. Thompson (1989) observed that both the ethic of care and the ethic of justice are important for long-term married couples who want to continue to maintain a vital relationship. Both partners need to be committed to equity and emotional intimacy, rather than having these qualities polarized in either person. The superior position of white males leads to their lack of experience in knowing how others feel. Their perspective is limited by their privilege (Tronto, 1987), whereas those with less status in the social structure must develop an understanding of individuals with more status (Collins, 1990). This is another example of how more oppressed members of a social system develop a double vision of reality (Westkott, 1979).

Dressel and Clark (1990) also critiqued the exclusive gender focus of the ethic of care. Based on an innovative qualitative methodology using self-report diaries, personal narratives about caregiving scenarios, and reflections on their own personal experiences with family care, they examined both the culture and the conduct of family care. Guided by symbolic interaction theory and a social constructionist perspective, they assumed that women's disproportionately greater involvement in the provision of caregiving may not be natural or chosen.

Dressel and Clark (1990) looked for meanings assigned to caregiving activities and sought to broaden the notion of care by incorporating diverse experiences of women and men within the family. They challenged the reification of care as solely a woman's activity. Conceptualizations of care typically presume a self-evident, unilateral, shared definition. This view is disadvantageous to women, leading to a separate and unequal mentality about women's work. Arguments that begin with a dichotomous assumption (e.g., women are expressive, men are instrumental; women work in the home, men work outside the home) force all human beings into gender categories.

Dressel and Clark (1990) found that both women and men viewed the culture of family care from a romanticized notion of family life. A great deal of variation was evident in the conduct of care, based on three themes: diversity of motives for caregiving; care as service; and emotive dissonance. Similarities and differences emerged from this analysis that cast gender distinctions in a new light. First, women were more motivated than men to make connections with other family members, based on their desire to benefit themselves and fulfill their own needs. This finding challenges popular ideas of who benefits from family care:

> Women may perform more apparent acts of care than men because their interpersonal needs are unfulfilled. If so, then what appear to be expressive behaviors (e.g., hugging, phoning) may instead by instrumental ones undertaken in the service of having one's own needs met. (Dressel & Clark, 1990, p. 776)

Women also were more likely to describe complex motives for their caretaking behaviors toward their children and spouses than were men. They had a more elaborated reading and vocabulary of motives in the family setting than men.

Second, in terms of the routine qualities of family care, many women found it difficult to list and describe all the caring acts they performed in a given day, because so much of their care is routine service to others. Women, much more than men, anticipated the needs of others. This finding supports Hochschild's (1983) work on the sociology of emotions: More research is needed to understand "to what extent anticipatory acts and other self-defined acts of care reflect deference and power differentials in addition to, or instead of, care" (Dressel & Clark, 1990, p. 778). An outstanding finding was the frequency with which women, in their roles as wives and mothers, provided services for others. Women constantly did things for others that those others could have done for themselves.

Dressel and Clark's (1990) findings on emotive dissonance debunk the assumption that acts of family care and caring feelings are inextricably intertwined. Hochschild (1983) defines emotive dissonance as a conflict between doing and feeling. Women, more than men, expressed ambivalent feelings about their acts of caring; dissonance was characteristic of the expressions of care of 75% of the women in the study. The majority of men did not report dissonance. Dressel and Clark (1990) reject an essentialist position on gender roles and offer two alternative explanations for men's more positive affect:

> They may feel, and indeed be, more rewarded by participation in family care precisely because it is not expected from them. Another explanation lies in the likelihood that they are not expected to anticipate, plan, organize, and coordinate family activities but only to participate in them, thereby relieving them of certain kinds of strain. (p. 779)

These recommendations for reconceptualizing family care inform a postmodern feminist perspective on caregiving. First, it is not possible to observe all the acts and behaviors associated with care. Some participants cited their own "nonactions" as acts of care, whereas others engaged in a process of reflection that included worry and anticipation about another's needs. Second, traditional dichotomies of care as gender based are inadequate because most family care scenarios are rooted multidimensionally in "internal family dynamics and the family's connections to the broader society" (Dressel & Clark, 1990, p. 780).

What is clear from Tronto (1987), Hare-Mustin and Marecek (1990), and Dressel and Clark (1990) is that a psychological explanation is not sufficient to explain the tension between caregiving as a choice (i.e., because caregiving is perceived by the caregiver as rewarding and personally meaningful) and caregiving as a manifestation of a woman's subordinate position in the social structure. To posit a female ethic of care does not allow examination of the conditions under which women might not provide care, such as when they are in more dominant positions themselves, or when they choose a lifestyle in which they are not in service of the typical recipients of care.

In addition to the need for a social-constructionist political perspective that is contained within our view of postmodern feminism, we must also remember the diversity among women over the life course. A woman may have chosen not to bear and rear children, but unexpectedly may be faced with caring for a frail, aging parent or a niece or nephew. Women's greater involvement in caregiving reflects the tension between their historically subordinate position (an aspect of coercion) and the power they achieve from meeting others' needs (an aspect of choice).

CARE RECIPIENTS: BURDENS OR PRIZES?

Having questioned compulsory caregiving as a natural or essential part of women's lives, we now consider why women may continue to "want" to care for children, spouses, aging parents, and others. Aside from their historic connection to caregiving, what do women get out of caring for others? If caregiving is such a burden, or simply the result of women's oppression and subordination, then why do women have children, take care of their spouses and partners, and care for aging parents? What are the benefits, or the rationalizations, of caregiving?

The relationship between the caregiver and the care receiver underlies much of women's motivations to care. In this section, we consider these motivations and the changing conditions under which the recipients of care are valued or devalued.

Maternal Thinking and Practice

Ruddick (1989) proposed a standpoint theory of caregiving, based upon the caring labor of mothers, about how women are motivated to provide care for fragile beings. Her description of maternal behavior and thinking offers a perspective on the relationship of a caregiver and a care receiver within a societal context. Caregiving is never carried out under ideal circumstances. The practice of maternal thinking provides the cornerstone for developing a more universal explanation of women's caring labor (Ruddick, 1989).

In Ruddick's (1989) view, mothers are charged with the responsibility of dependent children. When mothers are able to practice the best of maternal behavior, they respond with behaviors that are undergirded by the capacity for attention and the virtue of love. Ruddick (1982) describes attentive love as "a unity of reflection, judgment, and emotion" (p. 77).

Maternal thinking is motivated by three demands of children and the society in which children are raised. First, children demand that their lives be protected and preserved. Second, they demand that they be nurtured in order to grow. Third, a mother's social group demands that the mother raise a child who is acceptable to her society, and whom the mother herself can appreciate.

Ruddick proposed that maternal thinking arises from maternal practice. By analogy, maternal thinking develops in the same way as a scholarly discipline:

> I speak about a mother's thought—the intellectual capacities she develops, the judgments she makes, the metaphysical attitudes she assumes, the values she affirms. Like a scientist writing up her experiment, a critic working over a text, or a historian assessing documents, a mother caring for children engages in a discipline. She asks certain questions—those relevant to her aims—rather than others; she accepts certain criteria for the truth, adequacy, and relevance of proposed answers; and she cares about the findings she makes and can act on. (Ruddick, 1989, p. 24)

Maternal work is carried out in a society in which a mother's work is often compromised by competing demands. Mothers are relatively powerless in the economic structure, and yet mothers are required to be responsible for their children. Women's caring labor is devalued and misrepresented. In a 1975 government study that rated the difficulty of kinds of work in terms of complexity, child care attendant and nursery school teacher were rated less difficult than dog pound attendant, mud mixer helper, and shoveler of chicken offal (Ruddick, 1989).

Like Gilligan, Ruddick's work on maternal thinking has generated a great deal of critical response (hooks, 1984; Ruddick, 1989; Stacey, 1986). One issue is the choice of language: what about men or fathers? Ruddick (1989) counters that because women's work—and it is primarily women who care for children—has been misdescribed, sentimentalized, and obscured, her use of the word "maternal" is purposeful. In her view, one need not be a biological mother to practice maternal thinking: A child's father can preserve, nurture, and train a child as well as can an adoptive mother. Ruddick is careful to distinquish between fathers and Fathers, the latter being adherents to the patriarchal values of domination and control (Ruddick, 1989, 1990).

Instead, Ruddick insists on the child as a separate, unique individual whose care is entrusted to the parent. Her vision of a child is not a prize or commodity, or a burden, but a unique person worthy of parental investment. Loving attention to a "real child" underlies maternal practice, at least ideally. Mothers are required "to love a child without seizing or using it, to see the child's reality with the patient, loving eye of attention" (Ruddick, 1982, p. 87). Ruddick indicts not the parent–child relation-

ship, but the social context in which maternal labor and child development are compromised.

Parent and Elder Care

Women are the primary caregivers of the frail elderly (Gatz, Bengtson, &
Blum, 1990). Stone, Cafferata, and Sangl (1987) report that 72% of the
primary, informal caregivers to the frail elderly are women. Most caregivers are the wives of elderly men, but if there is no spouse, the next most
probable caregiver is an adult daughter or daughter-in-law. For the most
part, women care for aging parents, particularly their widowed mothers
(Finch & Groves, 1983; Lopata, 1979, 1987; Shanas, 1979). Thus,
wives, daughters, and daughters-in-law are most involved in adult
caregiving (Boyd & Treas, 1989).

As the lifespan continues to elongate, and parents continue to
survive into old age, a woman can expect to spend 20% of her lifetime
with at least one parent over the age of 65 (Boyd & Treas, 1989). For
women who were age 55 in 1980, almost 60% had a living parent in
comparison to only 6% of 55-year-old women in 1800 (Watkins, Menk-
en, & Bongaarts, 1987).

Currently, only a small proportion of middle-aged women care for
both aging parents and small children. However, more than half of the
women who care for their elderly parents also work outside the home, and
nearly 40% of these women still have children at home (Beck et al.,
1990). In the future, more women will face the simultaneous demands of
caring for dependent children and elderly parents because of postponed
childbearing, grown children returning home or never leaving the family
of origin, and the increased likelihood of chronic disease in old age (Boyd
& Treas, 1989).

There is little empirical support for the popular notion that because
more women are working outside the home, they will spend less time and
effort on caregiving (Hagestad, 1986). It appears, rather, that women are
accommodating their work plans and work schedules around the needs of
their aging parents, in much the same way that they used to plan around
their dependent children's needs (Hagestad, 1986). Because only about
3% of U.S. companies have policies or programs to assist employees who
are caring for elderly parents, women care for parents before and after
work, use their vacations to provide care, switch from full- to part-time
work, find work they can do at home, or leave the work force to meet the
demands of elder care (Beck et al., 1990). Thus, women are absorbing the
costs of caring for aging parents in ways that are like other forms of caring
labor: invisible, routine, and not rewarded with societal supports (Finch
& Groves, 1983; Hagestad, 1986; Stoller, 1990).

Women provide a variety of caregiving services to aging parents that depend upon factors such as the relative health or disability of the older person, the number of informal caregivers available to share the work of caregiving, and access to formal resources (Kahana & Young, 1990). Daughters typically provide services, such as housekeeping, transportation, meal preparation, laundry, personal care, or financial support, to assist an older relative to remain as independent as possible (Walker, Pratt, Shin, & Jones, 1990).

Interpersonal and subjective factors, such as the history of the relationship between caregiver and care receiver, affect the caregiving relationship. In an analysis of obligatory and discretionary motives for caregiving in a sample of 174 caregiving daughters and their elderly mothers, Walker et al. (1990) found that more than two thirds of the daughters reported high discretionary motives for caregiving, which included affection, closeness, and enjoyment of the relationship and the centrality of the mother–daughter bond in women's lives.

A major problem in caregiving research is defining who is the caregiver (Barer & Johnson, 1990). This problem derives from the conceptualization of "fragile beings" as wholly dependent upon a stronger and wiser figure (Ainsworth, 1982; Bowlby, 1969). Kahana and Young (1990) suggest that rather than looking exclusively to the care receiver's dependency on the caregiver, reciprocity and altruism should be included in the definition of caregiving relationships. A feminist approach would also respect the integrity of both participants in the relationship. To end this conceptual confusion, Barer and Johnson (1990) suggest that the most explicit definition of caregiver should be restricted to the term "primary caregivers," defined by Stone et al. (1987) as those having total responsibility for the provision of care. By contrast, three other types of caregivers are primary caregivers who have informal help, primary caregivers with both informal and formal help, and secondary caregivers who do not have the main responsibility. Again, the role of the care receiver should not be overlooked in the definition.

Although adult daughters are the primary caregivers to aging parents, sons are not wholly absent. Sons tend to be "on the periphery" of caregiving situations (Brubaker, 1990). Daughters provide comprehensive, routine care, whether they are employed outside the home or not (Matthews, Werkner, & Delaney, 1989), and sons provide care in specific or in narrowly defined situations (Matthews & Rosner, 1988; Stoller, 1990). The type of assistance provided by sons tends to be more instrumental and singular, such as helping an older parent financially, whereas daughters provide both instrumental and expressive kinds of care.

Findings from a study of 226 older white recent widows point to important ways in which gender, marital status, and sibling relationship mediate the provision of care. O'Bryant (1988) found that sisters contributed the most viable aspects of widows' support systems. Marital status of the sisters made a difference. Unmarried sisters provided unique and important forms of assistance. They served as a role model for getting along independently, they were helpful affectively with the recent widow's bereavement and grief, and they were the siblings who most often cared for the widow when she was ill. Married sisters shared their husbands with newly widowed sisters by offering their husbands' instrumental support such as household repairs, car care, and legal assistance. These brothers-in-law also served as escort for both their wives and widowed sisters-in-law. Brothers-in-law provided slightly more support than brothers did, probably because their support was an extension of the caring relationship between sisters. O'Bryant's (1988) findings regarding the lack of assistance from brothers corroborates other studies in which men are somewhat, but not completely, absent from the support networks of widows and older people in general (Adams, 1968; Gold, 1989; Lopata, 1979).

Much of the caregiving literature focuses on the negative outcomes of the caregiving experience, particularly the burden and stress accruing to caregivers (Mancini & Blieszner, 1989). The rewards of caregiving and the experiences of care receivers are often ignored (Walker & Allen, 1991). Positive outcomes of the caregiving relationship include companionship, concern and caring, and appreciation and gratitude (Allen & Walker, 1992b). Aging mothers are not just passive recipients of care, but derive their own set of rewards from receiving care and contribute to the rewards of their caregiving daughters. The quality of the relationship and the daughter's desire to attend to her mother's needs for care suggest that the fulfillment of instrumental tasks cannot account for why daughters care.

Ruddick (1989) suggested that the notion of "attentive love," originally applied to maternal caregiving, may underlie other forms of caring labor, such as parent care. In a study of 29 caregiving daughters, Allen and Walker (1992a) used Ruddick's theory of attentive love to examine the demands of aging mothers and the motivations of their adult daughters to care for them. Considerable evidence was found for the preservative and nurturant aspects of attentive love in parent care; daughters sought to prolong their mothers' independence and, therefore, their lives. The third demand of acceptability translates less well to another context. It may be that parents are responsible for how well their children turn out, whereas adult children are not held accountable for the acceptability of their parents. Still, some daughters felt responsible for their mothers' unacceptable behaviors.

The notion of attentive love is useful for understanding women's motivations in caring for aging parents because it considers the relational context of caregiving. The unit of analysis shifts from the concrete tasks of caregiving to an emphasis on the qualitative aspects of the caregiving relationship. Attentive love stresses the actions and thoughts required to support the care recipient as a unique person, to help retain her independence, and to provide a sense of appreciation for what she also contributes to her own care as well as to her caregiver's experience.

Lesbian Mothers and the Value of Children

Lesbian mothers provide another example of how women are deconstructing and demystifying caregiving and reconstructing a woman-centered perspective on caregiving. Lesbians have always raised children, but recent societal changes are allowing more openness among lesbians about their choices to mother (Weston, 1991). Changes include the emergence of the gay liberation movement, the feminist movement, and women's own disenchantment with traditional marriage and parenting arrangements (Falk, 1989).

The greater freedom lesbians have in claiming their right to bear and rear children is not without significant compromises. Lesbians who raise children, either singularly or with another woman, violate the way that women are allowed to be mothers in our society. They are outside male control, at least within the household and in the practical matters of childrearing (Falk, 1989). Thus, lesbian motherhood and, to some extent, single motherhood are stigmatized because they occur outside the context of heterosexual marriage (Falk, 1989).

The social sanction of lesbian mothers is evident in the legal system. Lesbians are often discriminated against by the courts when they petition for custody of their children. Court decisions are often based on general assumptions, stereotypes, and myths, rather than on expert testimony or empirical research findings. These myths tend to be about lesbians as a group, that is, the myth that lesbians are mentally ill or less likely to be child oriented than heterosexual women. Myths are also associated with children raised by lesbians, that is, that they will have more problems than those raised by heterosexual women, that they are more likely to be abused, that they are likely to develop a confused gender identity or become gay themselves, and that they will be harmed by the social stigma associated with their parents' homosexuality (Falk, 1989).

Falk (1989) counters each of these myths with empirical evidence and suggests, instead, the benefits a child may experience in being raised in a lesbian household. An important benefit is developing the ability to form independent moral convictions. From her review of the empirical literature, Falk (1989) concludes that a mother's lesbianism has little, if any, effect on child outcomes. In fact, living congruently with her homosexuality usually enables the mother to be a more secure parent. Instead of stereotypes and sanctions, social and legal supports for lesbian mothers would better serve the interests of their children.

Is the Value of Children Greater When Men Are Mothers?

Many scholars advocate that men should be more involved in caregiving (Chodorow, 1978; Gerson, 1985; Rubin, 1983; Ruddick, 1982). Male involvement would be beneficial to the interests of women, children, men, and society in general. In addition to relieving women of some caregiving responsibility, caring activities provide experiences that may transform men's thinking about the conditions under which caregivers labor in our society. These insights could then be translated into change within the family and advocacy for social supports for caregivers.

Complicating the issue of the gendered nature of care are recent investigations into the culture versus the conduct of fatherhood. Risman (1989) surveyed 141 single fathers, men who had at least one child under 14 years of age living within their home. Guided by a microstructural theory of limited gender differences, Risman concluded that single fathers provided the same kind of care as mothers, meeting both instrumental and expressive needs of their children. She took a minimalist position, finding no basis for inflexible gender behavior patterns in terms of mothering and fathering.

Although single-parent fathers may provide "mothering" to their children, the presence of a female caregiver leads to a traditionalization process in which the mother becomes the primary caregiver and the father merely helps (LaRossa & LaRossa, 1989). LaRossa and LaRossa's study of husbands and wives in the context of parenting is a reminder that gender differences in behavior cannot be easily dismissed. The fathers in this study provided far less child care than their wives; indeed, the mothers were responsible for the routine tasks of caretaking, like feeding, bathing, reading stories and the like, whereas fathers' interaction time was limited to brief periods of play or to being present in the house (babysitting) while the child slept. Risman's (1989) deconstruction of the female ethic of care revealed that single fathers can provide caregiving for their children, but reliance on female labor when a female is available remains a pattern that is resistant to change (Dressel & Clark, 1990).

In a historical analysis of fatherhood trends in the 20th century, LaRossa (1988) concluded that most fathers are functionally absent but technically present. This evidence deconstructs the current belief in greater caregiving by fathers for their children. The culture of fatherhood has become more accepting of a language of male nurturance, but the conduct of fatherhood—the actual man-hours spent taking care of children—has not changed over the course of this century (LaRossa, 1988). Having children may be culturally valued, but the provision of routine care remains the work of those in a subordinate position.

The only exception to the continued gender difference in the provision of child care may be occurring among middle-class couples (LaRossa, 1988). Ehrensaft's (1987) study of men and women who choose to "mother" together suggests that when women have greater economic power in a relationship, they can bargain for more equality in caregiving. A large number of these men were in child-related fields of work. This fact suggests that experience with caring activities might predispose men to have more interest in participating in the care of their own children.

Research indicates that fathers, too, are able to discover the intrinsic rewards of caring for their children. The message is clear, however, that the conduct of fathering is still resistant to change. More than good will and the romance of fatherhood is required for actual changes in routine behaviors.

A FEMINIST VISION OF CAREGIVING

Caregiving is a central aspect of human relationships. Although there is a growing proportion of young people who plan to have no children, the majority of women and men expect to be parents. Increasing numbers of elderly and those with chronic illnesses also require ongoing care. If caregiving is a responsibility that falls, by default, to those with less power in the society, an increase in women's social and economic power will create a crisis in caregiving. How can caregiving be reconstructed to maximize the pleasure and joy involved and minimize the laborious, demanding work required? What changes must be made so that women and men can share the burdens and the rewards of caregiving more equitably and without dominating another person?

A Further Deconstruction of Caregiving

To speak only of mothering is to ignore the great diversity that caregiving can encompass. The experiences of a new mother with an infant are very different from those of a mother of four raising her last adolescent. Race, class, age, education, religiosity, marital status, sexual orientation, and income, among other factors, influence caregiving. Continuing conceptual and empirical work needs to be done to challenge and clarify prevailing notions about caregiving and to examine the developmental dynamics of caring labor.

Providing care to individuals of different ages introduces different dynamics. Children, theoretically, become more independent and require less direct care and supervision, whereas aging parents require more attention as they become less able to meet their own needs. The effects on women's lives are likely to be different in each case.

Ideally, all care would be given voluntarily. Because this is not realistic, the degree of free choice in caregiving is an important variable to consider. If a person feels trapped into being a care provider, the experience will be very different than if the role is chosen freely and knowledgeably. Women who delayed childbearing and later made explicit decisions about becoming mothers come to mothering with a readiness and a williness to give time to their children, as a 32-year-old consultant explained:

> Because I made a conscious choice and I wanted very much to have a child, I value the time I have with my daughter, enjoy her accomplishments, and willingly devote the time and energy required. By waiting until I was ready, I can view the childcare responsibilities as an experience I consciously sought. This gives me more patience, understanding and happiness as a parent than I would have had if I were younger. (Baber, 1989, p. 7)

By further deconstructing caregiving, it is possible to identify and support both those aspects of caregiving that are rewarding and choiceful for women and men and those that are difficult or unpleasant and need to be shared equitably in families.

Instilling an Ethic of Care

People learn to care through practical experience (Tronto, 1987). Bronfenbrenner and Weiss (1983) advocate a "curriculum of caring" in the schools. At the very beginning of the life course, both boys and girls need the opportunity to experience what it is like to care for others' needs so that the caregiving scripts they develop will not be infused with gender restrictions about proper caregiving roles. This could be accomplished in a variety of ways.

One approach would be to structure formal courses for both boys and girls that provide information on caregiving. Females often take home economics and childcare courses in junior or senior high school, but usually only if they are not college bound. Such courses for males have been anomalies, but hold promise if they are introduced before such activities are considered "sissy." The Collegiate School in New York City offered a course on infant care to 11- and 12-year-old boys and found that it was the second most popular course after a computer course (Levine, Pleck, & Lamb, 1983).

More informal learning can be influenced in preschool. Such learning can be provided in day care, and it is up to parents to monitor programs for assumptions that may perpetuate traditional gender-based beliefs about caregivers. Centers that provide care for both children and elderly adults may be beneficial in nurturing a broader understanding of care in young children. Exposure to many models of caregiving will elaborate their understanding of individuals as both caregivers and care recipients. The opportunity to observe caregivers, particularly women, as the object of care may help challenge the notion of women as selfless nurturers whose primary responsibility is to take care of children and men.

Remedial programs for instilling an ethic and an understanding of care are needed, as well. The Fatherhood Project (Levine et al., 1983) is designed to critically examine policies and programs that permit and encourage men to take a greater role in child care. Programs like Fathers Inc. in Boston (Doten, 1991) have been developed to try to break the cycle of irresponsibility of adolescent fathers by supporting these young men's interest in helping them care for their children and learn basic parenting skills.

Developing Social Support for Caregiving

Innovative social programs can spread the responsibility of care and equalize the costs involved in caregiving. Large corporations have been more open to developing programs to assist in the care of elderly parents than they have been in assisting with child care, probably because the executive decision maker is often a 55-year-old male (Sit, 1989). Apparently, it is easier to make one's wife responsible for children than for elderly parents. Several hundred companies have developed some type of elder-care support such as adult day care, information and referral programs, flexible benefits, and family leave (Sit, 1989). As women become more valuable as employees, they can be assertive about expectations for family support benefits.

Most companies enact programs only when there appear to be economic benefits. Corporate America is unlikely to take the initiative to support families voluntarily if doing so does not seem economically profitable. More radical social interventions are needed to address caregiving inequities.

Douvan's (1980) proposal that both men and women take a mandatory work cutback when they have children is probably not likely to gain support during a time of economic recession and concern about the competitiveness of our national work force. In 1992, there is still resistance to implementing brief, unpaid family leave, not to mention subsidizing parents to take time off to be with their children. Uncompensated child care, apparently, does not appeal to men as an alternative to paid work.

Okin (1989) proposed a legal revision to compensate caregivers of either gender. This proposal avoids the intricacies of determining the dollar value of the work. By giving both partners in a family equal legal entitlement to all money coming into the household, both the wage-earning work and the domestic support work would be acknowledged. She suggests that employers write out checks to both partners, signifying that the income is jointly earned. There would be legal and social recognition of the work that the caregiving partner contributes, as well as a power shift resulting from equalization of control over income.

Such an approach offers an elegant solution to the problem of devaluation of caregiving and domestic work in our society. Resistance to such a measure would probably be an indication of the degree to which existing inequities are functional in retaining a subordinate class of caregivers. A plan such as this is not sufficient in itself to resolve all issues related to caregiving inequities. As long as women and men do not have equal access to work opportunities and other means of accumulating social power, there will be asymmetry in caregiving responsibility.

Increasing Women's Power to Arenas beyond Caregiving

Feminists face the dilemma of validating women's historic contribution to caregiving and deconstructing how women's limited access to other sources of power and reward have reinforced women's subordination. It is not enough for individual women to change. Men need to become more involved in the practical care of fragile beings (Chodorow, 1978; Rubin, 1983), indeed, in the responsibility for their own lives when they live with women who attend to their needs in countless, invisible, and unrecognized ways (Dressel & Clark, 1990). Yet, pleas for greater male responsibility in caregiving alone are not likely to change behaviors and social structures (Ferree, 1990; Goode, 1982; Thompson, 1991). Thompson (1991) points out that because women accept men's justifications for their small contributions to family work, women reduce their sense of unfairness at doing the bulk of the caring labor in the home, even when they, too, work outside the home.

It is important for women to recognize and respond to the injustice in their family arrangements and to push for change (Thompson, 1991).

Even more important, the structural conditions of women's wage work must change before family caregiving arrangements will change (Ferree, 1990). From a feminist perspective, changes need to occur in women's innermost awareness of their own oppression, in their relationships with their intimate partners, and, collectively, through changes in social structures that impinge on personal and family lives.

The Work Women Do

We have experienced a watershed in American family life. The majority of American women now work outside the home, whether they have young children or not. In 1970, 43% of all women aged 16 and over were employed; by 1989, 57% were working (U.S. Bureau of the Census, 1991). Black women are slightly more likely (59%) than white women (57%) or Hispanic women (54%) to be in the work force. Separation or divorce increases the likelihood that women will be working. In 1988, 61% of separated and 76% of divorced women worked. Even mothers of infants are likely to be employed out of the home. Fifty-one percent of all mothers of newborns were in the work force in 1988, up from 38% in 1980 and 31% in 1976 (U.S. Bureau of the Census, 1989). Most lesbians are in the work force; they are dependent on themselves for economic subsistence, and few ever rely on the financial support of another woman or a man (Schneider, 1984).

Feminist practitioners, scholars, and clinicians are collaborating to deconstruct traditional conceptions of work and construct a more valid picture of the range and complexity of work so that it incorporates the work of women. The concept of work no longer refers only to paid employment outside the home, but encompasses the variety of reproductive or caring labor that women do for which they receive no reimbursement—housework, child care, kin care, the nurturing of interpersonal relationships, and activities in the larger community. The new definition of work also accounts for the ways in which women's lives are circumscribed by the work they do. The result is an elaborated understanding of the richness and diversity of women's contributions to family life and society.

Incisive investigations of women's work generate controversy and conflict because evidence points to the fact that men, as a class, benefit more than women from the current system. In a carefully developed

theory of gender change, Chafetz (1990) claims: "All systems of stratification are, by definition, systems of power inequity. . . . By definition, a
system of gender stratification implies superior power for men" (pp.
32–33). Whether these inequities are unintentional vestiges of traditional
gender arrangements or more calculated strategies for perpetuating a
hierarchical social structure, they limit women's opportunities for growth,
fulfillment, and self-sufficiency. To achieve, at a minimum, the basic goal
of gender equality in families, the prevailing division of labor that over-
burdens and underrewards women must be revealed and changed.

Both paid and domestic work are stratified by gender. The most
controversial aspects of women and work relate directly to women's
reproductive role in society. Childbearing is unique to women. Most
women have children and become primary caregivers, thereby limiting
their employment options and experiences. Reciprocally, differences in
women's and men's opportunities and rewards in the marketplace translate into differences in expectations regarding housework and child care.
Likewise, differential involvement in family work results in differential
availability and interest in labor market participation. "A cycle of power
relations and decisions pervades both family and workplace, and the
inequalities of each reinforce those that already exist in the other" (Okin,
1989, p. 147).

Gender equality is unlikely until there is a change both in the
division of labor in families and in the existing male advantage in society
(Chafetz, 1990). According to Chafetz, change must occur in (1) the
division of labor in the household, (2) the way in which rewards and
opportunities are distributed in paid work, and (3) the dominance of
males in elite roles as makers of law and policy, distributors of rewards and
opportunities, and creators of social definitions. Change in the domestic
division of labor is a long-run, indirect result of change in "the gender
division of labor" (Chafetz, 1990, p. 38). Therefore, equality will be
achieved only through women's acquisition of the material and nonmate-
rial resources provided by paid work. These resources would offset the
power advantage that men have in family relationships so that women
may be more successful in renegotiating the division of household work.
Women could also use their resources collectively and strategically to gain
entrance into elite roles from which they would be able to advance
women's interests and develop policies that would redistribute rewards
and opportunities more equitably.

As in other areas of women's lives, dialectical tensions make the
achievement of gender equality more difficult than it might appear in
theory. The movement of significant numbers of women into the work
force has resulted in increased power and opportunities for women that
have far-reaching implications for both the workplace and traditional

family life. Women, intentionally or unintentionally, are effecting change in the workplace and transforming relationships in their families to better accommodate the roles of breadwinner, parent, and partner. Although there may be nostalgia about the demise of the traditional wife and mother role, few speak of turning back. Women have been changed by work, and work has been changed by women.

In this chapter, we explore the various aspects of women's paid and domestic work, the interconnections between them, the explicit effects of existing patterns of work on women's lives, and the ways that women are transforming the workplace. By deconstructing women's paid and unpaid work, a more comprehensive understanding of the nuances of women's work is revealed. Consideration of questions regarding the differences between women and men in the work force reveals the ongoing dilemma of "protective policies" that jeopardize women's work opportunities. We conclude the chapter with an agenda for change, including strategies for enhancing equity in paid and unpaid work.

THE CHANGING NATURE OF WOMEN'S PAID EMPLOYMENT

Deconstructing the Ideology of Dual Spheres

The notion of separate spheres—the public, male-dominated workplace and the private, female realm of home and family—is a perspective that has dominated explorations of women's work (Bose, 1987). Men have been associated exclusively with productive labor, which refers to working for pay outside the home. Women have been associated exclusively with reproductive labor, which refers to all of the work women do in the home, such as "the buying and preparation of food and clothing, provision of emotional support and nurturance for all family members, bearing children, and planning, organizing, and carrying out a wide variety of tasks associated with their socialization" (Dill, 1988, p. 430).

The dual-spheres approach attributes the traditional division of labor to industrialization, differential ability, preference, and/or socialization. Contemporary women are depicted as working hard to bridge the abyss between these two alien cultures as they break into the paid work force. This model is useful for organizing thinking about the often conflicting values and expectations of the family and the workplace. However, because family work is generally less valued than that in the public arena, a separate-spheres approach minimizes women's contributions and reinforces the subordination of women in society (Chow & Berheide, 1988).

Bose's (1987) historical analysis of women's paid work challenges the validity of the assumptions underlying the idea of dual spheres and argues that women's work roles were never as separated from the productive work sphere as is commonly believed. Women, particularly poor and minority women, have historically participated in productive work throughout their lives, but it was often invisible because it was done in the home, on the family farm, or in a husband's business. Dill (1988) argues that for African-American, Chinese-American, and Mexican-American women of the 19th century, there was a "double day." Their productive labor, required in order to "achieve even minimal levels of family subsistence" (p. 415), was often in conflict with their reproductive labor of bearing and caring for children and the emotional maintenance of their families. The double day continues for women today, as Hochschild (1989) found in her study of women's "second shift" of reproductive work after they return home from paid employment.

Inaccurate census enumeration also obscured information about women's work status (Bose, 1987). Census methods that encouraged women to report their primary role as housewife, even if temporarily employed, and those that excluded home-based labor unless it was the primary income, minimized women's involvement in paid work roles. Although men historically may have been able to maintain the separation between work and family experiences, this was an artificial distinction for all but white, middle-class women of the late 19th and 20th centuries. Even for this group of women, the separation of spheres was a transitory phenomenon (Bose, 1987; Rothman, 1978).

Women and men have exhibited different patterns of work, but women themselves have shown great diversity in work histories, interest in work, investment in their education and career development, and perceptions of work. The great variety in the contours of women's work lives is simultaneously a testament to their adaptability to sociohistorical change and the result of their activity as change agents. Women actively make choices that enhance their employment opportunities, resisting discrimination in the workplace and, albeit slowly, transforming the experience of work in the United States. Although great gaps exist between women's and men's income and status in the labor force, women have made impressive progress, considering the context of occupational segregation, pay inequities, harassment on the job, and primary responsibility for housework and child care.

Converging Work Patterns of Women and Men

Some women have chosen to move in and out of the work force or work part-time in response to changing demands of home and children. In a rare longitudinal study exploring women's labor force activity, Moen

(1985) investigated the complex patterns of women's work histories that tend to be obscured in cross-sectional studies. She used seven waves of data from a random sample of 3,586 women involved in the Michigan Panel Study of Income Dynamics. Within the 5 years covered by the study (1972–76), 42% of the women changed their labor force status. Only 23% had continuous full-time employment, and these women were likely to be unmarried or married with no children. Education was positively related to work attachment, and women with more education were more likely than those less educated to work continuously and full-time, except for college-educated mothers of preschoolers. Women with postsecondary education were more likely to move into and out of the labor force in response to changing family needs than were less educated women. However, there were no predominant employment patterns for women who were wives and mothers regardless of their age, education, or husband's education. Moen (1985) concluded that most women are "not either in or out of the labor force but, rather, in various transitional states during the transitional years and that this movement is especially pronounced for educated women" (p. 151).

These data support the conclusion that the demands of family life impact paid employment for women. Women, and not their male partners, have shaped their paid work lives around the needs of their families when possible. These data, however, reinforce the stereotype of women, particularly women with children, as uncommitted workers who will probably not remain in the work force full-time. These data characterize employed women of the early and mid-1970s, but they may be less relevant to women of the 1990s. Great changes have occurred in women's participation in the labor market over the last decade. It is important that descriptive findings are not generalized from one cohort of women to later cohorts in ways that may distort and obscure the current situation.

Women's labor market participation is in transition from being characterized by a "double-peak" to a "single-peak" pattern (Roos, 1985). A double peak represents women's participation in paid work prior to marriage and childbearing, a drop off during childbearing years, and another peak after the childbearing years. The single peak is similar to the male pattern, which reflects increased participation through the 30s and 40s and then trails off. The change in the pattern of female employment is due partly to the trend toward delayed childbearing or having no children. Women's tendency to remain in the work force even during their childbearing years is probably a greater influence (O'Connell & Bloom, 1987).

Cross-sequential studies that follow different cohorts of women over time could provide useful information about women's work patterns and preferences. Similar data on men should also be collected. As more women are moving into the full-time work force and making substantial contributions to the support of their families, men have more opportunities for variation and diversity in their work lives—working part-time, changing jobs, or even leaving paid work for other pursuits. Each of these decisions influences the opportunities and support available to their female partners. Women's and men's work patterns are converging—more women's work histories are becoming continuous, and more men's work histories are becoming discontinuous.

Women's Commitment to Permanence in the Paid Labor Force

It is unlikely that there will be a reversal of the movement of women into the work force. The proportion of single-parent families headed by women continues to increase (Dornbusch & Gray, 1988), and in two-parent families both parents usually work to provide adequate income (Strober, 1988). In addition, working provides both intrinsic and extrinsic rewards that women are unlikely to forgo to return to more traditional roles. Women work for the same reasons that men do—economic survival, financial rewards, personal fulfillment, a sense of identity, and the opportunity to interact with others and have one's efforts acknowledged. Contrary to the belief that most women would not work if they did not have to, the American Women's Opinion Poll in 1985 revealed that only 30% of women in all age groups indicated that they would stop working if they were financially secure—a proportion similar to that of men who said they would quit working in those circumstances (Walsh, 1986). The women most likely to want to leave their jobs were those without a high school education; women in households with the highest incomes were least likely to say they would quit. Women with higher incomes are more likely to have made significant investments in their careers and to have more rewarding work lives.

The results of interviews with 50 professional women who had left positions with Fortune 500 companies further challenges pervasive myths about women and work. Vicki Tashjian, the vice president of a Delaware-based research group, announced that their data revealed most of the women had left their jobs because of lack of challenge and opportunities for growth, not because of work/family issues (Skrzycki, 1990). Although day care and maternity leave are important to most women, they are not the only—or even the most—important benefits that women want in their jobs.

Women derive material security, a sense of control over their lives, and increased power in family decision making from having an income of their own (Okin, 1989). In a study of 300 white women, Baruch,

Barnett, and Rivers (1983) found that women with paid jobs had a higher sense of mastery or control over their lives than did women who were not employed. The more women enjoyed their work, the more positive they felt about themselves and their lives. The type of work that women did was important. Having a challenging and stimulating job with a variety of opportunities to learn and make decisions contributed more to women's sense of well-being than did positive social relationships experienced in the workplace. Dull jobs with little opportunity for personal growth and challenge were strongly associated with diminished well-being.

Confronting Resistance

Men appear to respect women more when they are employed than when they are not, and they may be more influenced by a partner who works. When men in Blumstein and Schwartz's (1983) study were asked if their partners were the type of person they would like to be, 35% of men with employed wives said no compared to 47% of men whose wives were full-time housewives. These men respected achievement for its own sake and admired people who did well in competition with others and in jobs requiring skill and discipline. They were sympathetic to the daily stresses of the workplace, but lacked appreciation for the demands of housework, minimizing its importance and the time that it requires. As one man said:

> I do not think there is anything about women's work that is demanding. I just don't think it takes all that much to do it. . . . If I am around the house and I feel like it, I can probably get done in half the time it takes her to do it. I think that she tries to mystify me with it. So I show her every once in a while just how easy it is to get it done. (Blumstein & Schwartz, 1983, p. 140)

Thus, having income of one's own may be necessary but not sufficient to give women power to make changes in relationship and family decision-making patterns (Ferree, 1990). As long as caring labor is defined as women's domain, and women do not confront the resistance of their male partners, few changes can be made at home (Thompson, 1991). Women and men must work together to challenge the broader structural mandates, such as institutionalized sexism, that reinforce the assignment of unrewarding and unrewarded work to women (Ferguson, 1991).

THE SEGREGATION OF WOMEN IN THE WORK FORCE

Women's segregation into lower-status, lower-paying occupations appears to be a cross-cultural phenomenon characteristic of industrial societies. In a comparative analysis of 12 countries, Roos (1985) found that men predominated in administrative and managerial positions and high- and medium-prestige production work, whereas women held high-prestige clerical, low-prestige service, and sales jobs. Female-dominated occupations were low paying in all countries, and individuals in those positions were underpaid relative to their average educational achievement.

Women in the United States are gaining entry into fields that traditionally have been male dominated. In 1970, for example, 10% of all physicians, 5% of lawyers, and 2% of engineers were women. By 1989, these percentages had risen to 18%, 19%, and 7% respectively (U.S. Bureau of the Census, 1986, 1991). Progress in decreasing gender stratification is reflected in increased numbers of women entering these occupations. However, women are still significantly underrepresented in these high-paying professions, and little information exists about either segregation *within* professions or retention of women in these occupations over time. For example, more women may become physicians, but they may be aggregated in pediatrics or obstetrics and may leave their jobs more frequently than their male colleagues (Menaghan & Parcel, 1990).

Reciprocal to women's underrepresentation in high-status professions is their overrepresentation in low-paying occupations that are associated with females. In 1989, women still accounted for 85% of the elementary schoolteachers, 95% of the nurses, and 99% of the secretaries in our society (U.S. Bureau of the Census, 1991). There is little evidence of a shift of men into female-dominated professions, which are generally seen as lower status.

An analysis of the gender distribution of teachers at different levels reveals the correlation between status and percentage of men in a profession. Ninety-eight percent of kindergarten and preschool teachers are women, as are 85% of elementary school teachers. Yet, only 51% of secondary school teachers and 39% of those at the postsecondary level are women.

Higher-status professions, generally those dominated by males, tend to pay better than do those traditionally filled by women. Therefore, the differential distribution of male and female workers contributes to the gender gap in income. The median income for males in 1988 was $18,908 and that for women was $8,884 (U.S. Bureau of the Census, 1991). Differences in median income among groups of women of different races and classes emphasize the hierarchical distribution of income in the United States. For example, although white women had a median income of $9,103, comparative figures were $7,349 for black women and $6,990 for Hispanic women.

A Census Bureau study conducted in 1989 and 1990 revealed persistent gender and race disparities in earnings, with white men earning more than women or black men (Bovee, 1991). College-educated white men averaged $41,090, a third more than black college-educated men's earnings of $31,380. The gap between black and white college-educated women was much narrower; their salaries were $26,730 and $27,440, respectively. For individuals who had 4 years of high school but no college, earnings showed the same pattern of differences. White men earned $26,510, and black men earned $20,280; white women earned $16,910, and black women earned $16,440.

Historically, maternal status provided a basis for occupational segregation, protective labor legislation, and direct discrimination that excluded women from higher-paying jobs (Huber & Spitze, 1983). As a result, men have traditionally monopolized higher-status, higher-paying jobs and controlled the economic resources in society. The demands of family work, particularly child care, constrain women's opportunities for work and increase the likelihood that women will interrupt their work lives. However, the results of Roos's (1985) cross-cultural study indicated that the economic disadvantage of women "cannot be attributed solely or even in substantial part to sex differences in marital responsibilities [but] . . . are certainly consistent with the expectation that women are limited in their access to high paying employment because of their sex" (p. 158).

Similarly, an analysis of data from the 1981 Study of Time Use from the Institute for Social Research (Shelton & Firestone, 1989) revealed that a relatively small portion of the variation in men and women's income was explained by time devoted to housework. Time spent in household labor, including child care, directly accounted for only 8.2% of the gender gap in earnings when years of work experience, hours worked per week, occupation, industry, union membership, and education were controlled. Even though clear differences exist in men's and women's domestic responsibilities, these differences cannot be used to explain away or rationalize men's income advantage.

Gender stratification, theoretically, should decrease as women become as educated as men and secure highly valued, economically productive roles in society (Chafetz, 1990). Women are currently surpassing men in educational achievement (U.S. Bureau of the Census, 1990). In 1950, 76% of all those receiving college degrees were men. This percentage decreased to 60% in 1970. By 1987 slightly more than 50% of all college degrees were awarded to women, and women outnumbered men in colleges and universities. Only at the Ph.D. level are more men than women currently receiving degrees.

The majority of women now have "economically productive" roles in society. In 1989, 57% of all women from 16 to 64 were in the labor force (U.S. Bureau of the Census, 1991), and it is estimated that 80% of women 25 to 44 years of age will be working by 1995 (Bernstein, 1986).

Black women are slightly more likely to be in the work force (59%) than are white (57%) or Hispanic (54%) women. Hispanic men are the most likely to be working (82%), with smaller proportions of white (77%) and black (71%) men employed.

A study released in August 1991 documented biases that discriminate against minorities and women (U.S. Department of Labor, 1991). In a review of nine randomly selected Fortune 500 companies, practices were found that hindered the advancement of all but white males. According to the report, each company had barriers to advancement for women and minorities based on attitudinal or organizational bias. Companies relied on word of mouth, employee networks, or executive referral firms that tend to favor white males rather than using a formal recruiting and hiring practice. Women and minorities had less access to special programs, and companies rarely monitored for pay, special benefits, or access to opportunities.

As the result of these findings, Labor Secretary Lynn Martin pledged to use her office's power to shatter the "glass ceiling" that keeps women and minorities from advancing (Ball, 1991). However, the essence of her plan is to encourage companies to develop their own strategies to promote women, a meager and employer-friendly response that holds little promise for addressing the underlying gender discrimination.

Barriers to Corporate Advancement

The corporate environment provides a microcosm for analyzing women's situations. Such an analysis is instructive because highly educated and career-oriented women have the best preparation for competing in a male-dominated work environment. In an article on women in business in *Fortune* magazine, Fraker (1984) revealed that even though women had made progress in entry-level jobs and middle management, they hit an invisible ceiling and were not making it to top positions in major corporations. Fraker cited evidence that women do not differ from men in their managerial styles, characteristics such as assertiveness or leadership, or the importance they attach to the psychic or monetary rewards of work. She concluded that it is subtle gender discrimination that results in men moving ahead of women.

A follow-up article 6 years later on "Why Women Still Don't Hit the Top" (Fierman, 1990) reemphasized the role of discrimination in keeping women from achieving in corporations. Although 40% of managers and administrators in this country are women, there are still few who have top jobs in American corporations. Mobility is a myth for all but a few token elite. In a review of 799 of the largest industrial and service companies in the United States, *Fortune* found that among the 4,012 people listed as the highest-paid officers and directors, there were 19 women—less than half of 1% of the total. One female chief executive officer (CEO) commented, "My generation came out of graduate school 15 or 20 years ago. The men are now in line to run major corporations. The women are not. Period" (Fierman, 1990, p. 40).

The Feminist Majority Foundation released data in August 1991 from a study of corporate jobs from the level of vice president up (Ball, 1991). Only 175 (2.6%) of the 6,502 corporate officers employed in the top jobs at the Fortune 500 companies were women; only 254 (4.5%) of 5,384 of the directorships were held by women. Five women were the chief executive officers among the Fortune 500 companies. Although a comparison with data from previous studies suggests that women are making some progress, Eleanor Smeal, who heads the Feminist Majority, noted, "At the current rate of increase in executive women, it will take until the year 2466—or over 450 years—to reach equality with executive men" (Ball, 1991, p. 13).

Structural and intergroup factors interact to keep women from achieving the highest levels in American corporations, but individual factors may be involved as well. Women may not be climbing as high on the corporate ladder because they are not willing to do what is necessary to continue moving up. In a reconsideration of Matina Horner's data indicating a fear of success in women, Georgia Sassen (1980) proposed that women have a greater awareness of the emotional costs of achieving success through competition. Because the relational context is important to most women, the competitive, hierarchical environment of many institutions may require difficult choices between success and close relationships. One woman who made it to the executive vice presidential level disclosed the relational cost when she explained how she manages: "I don't take care of the house. I don't cook. I don't do marketing. I don't take my children to malls and museums. And I don't have close friends" (Fierman, 1990, p. 58).

Both *Fortune* articles suggest that men do not feel as comfortable interacting with women as they do with other men and are conditioned to treat women co-workers more as they would wives, mothers, or secretaries. When a man is making a decision about advancement of subordinates, the choice is more likely to be another man. Women get conflicting messages about being more like one of the boys, but not being too shrill, aggressive, or hard-edged (Fierman, 1990). *Fortune's* recommendation to women wanting to get ahead in the 1990s is: "Look like a lady; act like a man; work like a dog" (Fierman, 1990, p. 72).

Overt discriminatory practices are prohibited by legislation, but covert—and perhaps inadvertent—practices may be even more insidious. Women's advancement is obstructed effectively if women are not given the same types of assignments as men, are not evaluated in the same way, are not included in leisure–business activities, or are not equally supported by senior management (Fraker, 1984). Although all women have faced discrimination in the work force, lesbians face additional difficulties because of discrimination linked to their sexual orientation.

Heterosexism in the Work Force

The relationship of women and work is further complicated by the assumption that the socioemotional climate of the workplace is heterosexual. The ideology of heterosexuality assumes that "every woman is defined by, and in some way is the property of, a man (father, husband, boss); thus a woman's work is secondary since she is, will be, or ought to be supported by a man" (Schneider, 1984, p. 227). There are societal and cultural pressures for lesbians to remain closeted in the workplace because they are not defined by their relationships to men. Sexual orientation becomes a major social issue for lesbians who "live openly as competent women, independent of male support and control (as most do today)" (Chafetz, 1990, p. 89).

With few exceptions, lesbians must support themselves; thus, a significant portion of a lesbian's life is devoted to work. The centrality of work for lesbians, however, is often obscured by the assumption that being a lesbian is solely about sexual behavior. Lesbians are much more likely to be preoccupied by their work than by their sexual or affectional relations (Schneider, 1984). On the one hand, lesbians and heterosexual women share a similar work culture. Most women are concentrated in workplaces that are occupied but not controlled by other women, thus creating a homosocial female environment (Schneider, 1984). In the primarily gender-segregated workplace, women tend to share the experiences of seeking supportive friendship networks, dealing with sexual harassment from primarily male supervisors, and using the workplace to meet intimate partners. On the other hand, lesbians alone face the discrimination that comes from their sexual identity difference. The workplace is just one more arena in which lesbians must manage and confront the consequences of disclosure, the fear of potential job loss, and the homophobia of co-workers and employers (Schneider, 1984).

Only a handful of studies have explicitly addressed the work culture of lesbians. Schneider (1984) examined the everyday experience of work for lesbians in comparison to heterosexual women in order to understand ways in which lesbians manage in a relatively hostile environment. She surveyed 228 lesbian workers, ranging in age from 21 to 58; 10% were women of color. All respondents were from the eastern United States, primarily New England and the Middle Atlantic states, thus avoiding a common problem in studies of lesbians, in which samples are taken only from major metropolitan centers such as San Francisco or New York City. Their employment status was as follows: 57% were in professional or technical jobs, 11% in clerical work, 10% in administrative and managerial jobs, 7% in crafts, 7% in service, 5% in operative, and 2% in sales.

Respondents were surveyed about their friendships, intimate partnerships, experiences of sexual harassment, and openness about being a lesbian. In terms of the degree to which they were open about their identity at work, more than half were at least somewhat open, with women at the upper end of the employment hierarchy more closeted than women working in lower-status jobs. Gender proportions in the workplace were crucial in determining whether lesbians could choose to be open. In workplaces in which 80% or more of the employees were men, only 10% of the lesbians were open, whereas in heavily female-dominated workplaces, 55% of the lesbians were open. Thus, lesbians tended to be open when their workplaces were primarily female, when they had a female supervisor, when their workplaces were small, when they had lower incomes, when they had fewer supervisory responsibilities, and when they were not dealing with children as students, clients, or patients (Schneider, 1984).

Levine and Leonard (1984) also found that lesbians anticipate and experience discrimination and develop coping strategies to avoid or deal with it. These authors gathered information from 203 white, middle-class, highly educated lesbians in metropolitan New York and found that 72% of the women remained at least partially closeted because they were concerned that disclosure of their sexual orientation would jeopardize their jobs. Thirteen percent had experienced direct discrimination through firing, not being promoted, being harassed, or not being hired for a particular job.

Actual discrimination probably occurs more frequently than reported here because lesbians often face job-related discrimination without knowing the exact source. An employee's sexual orientation usually is not the explicit reason why she is fired, not promoted, or demoted. An important question for future research is the extent to which work problems can be attributed to discrimination on the basis of sexual orientation or to the general condition of women in the workplace (Schneider, 1984).

Perhaps even more pernicious are the discriminatory costs of living a double life and the anguish of concealing personal relationships from co-workers (Blumstein & Schwartz, 1983). Not being authentic about one's life in the workplace can lead to "the appearance of being boring, unfriendly, sexless, or heterosexual" (Schneider, 1984, p. 214). The more closeted lesbians in Schneider's study reported a greater sense of powerlessness, strain, and anxiety at work, whereas lesbians who were more open felt they were treated with respect because of their honesty. Nevertheless, disclosure had some negative consequences for about a quarter of the sample who felt some co-workers avoided them and that they needed to work harder to retain the respect of peers (Schneider, 1984). Thus, the relationship of lesbians to work is extremely complex and contradictory because of sexist and heterosexist biases in the workplace.

Several companies have recognized the human costs of discriminatory practices resulting from heterosexist assumptions and have taken steps to correct these biases. In 1991, the Lotus Development Corporation of Cambridge, Massachusetts, became the best-known company to provide health insurance to domestic partners of lesbian and gay male employees (Bulkeley, 1991). Following an extensive investigation and comparison of married and same-sex couples, a Lotus personnel executive concluded that "long-term, committed homosexual couples are at no greater or less risk of catastrophic illness than married heterosexuals" (Bulkeley, 1991, p. B3). Lotus officials said that their equal treatment of same-sex couples reflected Lotus's reputation for embracing diversity, as well as their desire to attract top employees with the new benefits. In addition to Lotus's pioneering efforts, another private-sector employer, the American Psychological Association, offers health insurance benefits for all unmarried cohabitating couples, that is, same-sex and heterosexual couples. Municipalities that provide such coverage are Berkeley, Santa Cruz, and San Francisco, California, and Seattle, Washington (Bulkeley, 1991).

The leadership taken by such employers in the private and public sectors is necessary for change to occur in the workplace, but such leadership alone is not enough. Lesbians and gay men must take the risks associated with disclosing their relational and affectional preferences. Individuals who benefit from heterosexual privilege need to support the full integration of lesbians, gays, and bisexual persons in the workplace as well. Current challenges to full disclosure and acceptance in the work place come mainly from the resurgence of a climate of conservatism hiding behind a profamily rhetoric designed to "defend and preserve the sanctity of the family" (Schneider, 1984, p. 226). On balance, the emergence of the gay and lesbian liberation movement has challenged the assumed naturalness of heterosexuality, put gay and lesbian civil and legal rights in the fore of its agenda, and organized substantial efforts to confront the wisdom or the need for lesbians and gays to remain closeted (Boxer, Cook, & Herdt, 1991; Brown, 1989a; D'Emilio, 1989; Melton, 1989).

A recent *Fortune* magazine article reported that a survey of 4,000 gay men and lesbians found that "more homosexuals work in science and engineering than in social services; 40% more are employed in finance and insurance than in entertainment and the arts; and ten times as many work in computers as in fashion" (Stewart, 1991, p. 43). The major problem faced by lesbian and gay professionals is "the freedom to be visible" (Stewart, 1991, p. 43). The shroud of secrecy is becoming intolerable to a new generation of women and men in corporations.

Necessary changes must come from corporate leadership in the form of visible CEO support for workplace diversity and diversity training, confrontation and elimination of homophobia in the U.S. military, the continuing growth of grassroots lesbian and gay groups within coporations and across industries, and the determination of the gay men and lesbian women of corporate America to be themselves (Stewart, 1991). Lesbians as well must recognize and challenge the classism that separates women who otherwise share the common experience of sexual orientation. Oppression can result even when lesbians work for other lesbians unless they actively confront the greater power of the class who owns the means of production versus those who are paid a wage (Weston & Rofel, 1984). Lesbians earn far less than men who are gay and must confront the multiple stigmas of classism, sexism, and heterosexism. They can use their double vision as outsiders to challenge the oppression that results from these ideologies as they actively create a more livable working environment (Schneider, 1984).

THE DILEMMA OF DIFFERENCE

Many concerns about women and work stem from beliefs about whether women should be treated the same as men in the workplace or whether they should get special consideration because they are likely to be involved with the care of young children. In the following section, two topics highlight the dialectics of difference in the workplace. First, protective legislation historically has been used to provide "special accommodations" for women by stressing their *differences* from men. Second, the situation of women in the military provides an example in which regulations have been enforced to stress *similarities* between men and women.

Protective Legislation

Biological and social differences between men and women underlie some of the thorniest problems in the workplace. Women's childbearing capacity has been a double-edged sword. Should women be given special treatment that acknowledges biological differences and their maternal role, or should men and women be treated as similarly as possible? Alpha and beta biases (Hare-Mustin & Marecek, 1990) pervade both women's work experiences and social strategies for addressing documented inequities between men and women.

Protective labor legislation passed early in the 20th century provided special treatment for women by limiting their hours, prohibiting heavy lifting and night work, requiring rest periods, and outlawing their employment in certain professions so that they would be preserved for their primary function of childbearing (Kessler-Harris, 1987; Kirp, Yudof, & Franks, 1986). This legislation ameliorated the conditions under which women worked, but it also effectively limited women's opportunities and classified them as marginal workers. Because the legislation was designed to protect white, native-born women, it further marginalized racial–ethnic women such as African-American, Chinese-American, and Mexican-American women "who experienced the oppressions of a patriarchal society but were denied the protections and buffering of a patriarchal family" (Dill, 1988, p. 418).

The phenomenon of treating females as a special class of worker perpetuates the image of a woman as inferior—one who puts family before work and who is, therefore, less committed to the workplace, less dependable, and less likely to be continually available. Such a representation invites discrimination in treatment, opportunities, and rewards. If women are different than men and must be treated in a special way, their employment entails additional costs for the employer. Employers are tempted to avoid hiring the more costly special worker or, if it cannot be avoided, to hire the person for a less important position where special treatment will have less impact. If the expectation is that women should be given "extra" leave time to have and care for children or ill family members or need more flexible working hours, women may be passed over in favor of men in the hiring process. This emphasis on the differences between women and men and the implementation of social policies to institutionalize this difference carry the risk of putting women at a serious disadvantage in the workplace. The limitation of opportunity on the basis of gender constrains individual women's right to choose and dooms them to a marginal status in economic and political arenas (Kirp et al., 1986).

Beta bias may be equally problematic. Ignoring real differences and treating men and women exactly the same paradoxically result in inequity. Because women bear children, there must be some mechanism to ensure that their employment is not jeopardized, at least during the period of childbirth and recovery. A "gender-blind" workplace carries with it other risks for women who traditionally have had responsibility for, and derived fulfillment from, caring for children and meeting family needs.

The conventional work model in the United States is white, male-oriented, and based on the assumption of a wife being available to act as a support system for the family provider (Bernard, 1981). The burden has been on women workers to make the adaptations as they try to function in an environment that rarely acknowledges or provides solutions for conflicting work and family demands.

The controversy over the implementation of special legislation to "protect" female workers has not been resolved. Policies surrounding maternity leave and the exposure of women of reproductive age to toxic substances provide two examples that demonstrate the dialectical nature of protective legislation.

The Pregnancy Discrimination Act

Prior to Title VII of the Civil Rights Act and the Pregnancy Discrimination Act of 1978, pregnant women could be fired from their jobs and lose their benefits and seniority. Motherhood could be very costly for a woman who became pregnant while she was working and took time off to bear her child and recover from childbirth. This legislation protected women's rights:

> The underlying principle of Title VII is that applicants for employment or employees be treated equally without regard to their race, sex, color, religion, or national origin. This equality of treatment encompasses the receiving of fringe benefits made available in connection with employment. (*Federal Register*, 1979, p. 23804)

The Pregnancy Discrimination Act was introduced in Congress in 1977 in response to the Supreme Court's decision in *General Electric v. Gilbert*. In this case, the Court found that denial of benefits for pregnancy-related disability and illness was not discrimination based on sex (Gelb & Palley, 1982). Pregnant women were forced to take unpaid leave, losing benefits and seniority. The Pregnancy Discrimination Act, enacted into law on October 31, 1978, amended Title VII by outlawing discrimination on the basis of pregnancy and childbirth:

> The basic principle of the Act is that women affected by pregnancy and related conditions must be treated the same as other applicants and employees on the basis of their ability or inability to work. A woman is therefore protected against such practices as being fired, or refused a job or promotion, merely because she is pregnant or has had an abortion. She usually cannot be forced to go on leave as long as she still can work. If other employees who take disability leave are entitled to get their jobs back when they are able to work again, so are women who have been unable to work because of pregnancy. (*Federal Register*, 1979, p. 23805)

In 1982, a California bank receptionist, Lillian Garland, returned from pregnancy leave to find that her job had been filled by another person. Because California law guaranteed job protection and an unpaid leave, Garland filed a complaint with the state. Although her employer, California Federal Savings and Loan (CalFed), argued that hiring temporary replacements for pregnant employees placed an unfair economic burden on employers, the formal case revolved around the Pregnancy Discrimination Act (Press, 1987). CalFed went to the U.S. District Court, which agreed with the bank that the California state law contradicted Title VII because it gave pregnant women more protection than other temporarily disabled workers.

The case ultimately went to the Supreme Court, which upheld the California statute. In the interim, however, there were ongoing debates, even among feminists, regarding whether treating pregnant women differently was fair or detrimental to women. Friedan (1986) argued that pregnancy was not just like a hernia or prostate surgery and the difference needed to be acknowledged:

> Women should not have to forfeit the choice to give birth to children in order to keep their jobs. Real equity of women with men can only be enjoyed if that difference is recognized not as something special, but as a simple fact of life requiring some simple structural accommodation in jobs and professional training. (p. 10A)

The National Organization for Women and the American Civil Liberties Union, joined by the League of Women Voters, the National Women's Political Caucus, and the National Women's Law Center, filed separate briefs arguing that the California law conflicted with Title VII. A spokeswoman for the NOW Legal Defense and Education Fund said, "It is history repeating itself. It is an invitation to discriminate. What we're talking about is adopting employment laws that say, 'you pregnant women, you're different' " (Sege, 1986, p. 98).

The concern is not only that pregnant women will be treated differently, but also that protective legislation will result, ironically, in discrimination against all women. Don Butler, president of the California Merchants and Manufacturers Association, stressed this likelihood in his comments after the Supreme Court's decision: "If I'm an employer and I've weighed all the candidates, I'm going to hire either a male or an older woman. . . . And that is discrimination we don't want, but it will happen because business people are practical" (Press, 1987, p. 24).

Auto Workers v. Johnson Controls

The most recent Supreme Court case that sought to "protect" women was *United Auto Workers v. Johnson Controls Inc.* Johnson Controls barred all women of childbearing age from its battery manufacturing operations, claiming that exposure to lead might result in fetal abnormalities. They based their action on research that found a relationship among intrauterine exposure to lead, minor fetal malformations, and delayed cognitive development (Becker, 1990).

Gloyce Qualls was a 32-year-old woman who made $350 per week at Johnson Controls welding posts on batteries (Kaplan, Cohn, & Springen, 1991). As a result of the 1982 mandatory protection policy that Johnson Controls imposed, Qualls had to prove that she was sterile or be moved to another job. She was transferred to a $200-per-week job. An appeals court upheld the policy, concluding that such a regulation was "permissible under either a business necessity defense or as a bona fide occupational qualification for employment" (Supreme Court to Review, 1990, p. 3). In March 1991, the Supreme Court struck down the mandatory exclusion policy. According to Justice Harry Blackmun:

> Decisions about the welfare of future children must be left to the parents who conceive, bear, support, and raise them rather than to the employers who hire those parents. . . . Women as capable of doing their jobs as their male counterparts may not be forced to choose between having a child and having a job. (Kaplan et al., 1991, p. 56)

Gender-specific employment policies are discriminatory when there is insufficient information to warrant differential treatment. In the *Johnson Controls* case, only women, rather than individuals of reproductive age regardless of gender, were to have been excluded from certain jobs. Such a position would be insupportable because there is evidence that exposure to lead can have negative reproductive effects on men, including impotence, sterility, decreased sperm production, and effects on sperm. In addition, their female partners are more likely to have spontaneous abortions, stillbirths, or babies with abnormalities than are women in the general population (Becker, 1990). Excluding women from a hazardous workplace does not necessarily protect the future generation if potential fathers are continuing to be exposed. Women excluded from a "hazardous" but well-paying "man's" job may be forced to seek employment in a "woman's" job that might be equally hazardous but pay lower wages and have few or no benefits (Becker, 1990). Women and their fetuses, therefore, may be at increased, rather than decreased, risk as the result of exclusion.

Policies such as these are discriminatory and demeaning and perpetuate gender stereotypes. They also imply that, given accurate, valid information, women would not be responsible enough to make decisions that would protect themselves and any children they might be carrying. The fact that women might choose to take the risk anyway demands an analysis of the context in which such decisions are made. If the alternative is a "woman's" job that pays less or is otherwise less desirable, the costs associated with the risk may not outweigh the costs of the alternative. A structural solution to the issue of exclusion is changing the manufacturing process so that no worker would need to be excluded from any job because of potential health risks.

Women and War

The 1991 war in the Persian Gulf presented some work/family issues resulting from women's growing presence in the military. The call-up of active and inactive reservists led to the deployment of single parents, women with children only a few weeks old, and, in some cases, both parents in a two-parent family (Priest, 1991). Although the military requires that all personnel have a child care plan that designates a legal guardian and child care provider, many parents were forced to make last-minute arrangements and agonizing choices between their children and their jobs. Many women enlisted in the military as a way to improve their lives and probably did not anticipate that they would be called away to war, leaving their children behind (Quinn, 1991).

Faith Stewart received notice that she was to report for army duty on the day that she went into labor (Priest, 1991). Because her husband was already in Saudi Arabia, she had to take her 2-week-old son to elderly in-laws in Florida before reporting for active duty. Another woman, Malinda Davis, a single parent, was considered absent without leave after not reporting for active duty because she could find no one to care for her 16-month-old daughter (Caldwell, 1991). Harry Zentmeyer, an army public affairs officer, called her complaint "frivolous" and stated, "The people who have tried to stay home for one stupid reason or another are three out of 400" (Caldwell, 1991, p. 13).

Amid growing concern about parents being forced to go to war and leave their children in questionable situations, several bills were introduced in the House of Representatives to exempt single parents and one parent in a family where both the mother and the father served in the military (Frisby, 1991). In spite of concern about the effects on children, there was reluctance to treat women or single parents differently from other personnel. Assistant Secretary of Defense for Force Management and Personnel Christopher Jehn argued, "This legislation threatens to turn back the clock to the time when marriage and motherhood caused a discharge or discrimination in assignment" (Frisby, 1991, p. 3).

PROSPECTS FOR REDUCING GENDER STRATIFICATION

Persistence of Stratification

Several models have been used to explain the persistence of stratification. Most explanations and intervention programs fit one of the following models: an individual deficit model, a structural–institutional model, a sex-role model, or an intergroup model (Nieva & Gutek, 1981).

In the individual deficit model, the problem is located within women and men as individuals (Nieva & Gutek, 1981). This model portrays women as lacking the necessary assertiveness, motivation, and socialization to succeed competitively with men. Women "fear success," shirk challenges, and are more emotional than rational. Male attitudes, perceptions, and insecurities result in actions that impede the progress of women. Programs that "prepare" women for the realities of the market-place or try to sensitize men to women's concerns reflect the underlying assumptions of this model. For example, corporations such as Johnson & Johnson, Gannett, and Procter & Gamble provide mentoring and career counseling for "promising" but apparently deficit female and minority employees (*Opportunity 2000*, 1988).

The structural–institutional model has as a central focus the organization of work (Nieva & Gutek, 1981). Women's aspirations, expectations, and achievements are related to their adaptive adjustments to institutions where they tend to be powerless and in the minority. In this model, the problem is not with individual women, but with the organization. Thus, the organization, rather than women themselves, require scrutiny. By changing the characteristics of work, segregation and stratification would be minimized. Suggested structural adjustments include flexible work schedules, job sharing, equal pay, and child care programs.

A third approach is based on sex-role socialization and the effect of traditional role prescriptions on work patterns, occupational choices, and job performance (Nieva & Gutek, 1981). In this model, the problem lies in the inconsistencies between the demands and behaviors required by the male-oriented workplace and the socialization experiences of women. It also includes the differential responsibility that women and men have for family work. Minnesota Mining & Mfg.'s (3-M) Visiting Technical Women Program is an example of an intervention that derives from the socialization model and operates by educating women about opportunities in fields that have attracted primarily males (*Opportunity 2000*, 1988).

The fourth model, the intergroup model, focuses on the relationships between men and women as groups (Nieva & Gutek, 1981). Because of stereotypes that exaggerate between-group differences, treatment of women and their responses characterize them as subordinate. Males have more of the resources valued by society and therefore control women's entrance into and vertical mobility within the workplace. Du-Pont, for example, offers sessions on women and men working as colleagues to sensitize each other to gender issues (*Opportunity 2000*, 1988).

A comprehensive solution to the problems that women face in their paid work experience requires a perspective that integrates aspects of all four models identified by Nieva and Gutek (1981). No single model adequately addresses the factors that constrain women's employment opportunities and experiences. The patchwork of programs now in place offers only stopgap solutions.

Women still are more likely to alter their work life to accommodate the needs of their children than are men because there is no comprehensive strategy for change, and the realities of gender stratification prevail. In a national poll that included 1,153 parents in the sample, 50% of the women said that they had quit a job to devote more time to their children; only 12% of the men had done so (Morin, 1989).

Only women who are free of child care responsibilities or can afford to have help can meet the expectations of a gender-blind workplace without considerable sacrifice. For women who want to be married and raise children, the price of a successful career in a traditional male field may be costly. In a UCLA–Korn/Ferry study of executive women, 52% had never married, were divorced, or were widowed, and 61% had no children (Fraker, 1984).

Proposals for Alleviating the Work/Family Dilemma

There have been a number of recent attempts to resolve the dialectical tension produced by the conflicting demands of work and family for women. Three are discussed here.

Mommy Track

Felice Schwartz's (1989) article, written for executives in the *Harvard Business Review*, was surely the most controversial proposal offered. Schwartz is the president of Catalyst, a not-for-profit research and advisory organization whose stated purpose is to foster the career and leadership development of women. Noting that career interruptions, plateauing, and turnover are expensive costs of employing women, Schwartz suggested a two-tiered approach to dealing with women in management. This approach involves identifying and classifying women as "career-primary" or "career-and-family." Schwartz (1989) encouraged organizations to capitalize on career-primary women and "recognize them early, accept them, and clear artificial barriers from their path to the top" (p. 69), not because these women are just like men, but because they are "just like the *best* men in the organization" (p. 70).

Schwartz (1989) also proposed that career-and-family women, although talented and creative, are "willing to trade some career growth and compensation for freedom from the constant pressure to work long hours and weekends" (p. 70). She suggested that organizations offer these women flexibility and family supports to keep them in the work force and protect the company's investment in them because women's "primary responsibility for child care is a cause of distraction, diversion, anxiety, and absenteeism—to say nothing of the persistent guilt experienced by all working mothers" (p. 72).

Although its intent may have been to encourage employers to be more flexible in helping women integrate work and family responsibilities, Schwartz's (1989) approach implicitly proposed to institutionalize discrimination. Women who chose to be mothers and have family lives would be placed on a "Mommy track" that runs only as far as middle management. Women, in general, would still be deprived of the opportunity to have the same advantages and supports as men. Furthermore, there was no provision for women to participate in the tracking of their own careers. Rather than increase women's options, Schwartz's (1989) plan would only make the covertly discriminatory rules that exist in many corporations more explicit.

Mandatory Work Cutback for New Parents

Nearly a decade before the Schwartz article, Douvan (1980) suggested that a creative approach to the work/family issue would be for both parents to be subject to a mandatory cutback in work when they had a baby. For 5 to 10 years, parents would be employed part-time so that they could share the parenting of their children. Not only would they have the benefit of spending more time with their children, but also there would be a population of people who would have more time free from paid work to participate in community activities such as PTA, church groups, and play groups. Becoming a parent would have similar impact on men's and women's lives, and children would have the benefit of increased daily contact with both parents.

The risk in such a plan is that those individuals who chose to have children would be at a disadvantage for career advancement and income enhancement compared with those who chose to remain child free and continuously employed. The child free would accrue the advantages of the traditional "sociological" male: individuals who emphasize their public work lives and enjoy the resulting power and independence (Hunt &

Hunt, 1982). Parents, both men and women, would pay the occupational costs traditionally borne by women. Instead of a tension between men and women in society, the discrepancy would be between those with and those without children:

> While the old polarization combined careers and families in the same households, the new polarization implies more complete institutional separation. While old polarizations provided a structural base for families—albeit not symmetrical or often equitable—the new polarization is more clearly anti-family in its implications. (Hunt & Hunt, 1982, p. 504)

Integrating Gynocentric Values into the Workplace

An alternative approach to the work/family dilemma is one that has been identified as "gynocentric," or woman centered, and argues that ignoring differences between men and women tends to perpetuate inequalities. Kessler-Harris (1987) proposes that a more productive concept may be to revalue women's orientation to work and adapt workplace patterns for all workers to accommodate family life, nurturance, and sharing.

This approach assumes that the responsibility for family lives and childrearing should be shared, not just by mothers and fathers, but by society as a whole. Penetrating the workplace with an ethos of compassion, care, and responsibility, Kessler-Harris (1987) asserts, would address inequalities in both home and workplace, as well as stimulate innovative thinking about housing programs, child care, and the allocation of community resources.

Bronfenbrenner and Weiss (1983) suggested five "proposterous proposals for change" in the hope of improving family and work environments and enhancing the quality of life for children. First, they suggested the introduction of a "curriculum of caring into the schools, from the earliest grades onward" (p. 406). Children should be given hands-on opportunities to engage in caring and taking responsibility for others. Second, they suggested mutual support groups for parents to extend the curriculum of caring into the adult world. Third, the prevailing pattern of work for both women and men should be curtailed to three-quarters time to allow one-quarter more time for family relationships and friendships.

Fourth, major changes need to be made in public policy and practice in areas outside the family by involving significantly more women in positions of decision making and power. Women have the experience with and knowledge about care, but males are isolated from experiences of caring or from those needing care because current caregiving arrangements involve mostly women:

As a result, men are less able to understand the needs of such persons, the circumstances in which they live, their human potential, the necessity and nature of the support systems required to realize this potential, and the very practical social and economic gains that would be achieved as a result. (Bronfenbrenner & Weiss, 1983, p. 408)

Finally, Bronfenbrenner and Weiss (1983) advocated that federal job programs for parents be continued so that all families with young children have decent incomes.

Governmental Neglect of Family Policy: Costs to Women

The intersection of work and family is a potentially explosive situation that leaves intimate partners struggling to work out equitable arrangements, women struggling with conflicting demands of work and parenting, and employers struggling to meet the new expectations of a changing work force. The United States is unique in that it is the only industrialized nation that does not have some type of governmental support designed to facilitate women working and having children. American women and families have to resolve the often conflicting demands of paid work and child care on an individual basis. Because child care is still perceived to be the responsibility of women, and mothering the primary role of women, child care has been portrayed as a working woman's problem.

To reframe the issue of child care as a problem for men, women, and society, legislative proponents of family leave introduced the Parental and Medical Leave Act of 1986. This bill proposed an unpaid leave of up to 18 weeks for mothers and fathers after the birth or adoption of a child or in the case of a serious health problem of a dependent child or parent. The bill was defeated in various forms each time it was introduced in the 3 years following its initial introduction. In 1990, legislation that would have given a 12-week, unpaid leave to parents after the birth or adoption of a child or in the case of a family member's illness was passed by both the Senate and the House of Representatives. It was vetoed by President Bush.

The Family and Medical Leave Act of 1991 presented a further compromise of the original initiative. It would provide up to 12 weeks of unpaid leave for the birth or adoption of a child or during a serious illness of a child, parent, spouse, or the employee. "Key workers," the highest-paid 10% of employees in any company with more than 50 workers would be exempt, as would all workers in companies with fewer than 50 employees. This effectively excluded about half the work force and 95% of all companies from coverage (Anderson & Ledgard, 1991, p. 3). After being passed by both the House and the Senate, the Family and Medical Leave Act was again vetoed by President Bush.

A recent study by the Institute for Women's Policy Research assessed the costs and benefits of parental leave in the United States (Hartmann & Spalter-Roth, 1989). The situations of women who took leave to care for a child or a sick family member were compared with those who had not. In addition, the economic costs to women with some kind of parental leave were compared to women with no such leave. The analysis involved data from a study of 7,000 families and compared the situations of women under age 41 who had been employed for at least 600 hours in the calendar year prior to the arrival of their child. Some women were covered by leave programs; others were not. Comparisons were also made between new mothers and their husbands and between black and white women and men.

Although the earnings profiles of women who had babies and those who did not were very similar before the birth year, new mothers' annual earning losses were $3,232 during the birth year, $5,993 the year after birth, and $5,204 the second year after birth (Hartmann & Spalter-Roth, 1989). Mothers without leave benefits lost $1,088 more in earnings in each of the 3 years than did mothers with leave. Black women had lower earnings than white women before the birth, but earned more than white women in the years after birth because they worked more hours.

The difference between men's and women's hourly earnings increased from $3.91 per hour before birth to $6.23 per hour after birth (Hartmann & Spalter-Roth, 1989). Hartmann and Spalter-Roth warn that these high costs to women of having and caring for children without adequate leave policies will have negative consequences for women's lifetime earnings and economic status in old age.

In the absence of any comprehensive family policy, support for working families has been piecemeal. Individual states have been more progressive than the federal government in implementing family leave policies. As of 1990, 30 states have some type of maternal or parental leave policy (U.S. Department of Labor Women's Bureau, 1990). The parental leave policies in 15 of these states provide benefits for fathers as well as mothers. Allowable leave time varies from 6 weeks to 1 year. Only five states partially reimburse lost salaries, usually through temporary disability insurance. Policies in 13 states cover leave to care for sick children, spouses, or parents.

The lack of any federal policy means that there is no mandate for employers to be sensitive to the needs of families. A number of companies, however, have implemented relatively generous programs to support their employees. "Family-friendly" policies, designed to increase the proportion of female employees, may be motivated more by profit than by moral concern for women or families.

The Critical Importance of Child Care

The availability of child care services is essential to women's participation in paid work, and there has been a growing demand for child care policies. More than 60% of all Americans believe that the government has an obligation to provide some child care assistance to low- and middle-income working families (Morin, 1989). Somewhat fewer, 54%, believed that employers should provide child care assistance, preferably by setting up child care facilities at or near the workplace.

There is, however, a profound ambivalence in our society about nonmaternal child care as an acceptable alternative for children. Beliefs about child development and the biological mother's critical role in caregiving that are not supported by scientific evidence contribute to that ambivalence (Scarr, Phillips, & McCartney, 1990). The belief that mothers at home provide the best care ignores research indicating that some unemployed mothers are lonely, depressed, and dysfunctional; these mothers are unlikely to provide high-quality care for their children.

A deconstruction of the concept "child care" would reveal the diversity of possible environments a child could experience in such a setting. A child care center provides a very different experience than a family day-care home or care in a relative's home. Neither home care nor out-of-home care guarantees a positive outcome for a child (Scarr et al., 1990). Scarr et al.'s review of the research on child care revealed that, in fact, there are many advantages for children in out-of-home care. Children who have attended day-care programs are often more socially competent. Low-income children in child care settings experience better intellectual and social development than they would have in home care. Child care centers foster social and intellectual skills, give instruction in recognizing and following rules, and encourage independence and self-direction (Clarke-Stewart, 1991).

Policy debates about child care have moved from concern with whether child care is necessary to more pragmatic questions about delivery and funding (Scarr et al., 1990). The cost of child care is a burden, especially for low-income families who pay as much as 20–25% of their income for child care. High-income families may pay less than 5% (Hofferth & Phillips, 1991). The financial burden of child care for poorer families has been addressed recently by federal legislation.

Legislation passed by Congress in 1990 provided funding for care of children under age 13 whose family incomes are below 75% of their state's median income (Children's Defense Fund, 1990). The plan allows parents to select any licensed, regulated, or registered provider, and the government subsidizes the costs. Funds also have been included in the legislation to improve the quality and accessibility of programs. In addition, low-income working families receive a tax credit that provides an income subsidy. In 1994, it is anticipated that the credit would be $1,825 for one child and $2,013 for families with two or more children. This legislation provides support for working families and increases the availability of child care so that women who are mothers can pursue paid work.

How Women Are Transforming the Workplace

Women are transforming the workplace by bringing new expectations and skills into the labor force (Bernstein, 1986; Lenz & Myerhoff, 1985). Both personnel policies and the work environment have been affected. Many women bring their tendency to nurture and care for others into the workplace. Their approach to work reflects this orientation—even if the job requires significant assertiveness and leadership (Baruch et al., 1983). There is some evidence that employers are beginning to recognize the value of women's interpersonal skills in business as well as service occupations (Lenz & Myerhoff, 1985).

Lunneborg (1990) interviewed 204 women in male-dominated professions to explore how men and women may do the same job differently. Electricians, engineers, police officers, carpenters, and physicians were interviewed. Four dominant themes emerged from the interviews, revealing that the major changes women brought to these traditionally male occupations were related to stereotypical gender roles and attitudes. Women demonstrated a greater service orientation to clients and a nurturant approach to co-workers. They insisted upon a more balanced lifestyle that acknowledged the interwoven connections between work and family. Women used power in a way that ensured the equitable distribution of resources and helped empower others. Women's problem-solving attitudes emphasize coordination rather than control (Rudolph, 1990).

An approach that focuses on the differences between the ways that women and men do the same jobs carries with it the risk that women's ways will be devalued. The existing differences between men and women in the labor force, however, whatever their etiology, have resulted in a demand for change. The push for structural changes and the policies that have been implemented to equalize opportunities for men and women have forced companies to acknowledge the reciprocity between work and family life. As a result, more institutions are developing programs that support working parents. Flextime, job sharing, extended maternity leave, and on-site child care—programs that benefit both men and women—have been achieved partially because of the demands and persistence of women working for change.

Part of the power that women now have to elicit change in the workplace is related to sheer numbers and economic realities. Women now comprise half of the work force in the United States. It is estimated that two thirds of the new workers coming into the job market through 1995 will be women, and most of them will become mothers sometime during their work lives (Bernstein, 1986). If employers do not tailor the work environment to the needs of women, they risk labor shortages, lost productivity, and costly turnover of trained employees. The process of change may be accelerated as women reach positions of greater power in American business and as women start more of their own businesses. Businesses run by women are more likely to adopt innovative and supportive personnel polices than are those run by men, and it is anticipated that by the turn of the century, 50% of small businesses will be owned by women (O'Connell & Bloom, 1987).

Economic realities are forcing employers to attend to the needs and interests of women. Increasing competition for the most highly qualified employees, more and more of whom are likely to be women, means that companies have to change policies to remain competitive. Employers who have restructured to address family-related issues are reporting higher employee retention rates, fewer absences, less tardiness, higher morale, and higher productivity as a result (*Opportunity 2000*, 1988).

Most of the changes that have occurred were likely to have been motivated at some level by the employer's self-interest. George Harvey, chief executive of Pitney Bowes, was quoted in an article in *Time* magazine as saying, "If we're known as a good place to work, more people will want to work here. That will make us more competitive, which means more sales and higher stock prices" (Castro, 1990, p. 51). Regardless of the motivation, these changes do facilitate the integration of work and family responsibilities. However, because demographics and profit concerns, rather than a commitment to gender equity, drive these changes, they may alleviate some of the peripheral issues without addressing the underlying problems. Such actions and benefits can be reversed quickly if doing so becomes expedient. Structural changes must be made that challenge the interlocking ways in which class, race, gender, and heterosexism serve to benefit certain groups over others so that more of the population benefits from the work environment (Ferguson, 1991).

Without broad-based structural changes, many of the work/family issues will continue to be perceived as "women's special concerns"

(*Opportunity 2000*, 1988, p. 62). If innovative work policies are marketed to and used primarily by women, it is likely that utilizing these "opportunities" will only perpetuate women's position as second-class employees. Often, the cost of using flextime, job sharing, or parental leave is the loss of benefits, seniority, and one's place in the promotion track (Bernstein, 1986). The real revolution for gender equality in the workplace will have occurred when issues at the interface of work and family are perceived to be as much the responsibility of fathers, men, and society in general as they are of mothers and women.

HOUSEHOLD WORK

Housework has been synonymous with women's work. Little seems to be happening to change that perception, even as women move into full-time jobs in the paid labor force. Housework, particularly cleaning and laundry, is generally conceptualized as a necessary evil—work that must be done but is relatively unrewarding and unpleasurable. This approach negates an important part of family life and devalues the significant social contribution women make through day-to-day care of the home (Lein, 1984). The market value for a homemaker's labor is estimated to be more than $50,000 a year (Strong & Devault, 1992).

The low status of housework has been attributed to the fact that it is unpaid labor (Lein, 1984). Even when it is paid, however, housecleaning and doing laundry are low-prestige, poorly paid jobs. In spite of the complexity and variety of skills required to run a home smoothly, many of the individual tasks (e.g., washing floors, ironing shirts, vacuuming) are labor intensive, but relatively simple to do. For those who merely "help out" with individual tasks, the job of maintaining a home may not seem very difficult. The rewarding aspect of household work comes primarily from the successful integration of the multitude of tasks, each completed with attention to standards of quality, that results in a smooth-running, comfortable environment for the family (Dressel & Clark, 1990; Lein, 1984).

A paradoxical aspect of housekeeping is that the better one is at it, the more invisible one's work becomes. Because most housework is done in isolation, a consistently spotless home, full cupboard, and endless supply of clean laundry obscure the time and energy that are spent to maintain these comforts. Such service tends to be expected as a matter of course, rather than being valued as a significant, personal contribution that a woman makes to the well-being of the family.

The development of labor-saving devices, manufactured products, and easily purchased services may be a mixed blessing to women. There is no question that technological developments like automatic washing machines, gourmet frozen food, and microwave ovens make it possible to complete certain household work more quickly and efficiently. Their availability, however, contributes to the myth that housework is really not much work anymore. Women, too, may buy into this attitude, underestimating the time it takes to do a particular task, allocating too little time, and then feeling rushed and frustrated.

Research on household labor has displayed little consistency in conceptualization, method, or analysis (Berk, 1985). The pattern of results, however, has been remarkably consistent. Women do the majority of household work whether they are employed out of the home or not (Berardo, Shehan, & Leslie, 1987; Blumstein & Schwartz, 1983; Coverman, 1985; Coverman & Sheley, 1986; Fox & Nichols, 1983; Robinson, 1988). Men whose wives are employed outside the home do not put significantly more time into household work than those whose spouses are housewives. Men in dual-career marriages have been reported to put only about one third as much time in household work as do their wives (Berardo et al., 1987; McKenry, Price, Gordon, & Rudd, 1986). These men appear to do more than other men because less total household work tends to be done in dual-career families (Pleck, 1983). Even men in allegedly role-sharing marriages devote less time to family work than do their wives, and this time is more likely to be spent in parenting than in other household responsibilities (Gilbert, 1985).

Research on housework is a "methodological morass" (Ferree, 1990). Valid data on the amount of family work that men and women actually do are difficult to come by and often plagued by methodological problems. The Survey Research Center at the University of Maryland gathered data in 1965, 1975, and 1985 about the amount of time women and men contribute to housework (Robinson, 1988). The 1985 data included responses from approximately 5,000 men and women aged 18 and older. Generally, over the 20-year period, women have cut back the amount of household work they are doing, and men have increased somewhat the hours they contribute to housework. Women, however, continue to do most of the housework, particularly if they have children. Although women with children cut the number of hours spent in housework by 8 hours between 1965 and 1985, they did 81% of the cleaning, cooking, and laundry if they had children 5 or older, and 85% if they had children under 5.

Surprisingly, unemployed women have cut back the number of hours they spend in housework even more than have women who work out of the home (Robinson, 1988). Although there is less total work done in families where the woman is employed, these woman do a greater proportion of the work that does get done. In 1985, employed women did 79%

of the traditional "female tasks" like cooking, cleaning, and laundry and 36% of the traditional "male/shared tasks" such as outdoor chores, paying bills, repairs, and gardening. Unemployed women did 70% of the "female" and 30% of the "male/shared" chores.

In interviews with 50 working couples who were predominantly white and middle class, Hochschild (1989) found that 20% of the men shared housework equally, 70% did less than half but more than one third of the work, and 10% did less than one third. Almost all of the men who shared were urged to do so by their wives. Many men alternated between cooperating and resisting; resistant strategies included doing tasks in a distracted way, waiting to be asked to help out, making "substitute offerings" of support in other areas, or reducing their needs so they could rationalize not doing the work. Hochschild attributed these resistant strategies to men's fear of losing status, fear of losing control if their wives became economically independent, and fear of losing the male privilege of being cared for by a wife.

Men who were most likely to share were those whose wives earned about the same incomes as did they. Women with advanced degrees and careers who had "cultural capital" were most likely to have husbands who shared (Hochschild, 1989). The 20% of men who did share housework expressed a genuine desire to share the responsibilities of family work, exhibiting what Hochschild called a "deep ideology" of egalitarianism— one in which beliefs and deep feelings reinforce each other.

It is revealing to look at the division of labor in same-sex couples for whom traditional gender arrangements are absent. These couples generally are committed to an egalitarian approach to both paid and family work. Lesbians expect to work to take care of themselves and are especially careful to divide household tasks equitably to avoid casting either partner in the stereotypical housekeeper role (Blumstein & Schwartz, 1983). Lesbian mothers gain more personal time if another woman lives with them because both women tend to be committed to dividing housework and child care (McGuire & Alexander, 1985).

Understanding the politics of housework requires an analysis of the work itself. Lein (1984) proposed that housework has at least three dimensions: the allowable flexibility, the opportunity for socializing, and the relative "dirtiness" of the work. She identified the flexibility of scheduling as most related to satisfaction and pleasure experienced in completing a task. Many of the responsibilities that men are accepting in families as the result of pressure for them to participate in family work are those that allow the opportunity to socialize.

Other dimensions of household work that should be considered are the repetitiveness of the task and the visibility of the completed work. Some chores such as cooking, doing dishes, changing diapers, and doing laundry need to be done over and over again. Other household work such as repairs, new projects around the house, and outdoor work are often done once or at relatively infrequent intervals. A new screen door or a television that is repaired, an addition to the house, or a new tree planted in the yard have more visible impact than a clean kitchen or an empty laundry basket; because they are unique events, they are less tedious and more satisfying when they are completed.

Comparisons of time spent in housework by men and women are even more disturbing when these five dimensions are used to look at the distribution of tasks by gender. Men do chores that allow more flexibility in timing, allow simultaneous socializing, are more visible, and are less repetitious. The University of Maryland Survey Research Center report (Robinson, 1988) documented that in 1985 women did 77% of the cooking, 83% of cleaning up after meals, 88% of the laundry and ironing, and 78% of the housecleaning that was done. Men did 74% of the outdoor chores and 82% of the repairs around the house. Men and women participated almost equally in garden and animal care and managerial tasks like bill paying.

Some of both traditionally male and female chores are "dirty," but there are qualitative differences even in dirt. Some types of dirt may actually enhance a sense of traditional masculinity. Grease from servicing a car or dirt from plowing a field are indicators of hard work and expertise and are somehow different from the dirtiness of jobs that are usually relegated to women, such as cleaning a toilet, scrubbing a floor, or changing a diaper. It is unlikely that cleaning up after other people in such a way is rewarding.

The contrasting division of men's and women's household work clearly supports the notion that women bear the burden of family work, particularly when they are employed (Berheide, 1984; Mainardi, 1972). Statistics do not reveal why this division persists. Little information is available about the negotiation process between partners as decisions— either explicit or implicit—are made about who should do what. The current approach of feminist family scholars is to see the gendered distribution of labor to be the result of a complex pattern of rules constructed and maintained through daily interactions in the home (Ferree, 1990; Thompson & Walker, 1989). Although there are numerous theories that seek to explain conceptually the division of household work, there has been little empirical research testing these theories or exploring the negotiation process; such research is essential.

Individuals' gender role beliefs are undoubtedly a powerful factor in determining their perceptions of equitable distribution of work between partners; however, Lein (1984) found that what actually goes on in families may diverge from the ideology. Using data from 23 families with children under 12 and in which the wife was employed at least part-time, she described four different family models for the allocation of tasks and responsibilities, based on variation in practice and ideology: the "add-to," the "helping-out," the "specialist," and the "partners" models.

In the *add-to* model, which is based on a strict sex segregation of responsibilities, women who work in the labor force merely add paid work to their other responsibilities. Because the male is defined as the bread-winner, the woman's income is not seen as essential to the support of the family. Women are responsible for household tasks; even if they are working, a basis for renegotiating family responsibilities is not seen. Therefore, women increase their overall amount of work, leading to a sense of overload. The women in Lein's (1984) study whose families operated on this model blamed the resulting fatigue on their lack of ability to organize their responsibilities, their low stamina, or lack of creativity in scheduling. Women's work in these families was doubly devalued. Their paid work was seen as nonessential and not particularly valuable. Because they continued to take full responsibility for household work with little or no help from other family members, this contribution to family comfort and well-being remained invisible.

The *helping-out* model acknowledges that women's paid work makes an important contribution to a family's support and that it consumes a considerable amount of time and energy. Even though housework continues to be the primary responsibility of women, men are expected to contribute and help out around the house. Women's income is essential to maintain the family's standard of living, so they can negotiate for help from other family members. Lein (1984) notes that the advantages to this model are increased flexibility for the family and decreased isolation and fatigue for the woman. In addition, both partners have an opportunity to increase their awareness of each other's contributions through paid and household work.

Families that operate on the *specialist* model believe that men and women should share responsibilities for both paid and household work, but tend to allocate tasks in a sex-segregated way. Paid work is important to women in these families because it contributes to the family's financial stability and to their own growth and development. Men in these families share responsibility for domestic work, which then becomes seen as skilled and valuable.

Lein (1984) identified only 2 in her sample of 23 couples that followed the fourth pattern, the *partners* model. Men and women in these couples believed that each should have equal opportunity to participate in paid and family work and should assume equal responsibility for these tasks. This pattern results in greater flexibility for individuals in these couples, but also requires considerable ongoing negotiation to sort out who makes decisions and who does what work.

The slippage between ideology and practice in families may be explained by a more sophisticated model that considers both micro- and macrolevel variables. Coleman (1988), using a model of gender stratification in heterosexual couples, proposes that the ratio of husband's housework relative to wife's is dependent on the woman's "net economic power." A woman's economic power is affected by both macrolevel variables, such as the male-dominated hierarchy of the economy, societal beliefs regarding gender, and birth cohort, and microlevel variables like partners' commitment to the relationship, gender ideology, and the husband's perception of the need for the wife's income. Two variables that intervene are class and the stability of the economic balance between the husband and wife. Class is important because of earnings and ideology. Because of the limited range of earnings for both women and men in unskilled, lower-status jobs, husbands' and wives' earnings are more likely to be similar than they are in middle- or upper-middle-income families. Ideology is correlated with social class in that upper-socioeconomic-level couples tend to hold more liberal and egalitarian ideals.

Based on this model, Coleman (1988) predicts that the greater a woman's net economic power, (1) the more likely her husband is to be involved in housework and child care, (2) the more likely her husband is to see himself as responsible for rather than "helping out" with chores, and (3) the more likely there is to be a more equitable distribution of the "dirtier" tasks. In Lein's (1984) typology, as women move into the provider role, their husbands are more likely to take some responsibility for housework. It may be impossible to tease apart the reciprocal effects of gender ideology and paid work to determine the direction of causation. Smith and Reid's (1986) work on role-sharing couples indicated that "the breadwinner role is the pivotal role in the role-sharing relationship. It is only when the wife shares this role that any serious consideration is given to sharing the family roles" (p. 47). However, Ferree (1988) asserts that women's actual breadwinning is a necessary but not sufficient condition for reallocating domestic responsibilities. Women must believe that they are entitled to equality and be willing to negotiate household work for change to occur.

Hochschild (1989) found, for example, that the economic logic regarding the distribution of work went only so far. Of the men in her study who earned more than their wives, 21% shared housework. If spouses earned about the same, 30% shared; if men earned less than their wives, however, none of the men shared the housework. Hochschild used the principle of balancing to explain this phenomenon. Men who lost power through having a lower salary tried to balance this loss by avoiding housework, thereby maintaining dominance over their wives. Wives participated in balancing when they felt they had too much power by virtue of their income. They restored power to their husbands by excusing them from housework so that the men would not get depressed or feel their male egos threatened.

In addition to being concerned about having too much power in the relationship, some of the traditional women in Hochschild's sample did not feel it was right for their husbands to share housework. Other women wanted a more egalitarian relationship, but sacrificed equity for fewer marital tensions—even if they had to absorb the extra work. Some of the women resisted pressing for a more equitable distribution of work because they feared conflict, the threat of divorce, and the difficulty women have supporting themselves outside marriage.

The complexity of Coleman's (1988) model suggests the difficulty in understanding and predicting the division of household work for any particular couple. It also emphasizes the importance of the continual interaction between micro- and macrolevel variables. Focusing only on macrolevel, structural variables minimizes the effect of microlevel variables and obscures women's struggle for change (Scanzoni et al., 1989). As Ferree (1988) stated:

> The changes that do occur in the household division of labor are not the automatic result of impersonal social processes, but take place in a context of ongoing roles and relationships in which individuals negotiate more or less satisfactory arrangements. (p. 10)

Like Smith and Reid (1986), Ferree (1988) proposes that change in the household division of labor is a multistage process that only begins with women's labor force participation. Change is dependent on the alteration of women's own domestic aspirations, work expectations, and active negotiation between partners. We know little about what women want in regard to the division of household labor and the extent to which they have tried to bring about change through explicit negotiation (Ferree, 1988). Women who support their families and whose work is seen as an essential contribution are empowered to renegotiate the division of housework if they are dissatisfied and want change.

Women in relationships characterized by both partners participating in breadwinning and ideological commitment to equal opportunities and responsibilities are the most likely to negotiate a satisfactory division of labor (Baruch et al., 1983; Hochschild, 1989; Lein, 1984). Power negotiations are equalized because males can no longer exploit the privilege that goes with the role of breadwinner and because women's economic dependency is not an issue (Scanzoni et al., 1989). Women with adequate personal and financial resources can bargain explicitly for their preferred outcome. They have voice in the relationship, can raise conflictual issues for negotiation, and can make a satisfactory exit from the relationship if necessary (Okin, 1989).

Paradoxically, women sometimes negotiate an unequal burden of work for themselves. The explanation for the unequal distribution of household work among heterosexual couples may be more complicated than just men's resistance to taking on additional responsibilities. Women's ambivalence about giving up family work must also be considered (Rubin, 1983). An understanding of women's preferences would help clarify, too, why women do not necessarily expect men to share household work equally, even when women are employed outside of the home. Yogev (1981), for example, reported that even though the professional women in her sample spent 60 hours each week in family work compared to the 21 hours that their husbands spent, the majority of the women believed that their spouses were doing as much as they should be. In a survey of 103 women, Ferree (1988) found that 81% believed that their husbands' share of household work was either at least fair or only a little less than they had a right to expect.

A number of factors could provide partial explanations for these paradoxical findings. Ferree (1990) proposed that housework is socially constructed as "women's work" and is simultaneously an expression of both love and subordination. Several studies have suggested that some women may be unwilling to give up control over traditional female responsibilities, even if they are overburdened (Berardo et al., 1987; Grossman et al., 1988; Haas, 1980; Hochschild, 1989; Perrucci, Potter, & Rhoades, 1978). They may be reluctant to relinquish traditionally female roles because they fear tasks may not be performed up to their standards, because of guilt feelings about abandoning what they see as their responsibilities, because they are giving up a role that is valued, or because of perceived peer pressure. This may be particularly true in regard to child care.

Women may not want to give up control over the only sphere in which they clearly have power (Rubin, 1983). Mothering places women at the center of the family by virtue of the investment of care, attention, and connection (Kranichfeld, 1988). This is a position of power and influence. Some women may be doing a greater share of child care, not just because their partners resist so much, but because it means retaining control of the internal domain of the family. This may be true of high-achieving women as well as women in more traditional occupations. Women who are highly autonomous, older, and of higher occupational status were found to have husbands who spent less time in the care of their 5-year-old children (Grossman et al., 1988), leading the researchers to speculate that these mothers might be gatekeeping, "not allowing or inviting their husbands to spend large amounts of time with the child" (p. 89).

Another reason that women may not be motivated to push for men to do more may be because men tend to take the jobs for themselves that are clean, social, and flexible (Coleman, 1988; Lein, 1984), leaving women with a greater proportion of the dirty work. In addition, because family work has always been the responsibility of women, the condition of a family's home and children are seen as a reflection on the mother rather than on the father. Women, therefore, may have higher standards for *how* tasks are done. Ferree (1988) suggests that learning to lower one's standards may be the first step in employed women's renegotiation of household work. As long as women care more, they are unlikely to be willing to share the tasks if doing so means loss of control over setting standards.

A FEMINIST VISION FOR CHANGE: TOWARD GENDER EQUALITY

Achieving equity in the work that women do is an ongoing struggle, both in the home and in the labor force. A powerful legacy of gendered expectations about responsibilities and rights continues to influence the dynamics of both paid and unpaid work. Traditional beliefs and attitudes often pervade even the most progressive thinking about how to bring about change. As a result, the variables that affect the roles and opportunities of women and men in our society are numerous and complex.

The diversity of women's life experiences, interests, and needs makes it difficult to develop a coherent action plan that will benefit women and their families without exacerbating problems in their lives (Gerson, 1985). It is clear that empowerment programs should start early in life. Gerson (1985) found in her research that women differ in their early expectations about life trajectories. Aspirations regarding domesticity or career involvement were affected by constraints and opportunities encountered in adulthood. Many women Gerson studied choose motherhood as the best option among unappealing alternatives. The apparent erosion of motherhood as an acceptable choice was viewed as a threat by women who saw their paid work as unrewarding and dead-end.

No single approach can be rigidly prescribed for all women. Sociohistorical influences provide different contexts within which women live their lives, as Stacey (1990) revealed in her ethnography of downward economic mobility in the families of working-class women in the late-20th-century postindustrial era. Further, as feminists in the United States work to facilitate the entry of more women into the labor force, women leaders in Eastern European countries are working to allow women to stay home. According to Izabella Cywinska, Poland's minister of culture and the arts, women in these countries dream "of reaching the point where they have the choice to stay home" (McGeary, 1990, p. 32).

Although there are many perspectives and stories about women's work and what women want or should have, a slide into relativity is not inevitable. Radical socialist solutions are aimed at undermining the existing system and replacing it with a new form of decentralized democractic socialism (Ferguson, 1991); more liberal solutions aimed at gender equity have also been proposed (Chafetz, 1990). Thus, informed judgments can be made about what steps are likely to benefit the greatest number of women.

We assert that a reasonable and desirable goal for feminist action is to ensure equal opportunity for both women and men to make informed choices about critical aspects of their lives. In addition, both women and men should be afforded equal access to resources that will give them the power to act on their choices. Lesbians, gays, and bisexual persons should not be discriminated against because of lack of legal marital status. A policy approach should acknowledge the diversity and heterogeneity of women and families and avoid elitist and paternalistic (or maternalistic) prescriptions about what are the "right" solutions to the dilemmas of work and family.

General objectives must be translated into specific suggestions for change. Action must be taken at both public and private levels to advance a policy agenda based on maximizing choice. Structural changes may be among the most difficult to achieve. Institutions may oppose them because of the potential cost to the employer. Those in elite positions may oppose them because they feel threatened or disenfranchised by a change in the status quo. Although existing legislative policies designed to improve the status of women have had some inadvertent costs, legal actions are an important and highly visible route to securing equity. They provide a basis for legitimizing women's claims for equal opportunity, compensation, and benefits and an avenue of redress in cases of discrimination. Among the major identified structural goals yet to be accomplished are parental leave, pay equity including equal pay for comparable work, and revised opportunity and reward structures within work organizations (Nieva & Gutek, 1981).

Structural changes may be difficult to effect, but demographics are currently in women's favor, and the opportunity for change must be seized. Employers are now disposed to enact policies that attract skilled women. By carefully analyzing the policies of various companies and making an explicit choice to work for those with the most supportive structure, skilled women can reinforce the importance of such benefits in attracting the best employees. If supportive men use the same strategy, the effect can be increased significantly.

Change at the structural level will influence, as well as be influenced by, changes in sex-role socialization. Sex-role redefinition must proceed both at the levels of childhood socialization and in ongoing adult socialization for both long- and short-run benefits for women (Nieva & Gutek, 1981). Each young woman must be educated to believe that, as an adult, she will be inherently responsible for herself and must develop the abilities to ensure her own safety and financial well-being. Young women and men must be educated about the politics of gender, the stratification of the workplace, and the assymetrical costs women pay in traditional marriages (Okin, 1989).

There is ample evidence (Weitzman, 1988) that divorce impoverishes most women who have been financially dependent on men. Although welfare may provide some relief, families for whom it is the sole income live in poverty, regardless of the state in which they live (Plotnick, 1989). The reality of contemporary life is that no woman can assume that a man, another woman, or the state will provide adequately for her welfare or that of her children.

This revelation is not particularly startling, yet young women often have a magical view of what their lives will be like, and they think that somehow everything will turn out fine (Baber & Monaghan, 1988; Baruch et al., 1983). Baruch and colleagues (1983) concluded that "if women are to be spared the consequences of an 'accidental' life, a vision of themselves as part of the world beyond home and hearth is critical" (p. 134). Women can no longer afford the luxury of not planning for their own support. For all women, the notion of paid work must become a "normal" part of their life plans. As more occupational opportunities become available to women, and they are rewarded in the same way as their male colleagues, more women will aspire to expand the traditional female role and invest in the education and training that will prepare them to compete favorably for these positions.

The most effective way of developing the ability to care for oneself is through education. Young women must be convinced that they need to educate themselves to the point that they can provide adequately for themselves. Obstacles to receiving such an education must be removed. The movement of women into higher education implies an awareness of the importance of education in achieving career goals. Increased participation in the work force means that women can be more agentic in making life choices and are less likely to be dependent on men. The possibility for interdependent relationships among partners who freely choose to be together and negotiate the responsibilities of their lives together becomes more likely.

Young women, however, seem naive about the dilemmas involved in integrating work and family roles. Most college women expect to have children, even if they are planning careers in highly demanding, male-dominated professions (Baber & Monaghan, 1988; Hare-Mustin, Bennett, & Broderick, 1983; Komarovsky, 1985). Although females are now more likely to receive counseling and advice about career-related issues, there is no formal preparation regarding choices related to parenting and work/family issues. Now that there is a critical body of women with diverse experience in making these choices, their stories can provide guidance to young women following them. The truth needs to be told about the costs and benefits of various strategies so that young women can make knowledgeable decisions and formulate workable life plans. Experienced women need to take a generative role with girls and young women.

To free young women to consider all possibilities, there must be a public deconstruction of the notion that women are primarily biological actors not responsible economically for their families, and men are primarily economic actors without biological connections and responsibilities to their families (Becker, 1990). Women and men themselves and their employers need to see both paid and domestic work as the legitimate responsibility of both genders. This attitude will allow more flexibility for both women and men in making choices that will enhance both their work lives and their family relationships.

If both partners in relationships have more equal resources, decisions are unlikely to be coerced, and partners can negotiate arrangements that they feel are truly equitable. A woman might still choose to stay home with a child for a time after his or her birth, but the family might construct such an action as a sacrifice of her work that she makes for the family, rather than her responsibility to parent (Smith & Reid, 1986). If both partners want to have children, the negotiation commences prior to pregnancy for a commitment to an equitable distribution of paid and family work or whatever allocation is desirable. Such an approach deviates from the current norm because there is explicit negotiation and counting of all types of work in the family.

A postmodern feminist perspective requires the consideration of the great diversity among women in their thinking about, interest in, experiences with, and meaning of both paid and unpaid work. Much of the existing research tends to treat women as a homogeneous group and obscures data that might help untangle some of the dilemmas that result from setting up women and men, heterosexuals and lesbians, black women and white women, and everyone else as dichotomous groups. Only sophisticated ongoing research will document accurately the true advances that women—both generally and as heterogeneous subgroups—

are making to address the existing inequities. A variety of innovative advocacy programs and social policies are needed to help families make equitable choices about work and family roles that fit their own needs.

For women who are currently experiencing the conflicting demands of work and family and are overburdened by carrying primary responsibility for housework and child care, the changes proposed might seem too little, too late. Change, unless it is revolutionary, takes time. As with any other complex and strongly entrenched social phenomenon, it may take two or three generations before we can realistically assess the effectiveness of efforts currently being made to change existing gender arrangements (Chafetz, 1990). We look to the diversity in women's lives on a daily basis to see the signs of change and the ways in which women are actively leading the transformation of social and economic practices for themselves and their families.

Empowered Women,
Empowered Families

In this book, we have conceptualized families from the point of view of women. We have examined family experiences for women by deconstructing assumptions about families as bounded units under the control of a man. We have challenged myths about intimate adult relationships, caregiving, paid and unpaid labor, reproductive concerns, and the varieties of sexual experiences among women. Our work is unconventional because we consciously have omitted a malecentric view that places dualisms such as work versus family, marriage versus alternative lifestyles, and parenthood versus childlessness in the center of analysis. Instead, we have attempted to go beyond the dichotomies that reify individual and family development.

The theoretical perspective of postmodern feminism has allowed us to take a more fluid approach to our goal of contributing to the dialogue about reconstructing families for women. Several characteristics of this perspective bear repeating. First is the issue of deconstructing boundaries and exposing them as analytic devices, not as real things. By doing this, we see that women actually have greater autonomy and more varied life experiences than can be captured by a focus on the patriarchal family, which casts women in the limited roles of wife and mother.

Second, we have described tensions and debates among some of the most important thinkers of our time: feminists. Feminists have taken on the project of deconstructing prevailing ideas about every subject, adding women's experiences into the empirical descriptions and theories, and creating new knowledge. We talk about disagreements among feminists not to problemize a feminist perspective, but to show how innovators who allow a multiplicity of viewpoints advance more adequate knowledge and ways of knowing. Perhaps the debates and tensions revealed in feminist analyses are a reaction to the secrecy and exclusion that women and their experiences have been subjected to for centuries. Freeing ourselves from boundaries and silences, feminists are speaking in multiple voices and saying contradictory, innovative, and previously unheard ideas. Third, this perspective allows us to see gender as socially constructed, not an essential quality or a rigid, dichotomous category. Rather, women's and men's experiences are mediated by pluralistic intersections of race, class, sexual orientation, age, and family connections. There is no one woman's voice or experience.

FEMINIST RECONSTRUCTIONS OF FAMILIES

What do families look and feel like when women and their concerns are taken seriously? We believe that in such families women are recognized as leaders; they are heads of households or coequals with their partners. As such, they are leading the postmodern feminist revolution in families (Stacey, 1990). These women and their partners are "people in process" (Rubin, 1983). They are deconstructing traditional scripts that are rigidly tied to gender psychologies (Okin, 1989, 1990), living in ways that are unique to late-20th-century experience (Stacey, 1990), and charting a course for a more egalitarian, less oppressive future (Ferguson, 1991).

Here are some stories of empowerment. These stories focus on how women negotiate the dialectical tensions of integrating the needs and interests of self and loved ones in a society where social and behavioral scripts are in flux. These women are writing their own future stories (Witherell & Noddings, 1991), and their experiences provide a context for our closing observations and suggestions. In the following examples, we describe aspects of the lives and families of several women, composites of women we know, who have been influenced by feminist beliefs and practices.

Marcie is a secretary for a public agency. She has three children, two of whom are under age 12. She has always worked as a secretary and returned to work 6 weeks after each child was born. She enjoys her work; the benefits are good, and she feels connected to co-workers and clients. She has seniority at her job in her grade level, takes pride in her work, and takes every opportunity to learn new skills.

Through a women's support group at her office, she came to realize that she was working a double shift—carrying a full-time workload at home and at the office. Her husband, Tony, whom she loves deeply, did little around the house and believed childrearing and housekeeping to be his wife's domain. After almost a year of trying to get him to take more responsibility for family work, Marcie finally gave Tony an ultimatum—either they get help in working out a more equitable distribution of labor or she was filing for divorce. He was shocked but realized that she was serious and would follow through.

Marcie and Tony are working with a therapist through an employee assistance program at her office. Together they are working on both pragmatic issues and the stress of trying to change well-practiced patterns of interacting. Although they still have a long way to go before their relationship could be considered equitable, Tony now does half of the housework and has primary responsibility for the children two nights a week and on Saturday, which allows Marcie to take an accounting course that she hopes will help her get a promotion. Because Marcie feels less overwhelmed by her responsibilities and is less angry at her husband, she has become more relaxed around him and feels closer and more loving toward him.

Sara and Lisa have recently bought a new house and are moving for the fourth time in 2 years. Buying a house is an important milestone in their relationship. As two women, they cannot legally marry, so the purchase of the house is a public declaration of their very personal commitment to each other. Sara's former husband has accepted a job in another state and is also moving. Although legally divorced, Sara and Jon remain connected to each other by sharing the parenting of their child. These moves are dislocating on many levels; Sara is losing a once-significant attachment as well as her ex-husband's ability to share in the daily parenting of their child. She is also losing time alone for herself and time alone with Lisa.

At the same time, all three adults feel pride and relief. Going through a divorce, rearranging households, and incorporating new partnerships and another parent for their child have been exacting experiences that now feel integrated. Divorce has settled an old question about marital struggle and power differentials and allowed formerly married partners to generate new ways of relating to each other. On the one hand, Sara and Jon are altered by the experiences of being married and divorced; old friends and relatives seem to have more problems adjusting to the relocations than they are. On the other hand, both Sara and Jon have found a new place of comfort with each other. They are friends again, and friendship is where their relationship began. Divorce has become a kinship extension, not a rupture (Stacey, 1990). Former spouses have become more than survivors of each other. A feminist model of friendship allows Sara, Lisa, and Jon to become allies in establishing nurturant homes for themselves and their child.

Loren is a child-free woman who has just completed an advanced degree. After 2 years in a commuter marriage, she has returned to live with her husband, Tom, of 10 years. She feels she is a very different person now than when she first came to graduate school and more articulate about her feminist views. Tom has become more appreciative of her feminist ideas, although his beliefs are still somewhat more conservative than hers. As she has reestablished a full-time living arrangement with him, she is less afraid than before of their differences and ready to connect again, this time as more equal partners.

Separations from loved ones lead to new ways of thinking and the ability to imagine new ways of living. As Loren prepared to end the experience of intensive study and reflection, she talked with friends in her women's group about sexuality, marriage, and commitment. She had contemplated the possibility of becoming intimate with another woman. As she tentatively processed her feelings, she clarified and confirmed her choice to remain committed to her husband in a heterosexual marriage. One friendship, in particular, with a lesbian friend, Gina, allows both to talk across their differences from a place of mutual respect and to recognize what it is in the other's life that each is not choosing for herself. Their respective choices are not about rejecting the other but about choosing what seems best for each woman. A feminist model of sisterhood guides their relationship.

Alicia is the mother of two young children. She has a Ph.D. in biology. Her husband, Paul, is also a biologist. When they were students they agreed that whoever got the best offer would take the lead in relocating the family. Their first move was for Alicia's employment; she accepted a faculty position in a nearby state while Paul worked on his degree. Then she became pregnant with their first child when he was ready to go on the job market, so their second move was for his career.

It all seemed fair and equitable. The state to which they moved, like many during the recession of the late 1980s and 1990s, experienced extreme budget cuts in higher education, however, and the position promised to Alicia in the same department did not materialize. She felt lucky that at least her husband still had a job. Their second baby was born soon after they moved, and job prospects for her in this isolated college town are grim. For the first time, Alicia began to understand that she must take her career into her own hands and look for work, no matter where it takes her. She and her husband have had continuing arguments about how to accommodate both partners' careers. Alicia proposed that they move to a larger city with more job possibilities for both of them, but Paul is resisting moving because of the advantages to him of his current position. She contemplates daily what life as a working mother with an academic career will be like and realizes that she may have to make the decision to leave the town where they live, even if her husband chooses to stay.

Terry is in her early 40s and is thinking about returning to school
to work on a degree for the first time in 20 years. Terry lives with a
man, Keith, she has known for about 8 years. They have been
together for 4 years. He moved into her house only after they had
thoroughly negotiated all aspects of the relationship. Both partners
are clear about their expectations of the relationship and are committed to each other's continuing growth and development. Terry
had been married previously to a man who had been abusive to her
and her children Kim and Scott. She left the marriage as soon as she
was able and never wants to be in a dependent relationship again.
Her daughter, Kim, is finishing high school, and Terry is ready for a
new challenge. She feels proud of her children and their relationships. She is proud that they feel close to her, solicit her advice,
and seem to be making wise choices. Together, Terry, Keith, Kim,
and Scott have chosen to become the family each has always wanted.

Yet, Terry is well aware of the threats to the lives of young women and
men that are now on the horizon. She is active in the prochoice
movement in her community and state. Her activism is guided by a vivid
memory of the 1960s, that of arranging for a friend to have an abortion
in another state. The secrecy, terror, and uncertainty of those times
remind her of the potential erosion of women's rights to reproductive
freedom. Terry, her partner, and her children feel responsible and
committed to working to ensure that those rights are retained.

The stories of Marcie, Sara, Lisa, Loren, Alicia, and Terry offer
glimpses of families working to become more egalitarian. Such families
take the needs and interests of all family members seriously. Feminist
families are those in which women's voices as well as men's, are spoken,
heard, and respected. Feminist families are safe, nurturing, and empowering to all family members; both women and men have equal access to
opportunities and resources. These families protect the rights and ensure
the well-being of the vulnerable. They challenge the arbitrary awarding of
power and privilege to certain members strictly because of gender, race,
class, sexual orientation, and age. They provide a shared understanding
and worldview about structural constraints that inhibit the well-being and
advancement of people on the basis of characteristics over which they
have little control. As these stories reveal, feminist families are locations
of struggle, change, and resolution for women and their loved ones.

Feminist families allow for multiplicity in family configurations and
relationships; they are not prescriptive about structure or process. By
placing women in the center of vision and examining families from their
perspectives, as we have attempted to do in this book, we can now define
families as changeable collectivities in which intimate associates come
together, come apart, and reconfigure across lifetimes.

Our view of feminist families differs from a traditional definition in that we do not construe the family to be a closed or semiclosed system. We know from the literature assessed in this book and our own experiences that family boundaries are far more permeable than prevailing family theory suggests. Public and private experiences are not distinct. What happens to women in society also happens to women in families (e.g., Ferree, 1990 ; Glenn, 1987; Gravenhorst, 1988; Hare-Mustin, 1978; Thompson, 1992; Thompson & Walker, 1989; Thorne, 1982).

The notion of traditional family boundaries is problematic because it allows myths to persist about how families are supposed to be and obscures what actually goes on in families. Privacy can be a mask for secrecy. A system that is shrouded in secrecy is not safe. "The protection of the privacy of a domestic sphere in which inequality exists is the protection of the right of the strong to exploit and abuse the weak" (Okin, 1989, p. 174).

From a postmodern feminist perspective, it is clear that family structures or memberships are not necessarily permanent or fixed. No unitary family form is universal or most functional (Collier, Rosaldo, & Yanagisako, 1982). In late-20th-century America, new family forms are evolving. The lack of certainty associated with "what is new" is unsettling for those who wish to return to a past time when life seemed simple and more stable.

Still, there is no turning back, no return to an outdated, mythical past (Cheal, 1991). The new families, in which women have been leaders, innovators, and creators of change, continue to proliferate (Dornbusch & Strober, 1988; Stacey, 1990). What is needed is not rejection of contemporary change but the development of creative strategies to encourage diverse groups to build bridges of understanding and common ground. Friendships, intimate partnerships, and political coalitions across gender, race, class, and sexual divisions are needed to challenge elitism and essentialism and to create a more democratic and just society for all (Ferguson, 1991).

BASIC REQUIREMENTS FOR FEMINIST FAMILIES

Our agenda for feminist families includes four critical components, which we have addressed throughout this book. These components are ideal characteristics, not yet achieved by, or for, all women and their loved ones. Yet, we believe that they are essential for women's well-being and for preparing young people to sustain well-being across the life course. They are: economic autonomy, relational equality and choice, reproductive freedom, and lifelong education for a critical consciousness.

Women's Economic Autonomy

All women need to develop the capacity to be economically autonomous. Women who are economically autonomous have a voice in their intimate relationships, can more successfully resist abuse and domination, can leave an oppressive relationship, and are more likely to achieve positions from which they can influence policies and programs that will improve the lives of women and their families (Chafetz, 1990; Okin, 1989).

Poverty is a critical issue for women and their children. The poverty rate for all families in the United States in 1990 was 10.7%; the poverty rate for female-headed families was 33.4% (U.S. Department of Commerce, 1991). Female-headed families make up 12.7% of nonpoor families, but 53% of poor families. The situation for black and Hispanic families headed by women is even more desperate. Of these families, 48% lived below the poverty level.

Those who are the least enfranchised in our society suffer the most. White, educated, elite women have been able to make the greatest strides and to retain most of the ground they have won over the past three decades; women with fewer resources have not fared as well (Piven, 1985; Sidel, 1992).

Working is, and always has been, a necessity for all women. Indeed, assessments of paid and unpaid labor show that many women work at least double shifts (Hochschild, 1989). But, how can economic autonomy be achieved when social supports are lacking for all but the most elite women? How can a woman with little control over her work environment and lack of adequate, affordable child care get ahead in a male-dominated system at home and at work? At the very minimum, government-subsidized, high-quality day care must be available to families with young children so that women are as free as men to pursue paid work (Okin, 1989).

Relational Equality and Choice

A second major requirement is that intimate relationships are reconstructed so that they are characterized by equality between partners and choice in the selection of partners. Traditional patriarchal marriage, considered to be the bedrock of stable family relationships, is not in women's best interests. Patriarchal marriages are not always characterized by outright oppression, but rather by the preeminence of men's interests and desires and the subordination of women's (Hare-Mustin, 1991). As Okin (1989) points out, women are vulnerable by marriage, and their vulnerability increases when they have young children, when they are not employed full-time, when they are not employed long-term, and when they divorce. Women in traditional relationships do more than their share of home work; working outside the home usually results in a double burden (Dressel & Clark, 1990; Ferree, 1990; Hochschild, 1989; Thompson & Walker, 1989).

Women's growing dissatisfaction with traditional marriage has led them to form and maintain intimate relationships in adulthood in alternative ways (Chafetz, 1990; Falk, 1989; Stacey, 1990). When women are economically autonomous, they need not form intimate partnerships based on dependence. They are free to choose partners who will enhance their lives, share their interests and concerns, and work with them to build a family founded on love, care, and mutual respect.

Feminists are reclaiming heterosexual marriage from its oppressive connotations (Blaisure, 1992). What does it take to reclaim marriage, a necessity that Bernard (1972) warned of two decades ago? At a minimum, it takes a profound recognition by both husband and wife of the wife's greater risk in patriarchal society. Long-term marriages that are healthy for women are based on a best-friends model (Baruch et al., 1983), in which the relationship is co-constructed by the participants and there is recognition of the interlocking systems of oppression that constrain individual lives (Blaisure, 1992; Thompson, 1989, 1991). Men who support feminist goals must be alert to this oppression and work to neutralize power imbalances both in their relationships and in society as a whole.

Women's vulnerability by marriage must be recognized and acknowledged in a profound way, not just given lip service as to awareness of inequality (Okin, 1989). Given the vulnerability that children bring to heterosexual marriage for women, men and women must recognize and overcome socialization and structural opportunities that privilege males, particularly white, heterosexual, educated, married males.

Another way in which women resist patriarchy and choose self-determination is through a committed partnership with another woman. Historically, women have always relied on other women to supplement and enhance their lives; female-centered existence is not unique to the late 20th century. What seems to have changed, however, is the openness with which women may now choose to live as lesbians (Aptheker, 1989). Lesbian partnerships are more feasible today because of various liberation movements, women's dissatisfaction with traditional marriage, and changes in law and custom (Falk, 1989).

An abiding question for feminists concerns the continuing vitality of heterosexuality for many women in spite of the knowledge that traditional marriage puts women at risk (Stacey, 1986). Although most women continue to choose intimate partnerships with men, we have argued that homosociality is central to women's lives. In the current climate of repression, denial, homophobia, and secrecy regarding sexuality, statistics about women's intimate and sexual interactions with each other and with men are inconsistent and confusing. Knowing just how vital any forms of sexuality and intimate expression are for women may not be possible. Thus, intimacy and sexuality need continual deconstruction if we are to understand relationship equality and choice from the perspectives of women.

Reproductive Freedom

Women's ability to achieve economic autonomy is constrained by lack of reproductive control. If women are to enjoy the same educational and occupational opportunities as men, they must be able to plan the timing and the number of the children they bear. Continuing threats to women's reproductive freedom not only limit their ability to control the number of children they have, but also use up an incredible amount of women's time and energy as they fend off emotional, physical, and legal attacks by those who would limit women's right to choose.

Contemporary women now understand that reproductive freedom will not be *given* to them; instead, it is a right they must actively work to secure and maintain. Activist feminists and their supporters not only need to advocate for reproductive rights, but also must take other action to ensure that women's reproductive health is given the attention it deserves. Women need to be encouraged to choose careers in women's reproductive health fields so that the necessary research and technological development is done in ways that will benefit women. A proliferation of women obstetricians, gynecologists, endocrinologists, and infertility specialists could add to the existing force of midwives, nurses, and nurse-practitioners working to give women more control over their reproductive lives.

Moen (1979) warned more than a decade ago that feminists do not fully recognize that control over reproduction is power, perhaps the ultimate power. She argued that reproduction is not just a private matter between women and their partners but in addition is a political and economic act with enormous public consequences. The heated political debates about abortion are not just about abortion, but about a tremendous power at women's fingertips. "The women's movement and feminist theory will not develop fully until the public significance of reproduction and the power implied by its control is taken into acount" (Moen, 1979, p. 134).

Lifelong Education for a Critical Consciousness

Education from preschool years—indeed from birth—is needed to prepare people for the realities of postindustrial society. Valid and far-reaching education is necessary for all young people. We must counteract the myth that young people who do not know the facts will not get into trouble. Teenage pregnancy could be reduced if "girls grew up more assertive and self-protective, and with less tendency to perceive their futures primarily in terms of motherhood" (Okin, 1989, p. 178).

As a society, we cannot afford to continue to allow each young person to learn the hard way. In Stacey's (1990) analysis of working-class family life in the late 20th century, adolescents and young adults were already pessimistic about their potential and opportunities. Many gave in to drugs and despair. More protected young people, perhaps from middle- and upper-middle-class homes, face an equally disillusioning reality, although perhaps at a later point in life.

Education about the pluralistic ways in which people configure their intimate associations is needed. Sexuality, reproduction, marriage, and parenthood are becoming disentangled. Can we afford to continue to teach a traditional view of the family as if sexuality, marriage, and parenthood go together in a neat, tidy package? New family forms need social support, not just tolerance. The legal protections provided in marriage, despite other oppressive aspects of marriage as an institution for many women, are still withheld from lesbians. We need to make marriage safer for women who live with men and offer legal protections to same-sex partners.

BEYOND ALPHA AND BETA BIAS

We turn now to the importance of transcending the false dichotomies of alpha and beta bias (Hare-Mustin & Marecek, 1990), emphasizing difference or similarity, and toward a way of thinking and living that accepts differences and similarities simultaneously. To think and live within this fruitful tension is one of the benefits of a postmodern perspective (White, 1991), particularly in terms of incorporating the ever-increasing diversity of our society. Rather than responding with fear and repression of difference, as some conservative individuals and social movements have done, we suggest, like Ferguson (1991), that postmodern women and men learn to build coalitions that respect the differences among us and, at the same time, create bridges of mutual support and assistance.

Toward the Goal of a Nongendered Society

The issue of gender difference must be addressed in any strategy that seeks to enhance the status of women in our society. This means confronting the tension between alpha and beta bias. Scott's (1990) strategy for resolving this tension requires a fundamental rejection of the categorical opposition of male/female. This rejection must be actual as well as philosophical. The most radical way of accomplishing this rejection is by moving toward a society where gender is irrelevant to opportunity, responsibility, and the ways in which lives are structured. Both theoretically and pragmatically, gender must be transformed from a central organizing principle of society to a characteristic that "would have no more relevance than one's eye color or the length of one's toes" (Okin, 1989, p. 171). In such a society, knowing whether someone was a woman or a man would tell you nothing about that person's life or responsibilities.

Lorber (1991) sketched a plan for a nongendered society in which women and men are socially interchangeable and all aspects of family life are nongendered, including sexuality, procreation, wage work, and family work. Each adult would be treated as a single unit for purposes of income, taxation, rights, and responsibilities. Permanent linkages and household arrangements would be negotiated among consenting adults. Not all women would be categorized as potential childbearers or childrearers, and responsibile adults could be involved in the care of children in a variety of other ways: egg or sperm donors, professional caretakers, educators, legal kin, or emotional supporters. All adults would get a support allowance for themselves and their children. Professional caregiving, like all work, would be compensated based on the skill involved. After the demise of the gender-segregated and stratified occupational structure, men would no longer have greater material resources and monopoly over positions of authority and political power. A plan such as this has the radical potential to challenge and disrupt the notion of difference. Although it would be a challenge to implement, it is not entirely without precedent, as the following example from Sweden indicates.

Sweden has developed a comprehensive social policy that has equality as an explicit goal of social, fiscal, and economic reform (Korpi, 1990). Principles of equality are incorporated into the Swedish constitution and there is a minister for equality affairs, an equal opportunities ombudsman, and a Commission for Research on Equality between Men and Women (Equality between, 1989). Legislation has been enacted in a systematic way to put women and men on an equal footing in marriage, lay a foundation for shared responsibility of children, and protect the financially weaker partner in the case of divorce or death of a partner.

Under the National Insurance Act, each individual is financially responsible for herself or himself and is taxed separately (Child Care in Sweden, 1990). As a result, almost the same proportion of women (82%) as men (90%) are in the work force, and women represent about half of those employed (Equality between, 1989). Sex segregation is a problem in Sweden's labor market also, but the government has funded specific programs, some beginning as early as the preschool years, to strengthen women's position in the labor market and encourage women to choose work in male-dominated occupations.

Family planning in Sweden is based on the assumption that every child should be a wanted child and that women themselves should decide on the spacing and number of children (*Equality between*, 1989). For those who choose to have children, liberal parental leave programs provide 18 months of paid leave after the birth of a child, which can be split in any way between the parents (*Child Care in Sweden*, 1990). Women can take up to 2 months of leave before delivery, and fathers have an additional 10 days of leave when a baby is born (*Equality between*, 1989).

A variety of other programs support children and families. Parents receive a child allowance for each child, regardless of the family's income (*Child Care in Sweden*, 1990). Parents are provided compensation for up to 90 days per child per year when the parent stays home to take care of a sick child 12 years of age or younger. Sweden provides public child care for children aged 18 months to 7 years and "leisure time centers" for children 7 to 12 years old.

The effects of gender have not been eradicated in Sweden, but there is greater equality between women and men than in the United States. Structural measures are not the complete solution, but they legitimate equal opportunity and provide a foundation for attitudinal and behavioral change. Policies that encourage greater participation by women in the work force and greater participation by men in family work also make it more likely that women will move into positions of power and authority in the society. In 1989, 38% of the 349 members of the Swedish Parliament were women (*Equality between*, 1989). In the United States in 1992, women fill only 6% of the 535 House and Senate seats.

Plans such as Lorber's (1991) or policies such as those implemented in Sweden are often seen as utopian or unworkable in a society as diverse as the United States. To make significant changes in social arrangements and opportunities in the United States, large numbers of people have to be motivated to work for changes that will disrupt existing power structures and reconstruct more equitable policies, programs, and relationships.

Mobilizing for Change

Paradoxically, to achieve the long-term goal of a society in which gender is irrelevant to rights, responsibilities, or opportunities, in the short run we may need to focus on and highlight gender differences. Techniques for building a coalition to advocate social restructuring toward gender equality will be of critical importance. These techniques include consciousness raising for awareness and action, electing women to political office, empowering women to gain the resources and strategies to make wise decisions, and fighting the backlash against feminist progress.

Consciousness Raising for Awareness and Action

A primary strategy for coalition building is social action to achieve critical awareness through consciousness-raising, a long-standing feminist strategy that begins at the grassroots level (Hawkesworth, 1990; hooks, 1989). In addition to intensive ongoing experiences among small groups of women, efforts would be made to raise awareness among other constituencies, including men and nonfeminist women. The goal is to stimulate critical reflection about the unquestioned acceptance of gender stereotypes and emphasize the issue of distributive justice and social remedies (Hawkesworth, 1990). The overwhelming evidence of gender inequality could be used to "articulate a feminist stand on the issues and to demonstrate the importance of public action to eliminate persisting sex inequities" (Hawkesworth, 1990, p. 188).

Okin's (1989) recommendation that children be exposed early in their educational experiences to information about existing gender inequities is consistent with the awareness-raising strategy. Research on similar consciousness-raising programs with young children suggests that well-designed interventions can be quite effective. Singer and Singer (1983) reported on a program designed to raise children's awareness of the effects of television. Lessons were designed to help children in third, fourth, and fifth grade understand the difference between fantasy and reality, how television influences feelings and ideas, and how television presents violence and to encourage children to monitor their own viewing habits. A variety of assignments explored the influence of television. Children in the program showed an increase in knowledge and discrimination skills. They learned to distinguish between real people, realistic people, and fantasy characters on television. They also learned how advertising was used to enhance products, how television programs are paid for, and where to write letters regarding programs and commercials. Programs have since been developed for children in kindergarten to second grade.

Such a model could be effective in raising gender awareness among children and teenagers. Children's ability to understand the subtle, "backstage" influences of television indicate that they would have little difficulty becoming more sophisticated in understanding the effects of gender in society. Even very young children could critically evaluate books, toys, or videos for gender bias if provided with age-appropriate analytic tools. Older children could be encouraged to generate ideas for resolving gender inequities and themselves take actions to minimize gender bias in the classroom or in their families. Parents who smoke whose children have been exposed to antismoking programs in school can attest to the passion that children and teenagers bring to their efforts to change risky behaviors to which they have been sensitized.

Consciousness-raising efforts might also target less formally organized groups. Activist feminists can take advantage of all opportunities to provide information that challenges accepted assumptions about gender and its impact. Religious groups, work groups, and social groups provide opportunities to talk about factual information that reveals gender inequities. Awareness of gender inequities is a matter of degree; those with greater awarenesss can act as facilitators for those with less awareness (Chafetz, 1990). The Swedish concept of "dig where you stand" (Eiger, 1988) might be appropriated to encourage activists to begin in their own communities and with the groups with whom they usually come in contact to raise critical gender awareness.

Activist feminists also can take advantage of current events to accelerate the consciousness-raising process. In 1992 the William Kennedy Smith rape trial, the Clarence Thomas Supreme Court confirmation hearings, and the March for Women's Rights in Washington, D.C., generated discussion and activity. The testimony by Anita Hill before the Senate Judiciary Committee regarding Thomas's alleged sexual harassment of her mobilized women across the nation and divided the current wave of the women's movement into two eras: before Anita and after Anita (Graham, 1992). Discussions of sexual harassment permeated the media after the hearings and generated broader discussions of male privilege and power. The structure of the hearings themselves, dominated by white, male senators, powerfully emphasized the absence of women in the decision-making institutions of government.

Electing Women to Political Office

There is a growing consensus that women can be assured of making sustainable progress toward social and occupational equity only by moving women into positions of political power. Hawkesworth (1990) proposed introducing a constitutional principle mandating that women hold 50% of all elective, appointive, and bureaucratic offices. In a country that could not even pass the Equal Rights Amendment, such a proposal is unlikely to be successful.

Chafetz (1990) also has argued that equal representation for women among decision makers in society is the single most important change required to bring about gender equality. She argues that equal access to these positions of power is the most intractable problem facing women, and yet, without it, all other improvements in women's status remain incomplete, fragile, and vulnerable. She asserts that women will probably have to use their resources collectively and coercively to gain representation in more than token numbers. Women may need to organize open and outspoken boycotts and strikes of institutions that do not have adequate representation of women on their boards and among their administrators. Resources also must be accumulated to support female political candidates.

Support for women candidates is gaining momentum. Within 6 months of the Clarence Thomas confirmation hearings, membership in EMILY'S List tripled, reaching 10,000 members (Loth, 1992). This group, whose name stands for "Early Money Is Like Yeast," is one of the most powerful fund-raising groups in Washington and supports Democratic women candidates who are prochoice.

Voters appear ready to elect women candidates. Several polls conducted during the months before the 1992 elections indicated that voters favored women candidates (Loth, 1992). A survey of 1,160 likely voters conducted by a Washington pollster found that voters would chose a generic woman over a man by a margin of 8 points on the issue of protecting abortion rights, 7 points on health care, 8 points on education, and 5 points on meeting the needs of the middle class. A Times-Mirror study found that 69% of the 2,022 adults polled agreed that the country would be better off with more women in Congress.

Just because a woman is in a position of power does not mean that she will act to enhance the status of women and their families. However, there is evidence that women and men have different legislative priorities. A survey of male and female state legislators conducted by the Center for the American Woman and Politics at Rutgers University found that women were more than twice as likely as men to name health care or specific women's issues like pay equity, sexual harassment, or rape counseling as their top priority (Loth, 1992).

Empowering Women to Make Wise Decisions

For women to have a sense of control over themselves and their lives, they need the ability to make decisions and to follow through in the actualization of those decisions. Because of the often inherent conflict between the needs and goals of women and those of other family members, the issue of power comes into play.

Power is a multidimensional concept that includes resources, processes, and outcomes. Most definitions of power imply that the more powerful individual is the one who prevails in some way over the other and is able to get the other to do something that she or he otherwise would not do. Most research on power in intimate relationships and families has focused on outcomes or the resources that provide the power. This focus, however, reveals little about how power really works in families. Power strategies must be explored, as well, to understand power in relationships and families.

Because resources provide the basis for power, much of the effort to increase women's power in society has focused on increasing their available resources, particularly their financial resources. Blumberg and Coleman (1989) have developed a complex model to show how a woman's net economic power affects the gender balance of power in her marriage. They consider not only the woman's income relative to that of her partner and how much control she has over any surplus, but also the various "discount factors" that tend to decrease the leverage derived from these financial resources. Among the most powerful discount factors are macrolevel variables such as societal ideologies about women's place in society, birth cohort, and class/ethnic effects. Among the microlevel variables, Blumberg and Coleman identify commitment to the relationship, personal ideology, and the perceived need for the wife's income. Their theory can be used to predict dynamics in the relationship and the way in which a woman's income affects how the couple negotiates fertility, sexual, household, and economic issues.

According to this model, a woman would have the most power if she had an income similar to that of her partner, had independent control over any surplus money available, and shared with her partner an egalitarian ideology that includes a perception that her income is as necessary to the family as the male's. In addition, both partners would be equally invested in and committed to the relationship.

Although Blumberg and Coleman (1989) offer the most comprehensive model available for considering how a woman's income relates to her relative power in the relationship, they do not explicitly include power processes in the model. They conceptualize conflict resolution strategies as consequences of the gender balance of power and refer to Chafetz's (1980) framework as a way of organizing information about power processes. Power strategies, in fact, may be consequences of the previously discussed variables, but they must be seen as more than mere outcomes. The process of power intervenes between the resources, attenuated as they may be by ideological or demographic variables, and the actual outcomes. The type of power strategy chosen—the way power is used—is one step in the process.

Chafetz (1980) proposed four strategies that individuals may use: authority, control, influence, and manipulation. Because power is a system property, there is a reciprocity in the power strategies that partners may use. Authority as a power strategy depends upon a norm accepted by both parties that supports one individual's right to prevail over the other—traditionally the husband over the wife. Control is based on the ability of one partner to bribe, threaten, or coerce the other partner into acceding. Influence means having the information, knowledge, or skills to convince or persuade the other to comply. Manipulation is a strategy that depends on having intimate knowledge about the other so that one can covertly get the other to do something without being aware of being influenced in any way. This approach stereotypically has been seen as a female way of influencing the behavior of others.

Kranichfeld (1988) proposed that the definition of power has been masculinized and that women are portrayed as powerful only when they hold the type of power that is characteristic of men. Women have been depicted as passive, dominated, and powerless—victimized by their roles in families. Although it is clear that women's educational, occupational, and political opportunities have been limited by our patriarchal society, women have nonetheless been powerful agents of change. If the concept of power is redefined as the ability to intentionally change and shape the behavior of others, women would be seen as tremendously powerful (Kranichfeld, 1988). However, many questions remain unanswered. Even if women's power based on relationships, nurturance, and connectedness is acknowledged, can it be as effective at empowering women as external, resource-based power? Is women's reluctance to give up "family power" contributing to the conflict they feel between work and family responsibilities?

Poverty, divorce, and child custody and support problems are related to women's relative lack of material resources and power in the external world. Laws now exist in all states that prohibit "wife battering," and women have banded together to provide shelter for battered women and their children. Women's groups have been instrumental in bringing about reconsideration of inadequate and unenforced child support legislation. Elaborate underground networks operate to assist women who feel the courts have failed to protect their children from sexual abuse. The result of such efforts has been empowerment for women through both legal and informal means.

Families will work better when women claim their right to live powerful lives. Power has been defined from a male perspective only (Miller, 1991). The caregiving labor of women, which is geared toward increasing the resources of others, empowering them, and facilitating their movement from fragile to strong, has gone unrecognized and unrewarded. Because the intersections of caring and power are rendered invisible in a patriarchal society, women come to experience the assertion of power in their own self-interest as potentially destructive of their relationships with others. We need to construct and sustain a dialogue about women being "powerful in ways that simultaneously enhance, rather than diminish, the power of others" (Miller, 1991, p. 205).

Fighting the Backlash against Feminist Progress

The escalation of attention to the women's movement is simultaneously exciting and chilling. As women continue to press forward in the struggle for equal rights and opportunities, there is ferment and challenge on every front. Reports in the popular press of the demise of feminism because of women's lack of interest are countered by descriptions of barriers and backlash perpetrated by those who will have much to lose when women do gain equality (Faludi, 1991).

The reports of the death of feminism are greatly exaggerated. However, the women's movement may be temporarily stalled as the opposition figuratively marshals forces to resist women's continuing demands for social and domestic equality and recognition. Faludi (1991) chronicled an antifeminist backlash fueled by the media spreading the message that the source of women's frustration and dissatisfaction is their push for independence and equality. Antifeminists promote the solution that women retreat to their homes and reinstate "family values," giving priority to their husbands' jobs and subsuming their own interests and needs to those of other family members.

There is no indication that women are giving up the struggle for equal pay, reproductive rights, equitable distribution of family work, or the right to live and work free of violence and harassment. Few women are retreating to their homes and traditional roles after they experience the potential for economic autonomy and increased social power that paid work and involvement in the public sphere offer.

There is evidence, however, that current feminist theories and ideology are not speaking to the vast majority of women. In a recent *Time* magazine poll (Gibbs, 1992), only 29% of the women contacted considered themselves feminist. Only 39% thought that the women's movement had improved their lives, and 54% said that it had had no effect. Half of the respondents did not think that the women's movement reflected the views of most women. These responses can be interpreted differently if considered in the context of replies to other questions, however. Almost all of the women (82%) believed that women today have more freedom than their mothers did, and half indicated that they enjoy their lives more than did their mothers. More than half agreed that there is a continuing need for a strong women's movement.

The continuing evolution of feminist theory and epistemology is critical as a guiding force in the development of effective strategies for bringing about change in women's lives. Action devoid of theoretical underpinnings risks missing targeted goals or degenerating into chaos. Likewise, theoretical formulations that either mystify feminism or are based on reductionistic explanations that simply pit men against women ignore the everyday realities and complexities of women's lives. Failure to make feminist theory accessible results in the academic elite talking to themselves and winding up in a theoretical and political cul-de-sac (Sassoon, 1987).

Our society is poised on what could be the verge of a new wave of feminism. Under the surface a tremendous ferment has been fueled by the Thomas/Hill hearings, the escalating assault on reproductive rights, the refusal of lesbians and gays to remain invisible, and women's slowly accumulating power to redress violations of their rights. If the energy and thrust of this activity coalesce, revolutionary change will occur. The likelihood of this struggle's success will be increased significantly if feminists join forces with other groups to resist not only sexism, but also racism, classism, ageism, and heterosexism (Ferguson, 1991).

FEMINIST COLLABORATION AND EMPOWERMENT

In many ways, the ideas we have discussed in this book reflect the world as we, the authors, are able to know it and experience it. They reflect the tensions we experience as two white, middle-class, educated women who are university professors at similar places in our careers. Even our private histories are similar in terms of age, family background, and early marital history. Although we have brought to our work differences that informed our selection of themes and ideas (e.g., early and long-term marriage, divorce, childbearing, coparenting, heterosexual and lesbian identities), our grounding in feminism provided a solidarity that allowed us to share a particular point of view.

We emphasize again that we do not speak for all women. The ideas we discuss do not represent some acknowledged truth that stands for the experiences of all women at this time in history. Yet, we have tried to be as conscious as we can of multiple experiences in order to enhance the applicability of the ideas we present. We have relied on the following methods to address multiple experiences:

1. Feminism has guided this project, with an emphasis on deconstructing myths about women's lives, critiquing much of what we know as androcentric, and working toward social change (Stanley, 1990). The politics of knowledge has been at the heart of our project, along with an explicit agenda to empower ourselves and others as we wrote—so that

the effect of our words and the ideas we raised serve an agenda of liberation rather than an agenda of mystification.

> What we find when we study women are parts of the total human potential that have not been fully seen, recognized, or valued. These are parts that have not therefore flourished, and perhaps they are precisely the ingredients that we must bring into action in the conduct of all human affairs. (Miller, 1991, p. 205)

2. We have relied on our earlier training in family studies and lifespan human development to see women not as discrete entities at one point in time, but as changing and growing in temporal contexts. The sensitivity to the multiple contexts of a life course perspective allowed us to examine continuities and discontinuities in women's lives, at the level of the individual, the group, and society in general (Bengtson & Allen, in press; Elder, 1981; Runyan, 1984).

3. We have allowed our own personal experience to guide and inform the ideas presented. Much of what we feel strongly about has been part of our own experience, and passionate scholarship is valid (Du Bois, 1983). Reflexivity and practical applications to women and their families are aspects of feminist research and scholarship that feminists, collectively, are now in a position to understand (Allen & Baber, 1992a; Thompson, 1992; Walker et al., 1988; Walker & Thompson, 1984). Feminist work is reflexive; it includes consciousness-raising, collaboration, and the understanding that not all aspects of a research project can be examined while one is conducting the study (Fonow & Cook, 1991). Feminist work attends to the affective component of research; deals explicitly with issues of caring, emotionality, and negative feelings; and is spontaneous and creative in response to the exclusion of women from androcentric scholarship (Fonow & Cook, 1991).

We end where we began: with our collaboration. Working together has helped to check our exclusionary biases and brought an exhilaration to the process of writing. Our collaboration has helped to define the ways in which we locate ourselves in the material as well as to distance us from our limitations in writing only about our own lives. Perhaps this is the greatest benefit of feminist collaborative work. Personal experience becomes a divining rod and our writing partner a guidepost in the discovery of the tensions, contradictions, and possibilities in women's lives.

Writing this book has been an empowering experience. The feminist processes of reflexivity, collaboration, spontaneity, and liberation that accompany feminist work have empowered us. By connecting personal experience with a practical agenda for change, we hope we have added to the dialogue about how women are changing and empowering their families in ever more inclusive ways.

References

Abel, E. K., & Nelson, M. K. (Eds.). (1990). *Circles of care: Work and identity in women's lives.* Albany: State University of New York Press.

Acker, J., Barry, K., & Esseveld, J. (1979). Feminism, female friends, and the reconstruction of intimacy. In H. Z. Lopata & D. Maines (Eds.), *Research in the interweave of social roles: Friendship,* (Vol. 2) (pp. 75–108). Greenwich, CT: JAI.

Acker, J., Barry, K., & Esseveld, J. (1983). Objectivity and truth: Problems in doing feminist research. *Women's Studies International Forum, 6,* 423–435.

Adams, B. N. (1968). *Kinship in an urban setting.* Chicago: Markham.

Adams, B. N. (1986). *The family: A sociological interpretation* (4th ed.). San Diego: Harcourt Brace Jovanovich.

Adams, R. G., & Blieszner, R. (Eds.). (1989). *Older adult friendship.* Newbury Park, CA: Sage.

Addelson, K. P. (1986). Moral revolution. In M. Pearsall (Ed.), *Women and values: Readings in recent feminist philosophy* (pp. 291–309). Belmont, CA: Wadsworth.

Adler, N. E., David, H. P., Major, B. N., Roth, S. H., Russo, N. F., & Wyatt, G. E. (1990). Psychological responses after abortion. *Science, 5,* 41–43.

Adult children of alcoholics: After the anger, what then? (1990, January/February). *The Family Therapy Networker, 14*(1).

Ainsworth, M. D. S. (1982). Attachment: Retrospect and prospect. In C. M. Parkes & J. Stevenson-Hinde (Eds.), *The place of attachment in human behavior* (pp. 3–30). New York: Basic.

Allen, J. (1983). Motherhood: The annihilation of women. In J. Trebilcot (Ed.), *Mothering: Essays in feminist theory* (pp. 315–330). Totowa, NJ: Rowman and Allanheld.

238

Allen, K. R. (1989). *Single women/Family ties: Life histories of older women.* Newbury Park, CA: Sage.

Allen, K. R., & Baber, K. M. (1992a). Ethical and epistemological tensions in applying a postmodern perspective to feminist research. *Psychology of Women Quarterly, 16,* 1–15.

Allen, K. R., & Baber, K. M. (1992b). Starting a revolution in family life education: A feminist vision. *Family Relations, 41,* 378–384.

Allen, K. R., & Chin-Sang, V. (1990). A lifetime of work: The context and meanings of leisure for aging black women. *The Gerontologist, 30,* 734–739.

Allen, K. R., & Walker, A. J. (1992a). Attentive love: A feminist perspective on the caregiving of adult daughters. *Family Relations, 41,* 284–289.

Allen, K. R., & Walker, A. J. (1992b). A feminist analysis of interviews with elderly mothers and their daughters. In J. F. Gilgun, K. Daly, & G. Handel (Eds.), *Qualitative methods in family research* (pp. 198–214). Newbury Park, CA: Sage.

Allen, W. R. (1978). The search for applicable theories of black family life. *Journal of Marriage and the Family, 40,* 117–129.

Amaro, H. (1990). Women's reproductive rights in the age of AIDS: New threats to informed choice. In M. G. Fried (Ed.), *From abortion to reproductive freedom: Transforming a movement* (pp. 245–254). Boston, MA: South End Press.

Andersen, M. L. (1988). *Thinking about women* (2nd ed). New York: Macmillan.

Anderson, C., & Ledgard, L. (1991, September 19). Compromise bill on family leave offered in Senate. *The Boston Globe,* p. 3.

Aptheker, B. (1989). *Tapestries of life: Women's work, women's consciousness, and the meaning of daily experience.* Amherst: University of Massachusetts Press.

Arendell, T. (1990). Divorce: A women's issue. In C. Carlson (Ed.), *Perspectives on the family: History, class, and feminism* (pp. 479–495). Belmont, CA: Wadsworth.

Arguelles, L., & Rich, B. R. (1989). Homosexuality, homophobia, and revolution: Notes toward an understanding of the Cuban lesbian and gay male experience. In M. B. Duberman, M. Vicinus, & G. Chauncey, Jr. (Eds.), *Hidden from history: Reclaiming the gay and lesbian past* (pp. 441–455). New York: NAL Books.

Associated Press. (1988, February 7). Excerpts from landmark surrogate ruling. *The Boston Globe,* p. 19.

Atwater, L. (1982). *The extramarital connection: Sex, intimacy, and identity.* New York: Irvington.

Baber, K. (1989, November). *Elaborating our understanding of motherhood: The experiences of delayed childbearing women.* Paper presented at the National Council on Family Relations annual meeting, New Orleans.

Baber, K. M., & Dreyer, A. S. (1986). Gender-role orientations in older child-free and expectant couples. *Sex Roles, 14,* 501–512.

Baber, K. M., & Monaghan, P. (1988). College women's career and motherhood expectations: New options, old dilemmas. *Sex Roles, 19,* 189–203.

Bachrach, C. A. (1984). Contraceptive practices among American women, 1973–1982. *Family Planning Perspectives, 16,* 253–259.

Ball, K. (1991, August 26). Study: Less than 3% of Fortune 500 top jobs go to women. *The Boston Globe,* p. 13.

Barer, B. M., & Johnson, C. L. (1990). A critique of the caregiving literature. *The Gerontologist, 30,* 26–29.

Barry, K. (1979). *Female sexual slavery.* Englewood Cliffs, NJ: Prentice Hall.

Bart, P. B. (1971). Sexism in social science: From the iron cage to the gilded cage, or, the perils of Pauline. *Journal of Marriage and the Family, 33,* 734–745.

Baruch, G., Barnett, R., & Rivers, C. (1983). *Life prints.* New York: McGraw-Hill.

Beck, M., Kantrowitz, B., Beachy, L., Hager, M., Gordon, J., Roberts, E., & Hammill, R. (1990, July 16). Trading places. *Newsweek,* pp. 48–54.

Becker, M. E. (1990). Can employers exclude women to protect children? *Journal of the American Medical Association, 264,* 2113–2117.

Bell, A. P., & Weinberg, M. S. (1978). *Homosexualities: A study of diversity among men and women.* New York: Simon & Schuster.

Belsky, J. (1990). Parental and nonparental child care and children's socioemotional development: A decade in review. *Journal of Marriage and the Family, 52,* 885–903.

Bem, S. L. (1987). Gender schema theory and its implications for child development: Raising gender-aschematic children in a gender-schematic society. In M. R. Walsh (Ed.), *The psychology of women: Ongoing debates* (pp. 226–245). New Haven: Yale University Press.

Bengtson, V. L., & Allen, K. R. (in press). The life-course perspective applied to families over time. In P. Boss, W. Doherty, R. LaRossa, W. Schumm, & S. Steinmetz (Eds.), *Sourcebook of family theories and methods: A contextual approach.* New York: Plenum.

Berardo, D. H., Shehan, C. L., & Leslie, G. R. (1987). A residue of tradition: Jobs, careers, and spouses' time in housework. *Journal of Marriage and the Family, 49,* 381–390.

Berheide, C. W. (1984). Women's work in the home: Seems like old times. *Marriage and Family Review, 7,* 37–55.

Berk, S. F. (1985). *The gender factory.* New York: Plenum.

Berkowitz, G. S., Skovron, M. L., Lapinski, R. H., & Berkowitz, R. (1990). Delayed childbearing and the outcome of pregnancy. *New England Journal of Medicine, 322,* 659–664.

Bernard, J. (1972). *The future of marriage.* New York: Bantam.

Bernard, J. (1977). Infidelity: Some moral and social issues. In R. Libby & R. Whitehurst (Eds.), *Marriage and alternatives* (pp. 131–146). Glenview, IL: Scott, Foresman.

Bernard, J. (1981). *The female world.* New York: Free Press.

Bernstein, A. (1986, October 6). Business starts tailoring itself to suit working women. *Business Week,* pp. 50–54.

Berrien, J. (1990). Pregnancy and drug use: Incarceration is not the answer. In

M. G. Fried (Ed.), *From abortion to reproductive freedom: Transforming a movement* (pp. 263–267). Boston, MA: South End Press.

Best, S., & Kellner, D. (1991). *Postmodern theory: Critical interrogations.* New York: Guilford Press.

Bianchi, S., & McArthur, E. (1991). Family disruption and economic hardship: The short-run picture for children. *Current Population Reports* (Series P–70, No. 23). Washington, D.C.: U.S. Government Printing Office.

Bianchi, S., & Spain, D. (1986). *American women in transition.* New York: Russell Sage Foundation.

Blaisure, K. R. (1992). *Feminists and marriage: A qualitative analysis.* Unpublished doctoral dissertation, Virginia Polytechnic Institute and State University, Blacksburg.

Blieszner, R., & Adams, R. G. (1992). *Adult friendship.* Newbury Park, CA: Sage.

Bloom, D. E. (1984). Delayed childbearing in the United States. *Population Research and Policy Review, 3,* 103–139.

Bloom, D. E. (1986, August). *The labor market consequences of delayed childbearing.* Paper presented at the annual meeting of the American Statistical Association, Chicago, IL.

Blumberg, R. L., & Coleman, M. T. (1989). A theoretical look at the gender balance of power in the American couple. *Journal of Family Issues, 10,* 225–250.

Blumstein, P., & Schwartz, P. (1983). *American couples: Money, work, sex.* New York: William Morrow.

Blumstein, P., & Schwartz, P. (1989). Intimate relationships and the creation of sexuality. In B. J. Risman & P. Schwartz (Eds.), *Gender in intimate relationships* (pp. 120–129). Belmont, CA: Wadsworth.

Blumstein, P., & Schwartz, P. (1990). Intimate relationships and the creation of sexuality. In D. P. McWhirter, S. A. Sanders, & J. M. Reinisch (Eds.), *Homosexuality/ heterosexuality* (pp. 307–320). New York: Oxford University Press.

Bograd, M. (1988a). Feminist perspectives on wife abuse: An introduction. In K. Yllo & M. Bograd (Eds.), *Feminist perspectives on wife abuse* (pp. 11–26). Newbury Park, CA: Sage.

Bograd, M. (1988b). Enmeshment, fusion or relatedness? A conceptual analysis. In L. Braverman (Ed.), *A guide to feminist family therapy* (pp. 65–80). Binghamton, NY: Harrington Park.

Bordo, S. (1990). Feminism, postmodernism, and gender-scepticism. In L. J. Nicholson (Ed.), *Feminism/ Postmodernism* (pp. 133–156). New York: Routledge.

Bose, C. E. (1987). Dual spheres. In B. B. Hess & M. M. Ferree (Eds.), *Analyzing gender* (pp. 267–285). Newbury Park, CA: Sage.

Boss, P., & Thorne, B. (1989). Family sociology and family therapy: A feminist linkage. In M. McGoldrick, C. Anderson, & R. Walsh (Eds.), *Women in families: A framework for family therapy* (pp. 78–96). New York: W. W. Norton.

Bovee, T. (1991, September 20). Wide gap found in earnings by white, black college grads. *The Boston Globe*, pp. 1, 7.

Bowlby, J. (1969). *Attachment and loss: Vol. 1. Attachment*. New York: Basic.

Boxer, A. M., Cook, J. A., & Herdt, G. (1991). Double jeopardy: Identity transitions and parent-child relations among gay and lesbian youth. In K. Pillemer & K. McCartney (Eds.), *Parent-child relations throughout life* (pp. 59–92). Hillsdale, NJ: Lawrence Erlbaum.

Boyd, S. L., & Treas, J. (1989). Family care of the frail elderly: A new look at "women in the middle." *Women's Studies Quarterly, 1 & 2*, 66–74.

Boyer, D., & Fine, D. (1992). Sexual abuse as a factor in adolescent pregnancy and child maltreatment. *Family Planning Perspectives, 24*, 4–11.

Boylan, A. M. (1978). Evangelical womanhood in the nineteenth century: The role of women in Sunday schools. *Feminist Studies, 4*, 62–80.

Bram, S. (1978). Through the looking glass: Voluntary childlessness as a mirror for contemporary changes in the meaning of parenthood. In W. B. Miller & L. F. Newman (Eds.), *The first child and family formation* (pp. 368–391). Chapel Hill, NC: Carolina Population Center.

Brick, P. (1989). Toward a positive approach to sexuality education. *SIECUS Report, 17*, 1–3.

Bridenthal, R. (1982). The family: The view from a room of her own. In B. Thorne & M. Yalom (Eds.), *Rethinking the family: Some feminist questions* (pp. 225–239). New York: Longman.

Bristow, A. R., & Pearn, P. L. (1984). Comment on Krieger's "Lesbian identity and community: Recent social science literature." *Signs, 9*, 729–732.

Bronfenbrenner, U., & Weiss, H. B. (1983). Beyond policies without people: An ecological perspective on child and family policy. In E. F. Zigler, S. L. Kagan, & E. Klugman (Eds.), *Children, families and government: Perspectives on American social policy* (pp. 393–414). London: Cambridge University Press.

Brown, L. S. (1989a). New voices, new visions: Toward a lesbian/gay paradigm for psychology. *Psychology of Women Quarterly, 13*, 445–458.

Brown, L. S. (1989b). Beyond thou shalt not: Thinking about ethics in the lesbian therapy community. In E. D. Rothblum & E. Cole (Eds.), *Loving boldly: Issues facing lesbians* (pp. 13–25). Binghamton, NY: Harrington Park.

Brown, L. S. (1990, Winter). What's addiction got to do with it: A feminist critique of codependence. *Psychology of Women* (Newsletter of Division 35, American Psychological Association), *17*(1), 1, 3–4.

Brubaker, T. H. (1990). Families in later life: A burgeoning research area. *Journal of Marriage and the Family, 52*, 959–981.

Bulkeley, W. M. (1991, October 25). Lotus creates controversy by extending benefits to partners of gay employees. *The Wall Street Journal*, pp. B1, B3.

Bumpass, L. L., & Sweet, J. A. (1989). National estimates of cohabitation. *Demography, 26*, 615–625.

Bumpass, L. L., Sweet, J. A., & Cherlin, A. (1991). The role of cohabitation in declining rates of marriage. *Journal of Marriage and the Family, 53*, 913–927.

Burch, B. (1987). Barriers to intimacy: Conflicts over power, dependency, and nurturing in lesbian relationships. In Boston Lesbian Psychologies Collective (Eds.), *Lesbian psychologies* (pp. 126–141). Urbana: University of Illinois Press.

Burgess, A. W., & Holmstrom, L. L. (1974). *Rape: Victims of crisis.* Bowie, MD: Brady.

Butler, J. R., & Burton, L. M. (1990). Rethinking teenage childbearing: Is sexual abuse a missing link? *Family Relations, 39,* 73–80.

Caldwell, J. (1991, January 3). Reservist, citing child, fails to report. *The Boston Globe,* p. 13.

Califia, P. (1988). *Sapphistry: The book of lesbian sexuality* (3rd ed., rev.). Tallahassee, FL: Naiad Press.

Cancian, F. (1987). *Love in America: Gender and self-development.* Cambridge: Cambridge University Press.

Castro, J. (1990, Fall). Get set: Here they come *Time* (Special Issue: *Women: The Road Ahead*), pp. 50–52.

Chafetz, J. S. (1980). Conflict resolution in marriage: Toward a theory of spousal strategies and marital dissolution rates. *Journal of Family Issues, 1,* 397–421.

Chafetz, J. S. (1990). *Gender equity: An integrated theory of stability and change.* Newbury Park, CA: Sage.

Chambers-Shiller, L. V. (1984). *Liberty, a better husband: Single women in America: The generations of 1780–1840.* New Haven: Yale University Press.

Cheal, D. (1991). *Family and the state of theory.* Toronto: University of Toronto Press.

Cheal, D. J. (1989). Women together: Bridal showers and gender membership. In B. J. Risman & P. Schwartz (Eds.), *Gender in intimate relationships* (pp. 87–93). Belmont, CA: Wadsworth.

Cherlin, A. J. (1981). *Marriage, divorce, remarriage.* Cambridge, MA: Harvard University Press.

Child care in Sweden. (1990). Stockholm, Sweden: The Swedish Institute.

Children's Defense Fund. (1990, October 30). *New federal child care legislation.* Washington, DC: Children's Defense Fund.

Chodorow, N. (1978). *The reproduction of mothering.* Berkeley: University of California Press.

Chow, E. N., & Berheide, C. (1988). The interdependence of family and work: A framework for family life education, policy, and practice. *Family Relations, 37,* 23–28.

Chu, S. Y., Buehler, J. W., & Berkelman, R. L. (1990). Impact of the human immunodeficiency virus epidemic on mortality in women of reproductive age, United States. *Journal of the American Medical Association, 264,* 225–229.

Clarke-Stewart, K. A. (1991). A home is not a school: The effects of child care on children's development. *Journal of Social Issues, 47,* 105–123.

Clunis, D. M., & Green, G. D. (1988). *Lesbian couples.* Seattle: Seal Press.

Cohen, J. B. (1985). *Parenthood after 30?* Lexington, MA: D. C. Heath.

Colby, A., & Damon, W. (1987). Listening to a different voice: A review of Gilligan's *In a different voice.* In M. R. Walsh (Ed.), *The psychology of women: Ongoing debates* (pp. 321–329). New Haven: Yale University Press.

Cole, R., & Cooper, S. (1991). Lesbian exclusion from HIV/AIDS education:

Ten years of low-risk identity and high-risk behavior. *SIECUS Report, 19,* 18–23.

Coleman, E. (1981/82). Developmental stages of the coming out process. *Journal of Homosexuality, 7,* 31–43.

Coleman, E., Hoon, P. W., & Hoon, E. F. (1983). Arousability and sexual satisfaction in lesbian and heterosexual women. *The Journal of Sex Research, 19,* 58–73.

Coleman, M. T. (1988). The division of household labor. *Journal of Family Issues, 9,* 132–148.

Colker, R. (1991). Feminism, sexuality, and authenticity. In M. A. Fineman & N. S. Thomadsen (Eds.), *At the boundaries of law: Feminism and legal theory* (pp. 135–147). New York: Routledge.

Collier, J., Rosaldo, J. Z., & Yanagisako, S. (1982). Is there a family? New anthropological views. In B. Thorne (Ed.), *Rethinking the family: Some feminist questions* (pp. 25–39). New York: Longman.

Collins, P. H. (1989). The social construction of black feminist thought. *Signs, 14,* 745–773.

Collins, P. H. (1990). *Black feminist thought: Knowledge, consciousness, and the politics of empowerment.* Boston: Unwin Hyman.

Collins, R. (1988). *Sociology of marriage & the family: Gender, love, and property* (2nd ed.). Chicago: Nelson-Hall.

Committee on Small Business. (1989, March 9). *Consumer protection issues involving in vitro fertilization clinics.* Transcript of hearing before the Subcommittee on Regulation, Business Opportunities, and Energy. Washington, DC: U.S. Government Printing Office.

Cook, B. W. (1979). Female support networks and political activism. In N. F. Cott & E. H. Pleck (Eds.), *A heritage of her own* (pp. 412–444). New York: Touchstone.

Corea, G. (1985). *The mother machine.* Boston: Harper & Row.

Coverman, S. (1985). Explaining husbands' participation in domestic labor. *The Sociological Quarterly, 26,* 81–97.

Coverman, S., & Sheley, J. F. (1986). Change in men's housework and childcare time: 1965–1975. *Journal of Marriage and the Family, 48,* 413–422.

Crawford, S. (1987). Lesbian families: Psychosocial stress and the family-building process. In Boston Lesbian Psychologies Collective (Ed.), *Lesbian psychologies* (pp. 195–214). Urbana: University of Illinois Press.

Crooks, R., & Baur, K. (1990). *Our sexuality* (5th ed.). New York: Benjamin-Cummings.

Cuber, J. F., & Harroff, P. B. (1965). *The significant Americans.* New York: Appleton-Century.

Dahlerup, D. (1987). Confusing concepts—confusing reality: A theoretical discussion of the patriarchal state. In A. S. Sassoon (Ed.), *Women and the state* (pp. 93–127). London: Hutchinson.

Daniels, P., & Weingarten, K. (1979, Spring). A new look at the medical risks in late childbearing. *Women and Health,* pp. 17–21.

Daniels, P., & Weingarten, K. (1982). *Sooner or later: The timing of parenthood in adult lives.* New York: W. W. Norton.

Davidson, J. K., & Darling, C. A. (1988). The sexually experienced woman: Multiple sex partners and sexual satisfaction. *The Journal of Sex Research*, 24, 141–154.

Davis, K. B. (1929). *Factors in the sex life of twenty-two hundred women.* New York: Harper.

Davis, M., & Kennedy, E. L. (1986). Oral history and the study of sexuality in the lesbian community: Buffalo, New York, 1940–1960. *Feminist Studies*, 12, 7–26.

D'Emilio, J. (1989). Gay politics and community in San Francisco since World War II. In M. B. Duberman, M. Vicinus, & G. Chauncey, Jr. (Eds.), *Hidden from history: Reclaiming the gay & lesbian past* (pp. 456–473). New York: NAL Books.

D'Emilio, J., & Freedman, E. B. (1988). *Intimate matters: A history of sexuality in America.* New York: Harper & Row.

Demo, D. H. (1992). Parent-child relations: Assessing recent changes. *Journal of Marriage and the Family*, 54, 104–117.

DeVore, N. E. (1983). Parenthood postponed. *American Journal of Nursing*, 83, 1160–1163.

Diamant, A. (1989, April 16). The baby quest. *The Boston Globe Magazine*, pp. 17, 57–59, 66–72.

Diaz, E. (1991). Public policy, women, and HIV disease. *SIECUS Report*, 19, 4–5.

DiLapi, E. M. (1989). Lesbian mothers and the motherhood hierarchy. In F. W. Bozett (Ed.), *Homosexuality and the family* (pp. 101–121). Binghamton, NY: Harrington Park.

Dill, B. T. (1983). Race, class, and gender: Prospects for an all-inclusive sisterhood. *Feminist Studies*, 9, 131–150.

Dill, B. T. (1988). Our mothers' grief: Racial ethnic women and the maintenance of families. *Journal of Family History*, 13, 415–431.

Dinnerstein, D. (1976). *The mermaid and the minotaur.* New York: Harper & Row.

Dornbusch, S. M., & Gray, K. D. (1988). Single-parent families. In S. M. Dornbusch & M. H. Strober (Eds.), *Feminism, children and the new families* (pp. 274–296). New York: Guilford.

Dornbusch, S. M., & Strober, M. H. (Eds.). (1988). *Feminism, children, and the new families.* New York: Guilford.

Doten, P. (1991, June 15). School for dads. *The Boston Globe*, pp. 6, 9.

Douvan, E. (1980). Toward a new policy for family. In D. G. McGuigan (Ed.), *Women's lives: New theory, research and policy* (pp. 391–396). Ann Arbor: University of Michigan.

Dressel, P., & Clark, A. (1990). A critical look at family care. *Journal of Marriage and the Family*, 52, 769–782.

Duberman, M. B., Vicinus, M., & Chauncey, G., Jr. (Eds). (1989). *Hidden from history: Reclaiming the gay & lesbian past.* New York: NAL Books.

Du Bois, B. (1983). Passionate scholarship: Notes on values, knowing and method in feminist social science. In G. Bowles & R. D. Klein (Eds.), *Theories of women's studies* (pp. 105–116). London: Routledge & Kegan Paul.

Duvall, E. (1971). Family development. Philadephia: J. B. Lippincott.

Dworkin, A. (1980). Why so-called radical men love and need pornography. In L. Lederer (Ed.), Take back the night: Women on pornography (pp. 148–154). New York: William Morrow.

Echols, A. (1989). The new feminism of yin and yang. In B. J. Risman & P. Schwartz (Eds.), Gender in intimate relationships (pp. 48–57). Belmont, CA: Wadsworth.

Ehrenreich, B. (1989). Fear of falling: The inner life of the middle class. New York: Pantheon.

Ehrensaft, D. (1983). When women and men mother. In J. Trebilcot (Ed.), Mothering: Essays in feminist theory (pp. 41–61). Totowa, NJ: Rowman and Allanheld.

Ehrensaft, D. (1987). Parenting together: Men and women sharing the care of their children. New York: Macmillan.

Ehrhardt, A. A. (1985). The psychology of gender. In A. S. Rossi (Ed.), Gender and the life course (pp. 81–96). New York: Aldine.

Eiger, N. (1988). Worker education in Sweden: A force for extending democratic participation. Scandinavian Review, 76, 81–89.

Elder, G. H., Jr. (1977). Family history and the life course. Journal of Family History, 2, 279–304.

Elder, G.H., Jr. (1981). History and the family: The discovery of complexity. Journal of Marriage and the Family, 43, 489–519.

Enarson, E. (1990). Experts and caregivers: Perspectives on underground day care. In E. K. Abel & M. K. Nelson (Eds.), Circles of care (pp. 233–245). Albany: State University of New York Press.

English, D. (1983). The fear that feminism will free men first. In A. Snitow, C. Stansell, & S. Thompson (Eds.), Powers of desire (pp. 477–483). New York: Monthly Review Press.

Equality between Men and Women in Sweden. (1989). Stockholm, Sweden: The Swedish Institute.

Evans, L., & Bannister, S. (1990). Lesbian violence, lesbian victims: How to identify battering in relationships. Lesbian Ethics, 4, 52–65.

Faderman, L. (1981). Surpassing the love of men: Romantic friendship and love between women from the Renaissance to the present. New York: William Morrow.

Faderman, L. (1991). Odd girls and twilight lovers: A history of lesbian life in twentieth-century America. New York: Penguin.

Falk, P. J. (1989). Lesbian mothers: Psychosocial assumptions in family law. American Psychologist, 44, 941–947.

Faludi, S. (1991). Backlash: The undeclared war against American women. New York: Crown.

Federal Register. (1979, April 20). Guidelines on sex discrimination; Adoption of final guidelines; Questions and answers, 44, 23804–23805.

Federal Register. (1988, February 2). Statutory prohibition on use of appropriated funds in programs where abortion is a method of family planning: Standard of compliance for family planning projects, 53, 2922–2923.

Ferguson, A. (1991). *Sexual democracy: Women, oppression, and revolution.* Boulder, CO: Westview.

Ferree, M. M. (1988, November). *Negotiating household roles and responsibilities.* Paper presented at the National Council on Family Relations annual meeting, Philadelphia, PA.

Ferree, M. M. (1990). Beyond separate spheres: Feminism and family research. *Journal of Marriage and the Family, 52,* 866–884.

Fierman, J. (1990, July 30). Why women still don't hit the top. *Fortune, 122,* pp. 40–42, 46, 50, 54, 58, 62.

Finch, J., & Groves, D. (Eds.). (1983). *A labour of love: Women, work and caring.* London: Routledge & Kegan Paul.

Fine, M. (1988). Sexuality, schooling, and adolescent females: The missing discourse of desire. *Harvard Educational Review, 58,* 29–53.

Finkelhor, D. (1979). *Sexually victimized children.* New York: Free Press.

Finkelhor, D., & Yllo, K. (1985). *License to rape: Sexual abuse of wives.* New York: Holt.

Firestone, S. (1970). *The dialectics of sex: The case for feminist revolution.* New York: William Morrow.

Fischer, L. R. (1981). Transitions in the mother-daughter relationship. *Journal of Marriage and the Family, 43,* 613–622.

Fishman, P. M. (1978). Interaction: The work that women do. *Social Problems, 25,* 397–406.

Flax, J. (1982). The family in contemporary feminist thought: A critical review. In J. B. Elshtain (Ed.), *The family in political thought* (pp. 223–253). Amherst: University of Massachusetts Press.

Flax, J. (1987). Postmodernism and gender relations in feminist theory. *Signs, 12,* 621–643.

Flax, J. (1990). *Thinking fragments: Psychoanalysis, feminism, and postmodernism in the contemporary West.* Berkeley: University of California Press.

Fonow, M. M., & Cook, J. A. (1991). Back to the future: A look at the second wave of feminist epistemology and methodology. In M. M. Fonow & J. A. Cook (Eds.), *Beyond methodology: Feminist scholarship as lived research* (pp. 1–15). Bloomington: Indiana University Press.

Fox, K. D., & Nichols, S. Y. (1983). The time crunch. *Journal of Family Issues, 4,* 61–82.

Fraker, S. (1984, April 16). Why women aren't getting to the top. *Fortune,* pp. 40–45.

Francoeur, R. (1987). Human sexuality. In M. B. Sussman and S. K. Steinmetz (Eds.), *Handbook of marriage and the family* (pp. 509–534). New York: Plenum.

Frankel, S. A., & Wise, M. J. (1982). A view of delayed childbearing: Some implications of a new trend. *Psychiatry, 45,* 220–225.

Fraser, N., & Nicholson, L. J. (1990). Social criticism without philosophy: An encounter between feminism and postmodernism. In L. Nicholson (Ed.), *Feminism/postmodernism* (pp. 19–38). New York: Routledge.

Friedan, B. (1963). *The feminine mystique.* New York: Dell.

Friedan, B. (1986, October 14). Women are 'special,' need special treatment. USA Today, p. 10A.

Frisby, M. K. (1991, February 20). Three house bills seek exemptions for single parents, military couples. The Boston Globe, p. 3.

Frye, M. (1990). Lesbian "sex." In J. Allen (Ed.), Lesbian philosophies and cultures (pp. 305–315). Albany: State University of New York Press.

Fullilove, M. T., Fullilove, R. E., Haynes, K., & Gross, S. (1990). Black women and AIDS prevention: A view towards understanding the gender rules. The Journal of Sex Research, 27, 47–64.

Gagnier, R. (1990). Feminist postmodernism: The end of feminism or the ends of theory? In D. L. Rhode (Ed.), Theoretical perspectives on sexual difference (pp. 21–30). New Haven, CT: Yale University Press.

Gatz, M., Bengtson, V. L., & Blum, M. J. (1990). Caregiving families. In J. E. Birren & K. W. Schaie (Eds.), Handbook of the psychology of aging (3rd ed.) (pp. 404–426). San Diego, CA: Academic.

Gavey, N., Florence, J., Pezaro, S., & Tan, J. (1990). Mother-blaming, the perfect alibi: Family therapy and the mothers of incest survivors. Journal of Feminist Family Therapy, 2, 1–25.

Gelb, J., & Palley, M. L. (1987). Women and public policies. Princeton, NJ: Princeton University Press.

Gelles, R., & Conte, J. (1990). Domestic violence and sexual abuse of children: A review of research in the eighties. Journal of Marriage and the Family, 52, 1045–1058.

Gelles, R. J., & Cornell, C. P. (1985). Intimate violence in families. Beverly Hills, CA: Sage.

Gelles, R. J., & Strauss, M. A. (1988). Intimate violence. New York: Simon & Schuster.

Gerson, K. (1985). Hard choices: How women decide about work, career, and motherhood. Los Angeles: University of California Press.

Gerstel, N., & Gross, H. (1987). Commuter marriage: A microcosm of career and family conflict. In N. Gerstel & H. E. Gross (Eds.), Families and work (pp. 422–433). Philadelphia: Temple University Press.

Gibbs, N. (1992, March 2). The war against feminism. Time, pp. 50–55.

Gilbert, L. A. (1985). Men in dual-career families. Hillsdale, NJ: Lawrence Erlbaum.

Gilkes, C. T. (1985). "Together and in harness": Women's traditions in the sanctified church. Signs, 10, 678–699.

Gilligan, C. (1982). In a different voice. Cambridge, MA: Harvard University Press.

Gimenez, M. E. (1983). Feminism, pronatalism, and motherhood. In J. Trebilcot (Ed.), Mothering: Essays in feminist theory (pp. 287–314). Totowa, NJ: Rowman and Allanheld.

Ginsburg, F. (1989). Dissonance and harmony: The symbolic function of abortion in activists' life stories. In Personal Narratives Group (Eds.), Interpreting women's lives: Feminist theory and personal narratives (pp. 59–84). Bloomington: Indiana University Press.

Glenn, E. N. (1987). Gender and the family. In B. B. Hess & M. M. Ferree (Eds.), *Analyzing gender* (pp. 348–380). Newbury Park, CA: Sage.

Glenn, N. (1991). The recent trend in marital success in the United States. *Journal of Marriage and the Family, 53,* 261–270.

Glick, P. C. (1977). Updating the life cycle of the family. *Journal of Marriage and the Family, 39,* 5–13.

Gold, D. T. (1989). Sibling relationships in old age: A typology. *International Journal of Aging and Human Development, 28,* 37–51.

Golden, C. (1987). Diversity and variability in women's sexual identities. In Boston Lesbian Psychologies Collective (Eds.), *Lesbian psychologies* (pp. 19–34). Urbana: University of Illinois Press.

Goode, W. J. (1982). Why men resist. In B. Thorne & M. Yalom (Eds.), *Rethinking the family: Some feminist questions* (pp. 131–150). New York: Longman.

Gordon, L. (1976). *Women's body, women's right.* New York: Viking.

Gosselin, P. J. (1991, July 24). Sullivan drops $18m teen-age sex survey. *The Boston Globe,* pp. 1, 14.

Gove, W. (1972). The relationship between sex roles, marital status, and mental health. *Social Forces, 51,* 34–44.

Graham, R. (1992, April 29). Why women are angry: Enough is enough they say. *The Boston Globe,* pp. 43, 46.

Grant, J. (1982). Black women and the church. In G. T. Hull, P. B. Scott, & B. Smith (Eds.), *All the women are white, all the blacks are men, but some of us are brave: Black women's studies* (pp. 141–152). Old Westbury, NY: Feminist Press.

Gravenhorst, L. (1988). A feminist look at family development theory. In D. M. Klein & J. Aldous (Eds.), *Social stress and family development* (pp. 79–101). New York: Guilford.

Green, J. E. (1988). Chorionic villus sampling: Experience with an initial 940 cases. *Obstetrics and Gynecology, 71,* 208.

Green, G. D., & Clunis, D. M. (1989). Married lesbians. In E. D. Rothblum & E. Cole (Eds.), *Loving boldly: Issues facing lesbians* (pp. 41–49). New York: Harrington Park.

Greenglass, E. R., & Borovilos, R. (1984). *Psychological correlates of fertility plans in unmarried women.* Unpublished manuscript.

Grossman, F. K., Pollack, W. S., & Golding, E. (1988). Fathers and children: Predicting the quality and quantity of fathering. *Developmental Psychology, 24,* 82–91.

Haas, L. (1980). Role-sharing couples: A study of egalitarian marriages. *Family Relations, 29,* 289–296.

Hagestad, G. O. (1986). The family: Women and grandparents as kin-keepers. In A. Pifer & D. L. Bronte (Eds.), *Our aging society: Paradox and promise* (pp. 141–160). New York: W. W. Norton.

Hall, M. (1978). Lesbian families: Cultural and clinical issues. *Social Work, 23,* 380–385.

Hall, R. (1928). *The well of loneliness.* New York: Coucici-Friede, 1934.

Halperin, D. M. (1989). Sex before sexuality: Pederasty, politics, and power in classical Athens. In M. B. Duberman, M. Vicinus, & G. Chauncey, Jr. (Eds.), Hidden from history: Reclaiming the gay & lesbian past (pp. 37–53). New York: NAL Books.

Hammond, N. (1989). Lesbian victims of relationship violence. In E. D. Rothblum & E. Cole (Eds.), Loving boldly: Issues facing lesbians (pp. 89–105). New York: Harrington Park.

Hanscombe, G. E., & Forster, J. (1982). Rocking the cradle. Lesbian mothers: A challenge in family living. Boston: Alyson.

Harding, S. (1987a). Introduction: Is there a feminist method? In S. Harding (Ed.), Feminism & methodology: Social science issues (pp. 1–14). Bloomington: Indiana University Press.

Harding, S. (1987b). Conclusion: Epistemological questions. In S. Harding (Ed.), Feminism & methodology: Social science issues (pp. 181–190). Bloomington: Indiana University Press.

Hare-Mustin, R. T. (1978). A feminist approach to family therapy. Family Process, 17, 181–194.

Hare-Mustin, R. T. (1989). The problem of gender in family therapy theory. In M. McGoldrick, C. M. Anderson, & F. Walsh (Eds.), Women in families: A framework for family therapy (pp. 61–77). New York: W. W. Norton.

Hare-Mustin, R. T. (1991). Sex, lies, and headaches: The problem is power. Journal of Feminist Family Therapy, 3, 39–61.

Hare-Mustin, R. T., Bennett, S. K., & Broderick, P. C. (1983). Attitude toward motherhood: Gender, generational, and religious comparisons. Sex Roles, 9, 643–661.

Hare-Mustin, R. T., & Marecek, J. (1988). The meaning of difference: Gender theory, postmodernism, and psychology. American Psychologist, 43, 455–464.

Hare-Mustin, R. T., & Marecek, J. (1990). Gender and the meaning of difference: Postmodernism and psychology. In R. T. Hare-Mustin & J. Marecek (Eds.), Making a difference: Psychology and the construction of gender (pp. 22–64). New Haven, CT: Yale University Press.

Hareven, T. K. (1987). Historical analysis of the family. In M. B. Sussman & S. K. Steinmetz (Eds.), Handbook of marriage and the family (pp. 37–57). New York: Plenum.

Hareven, T. K. (1991). The history of the family and the complexity of social change. American Historical Review, 96, 95–124.

Harlow, C. W. (1991). Female victims of violent crimes. Washington, DC: U. S. Department of Justice.

Hartmann, H. (1981). The family as the locus of gender, class, and political struggle: The example of housework. Signs, 6, 366–394.

Hartmann, H. I., & Spalter-Roth, R. M. (1989). Family and medical leave: Who pays for the lack of it? Washington, DC: The Women's Research Institute.

Hartsock, N. C. M. (1986). Feminist theory and the development of revolutionary strategy. In M. Pearsall (Ed.), Women and values: Readings in recent feminist philosophy (pp. 8–18). Belmont, CA: Wadsworth.

Harvard Law Review Association. (1990). *Sexual orientation and the law.* Cambridge, MA: Harvard University Press.

Hawkesworth, M. E. (1989). Knowers, knowing, known: Feminist theory and claims of truth. *Signs, 14,* 533–557.

Hawkesworth, M. E. (1990). *Beyond oppression: Feminist theory and political strategy.* New York: Continuum.

Hays, D., & Samuels, A. (1989). Heterosexual women's perceptions of their marriages to bisexual or homosexual men. In F. W. Bozett (Ed.), *Homosexuality and the family* (pp. 81–100). Binghamton, NY: Harrington Park.

Henshaw, S. K. (1991). The accessibility of abortion services in the United States. *Family Planning Perspectives, 23,* 246–252.

Henshaw, S. K., Koonin, L. M., & Smith, J. C. (1991). Characteristics of U.S. women having abortions, 1987. *Family Planning Perspectives, 23,* 75–81.

Henshaw, S. K., & Silverman, J. (1988). The characteristics and prior contraceptive use of U.S. abortion patients. *Family Planning Perspectives, 20,* 158–168.

Hertz, R. (1987). Three careers: His, hers, and theirs. In N. Gerstel & H. E. Gross (Eds.), *Families and work* (pp. 408–421). Philadelphia: Temple University Press.

Hill, M. (1987). Child-rearing attitudes of black lesbian mothers. In Boston Lesbian Psychologies Collective (Ed.), *Lesbian psychologies* (pp. 215–226). Urbana: University of Illinois Press.

Hite, S. (1976). *The Hite report: A nationwide study of female sexuality.* New York: Dell.

Hite, S. (1987). *Women in love: A new cultural revolution in progress.* New York: Alfred A Knopf.

Hoaglund, S. L. (1991). Some thoughts about "caring." In C. Card (Ed.), *Feminist ethics* (pp. 246–263). Lawrence: University Press of Kansas.

Hochschild, A. R. (1983). *The managed heart.* Berkeley: University of California Press.

Hochschild, A. R., with Machung, A. (1989). *The second shift: Working parents and the revolution at home.* New York: Viking.

Hofferth, S. L. (1984). Long-term economic consequences for women of delayed childbearing and reduced family size. *Demography, 21,* 141–155.

Hofferth, S. L., & Phillips, D. A. (1991). Child care policy research. *Journal of Social Issues, 47,* 1–13.

Hollibaugh, A., & Moraga, C. (1983). What we're rollin around in bed with: Sexual silences in feminism. In A. Snitow, C. Stansell, & S. Thompson (Eds.), *Powers of desire* (pp. 394–405). New York: Monthly Review Press.

Holmes, K. K., Karon, J. M., & Kreiss, J. (1990). The increasing frequency of heterosexually acquired AIDS in the United States. *American Journal of Public Health, 80,* 858–863.

Holten, J. D. (1990). When do we stop mother-blaming? *Journal of Feminist Family Therapy, 2,* 53–60.

Hook, E. (1981). Rates of chromosome abnormalities at different maternal ages. *Obstetrics and Gynecology, 58,* 282–284.

hooks, b. (1984). *Feminist theory: From margin to center.* Boston: South End Press.

hooks, b. (1989). *Talking back: Thinking feminist, thinking black.* Boston: South End Press.

Houseknecht, S. K. (1979). Childlessness and marital adjustment. *Journal of Marriage and the Family, 41,* 259–265.

Houseknecht, S. K. (1987). Voluntary childlessness. In M. B. Sussman & S. M. Steinmetz (Eds.), *Handbook of marriage and the family* (pp. 369–395). New York: Plenum.

Huber, J., & Spitze, G. (1983). *Sex stratification: Children, housework, and jobs.* New York: Academic.

Hunt, J. G., & Hunt, L. L. (1982). The dualities of careers and families: New integrations or new polarizations? *Social Problems, 29,* 499–510.

Hurtado, A. (1989). Relating to privilege: Seduction and rejection in the subordination of white women and women of color. *Signs, 14,* 833–855.

Jackson, M. (1987). "Facts of life" or the eroticization of women's oppression? Sexology and the social construction of heterosexuality. In P. Caplan (Ed.), *The cultural construction of sexuality* (pp. 52–81). London: Tavistock.

Jackson, R. M. (1989). The reproduction of parenting. *American Sociological Review, 54,* 215–232.

Jaggar, A. M. (1990). Sexual difference and sexual equality. In D. L. Rhode (Ed.), *Theoretical perspectives on sexual difference* (pp. 239–254). New Haven, CT: Yale University Press.

James, W. H. (1979). The causes of the decline of fecundability with age. *Social Biology, 26,* 330–334.

Janeway, E. (1980). Who is Sylvia? On the loss of sexual paradigms. In C. R. Stimpson & E. S. Person (Eds.), *Women: Sex and sexuality* (pp. 4–20). Chicago: University of Chicago.

Jeffreys, S. (1990). Eroticizing women's subordination. In D. Leidholdt & J. G. Raymond (Eds.), *The sexual liberals and the attack on feminism* (pp. 132–153). Elmsford, NY: Pergamon.

Johnson, S. (1989). *Wildfire: Igniting the she/volution.* Albuquerque, NM: Wildfire Books.

Jordan, J. V. (1991). The meaning of mutuality. In J. V. Jordan, A. G. Kaplan, J. B. Miller, I. P. Stiver, & J. L. Surrey (Eds.), *Women's growth in connection: Writings from the Stone Center* (pp. 81–96). New York: Guilford.

Jordan, J. V., Kaplan, A. G., Miller, J. B., Stiver, I. P., & Surrey, J. L. (Eds.). (1991). *Women's growth in connection: Writings from the Stone Center.* New York: Guilford.

Kahana, E., & Young, R. (1990). Clarifying the caregiving paradigm: Challenges for the future. In D. E. Biegel & A. Blum (Eds.), *Aging and caregiving: Theory, research, and policy* (pp. 76–97). Newbury Park, CA: Sage.

Kahn, A. S., & Yoder, J. D. (1989). The psychology of women and conservatism. *Psychology of Women Quarterly, 13,* 417–432.

Kanuha, V. (1990). Compounding the triple jeopardy: Battering in lesbian of color relationships. In L. S. Brown & M. P. P. Root (Eds.), *Diversity and complexity in feminist theory* (pp. 169–184). New York: Haworth.

Kaplan, D. A., Cohn, B., & Springen, K. (1991, April 1). Equal rights, equal risks. *Newsweek*, pp. 56, 59.

Kaplan, H. S. (1979). *Disorders of sexual desire.* New York: Brunner/Mazel.

Kassoff, E. (1989). Nonmonogamy in the lesbian community. In E. D. Rothblum & E. Cole (Eds.), *Loving boldly: Issues facing lesbians* (pp. 167–182). Binghamton, NY: Harrington Park.

Katchadourian, H. A. (1989). *Fundamentals of human sexuality* (5th ed.). Philadelphia: Holt, Rinehart & Winston.

Katz, M. B. (1989). *The undeserving poor: From the war on poverty to the war on welfare.* New York: Pantheon.

Kaufman, D. R. (1985). Women who return to orthodox Judaism: A feminist analysis. *Journal of Marriage and the Family, 47,* 543–551.

Kelly, L. (1988). How women define their experiences of violence. In K. Yllo & M. Bograd (Eds.), *Feminist perspectives on wife abuse* (pp. 114–132). Newbury Park, CA: Sage.

Kerber, L. K., Greeno, C. G., Maccoby, E. E., Luria, Z., Stack, C. B., & Gilligan, C. (1986). On *In a different voice:* An interdisciplinary forum. *Signs, 11,* 304–333.

Kerckhoff, R. K. (1976). Marriage and middle age. *Family Coordinator, 25,* 5–11.

Kessler-Harris, A. (1987). The debate over women in the work-place: Recognizing differences. In N. Gerstel & H. G. Gross (Eds.), *Families and work* (pp. 520–539). Philadelphia: Temple University Press.

Kilbride, P. L., & Kilbride, J. C. (1990). *Changing family life in East Africa: Women and children at risk.* University Park: Pennsylvania State University Press.

Kinsey, A. C., Pomeroy, W. B., & Martin, C. E. (1948). *Sexual behavior in the human male.* Philadelphia: W. B. Saunders.

Kinsey, A. C., Pomeroy, W. B., Martin, C. E., & Gebhard, P. (1953). *Sexual behavior in the human female.* Philadelphia: W. B. Saunders.

Kirp, D. L., Yudof, M. G., & Franks, M. S. (1986). *Gender justice.* Chicago, IL: University of Chicago Press.

Kitzinger, C. (1987). *The social construction of lesbianism.* London: Sage.

Klatch, R. (1987). *Women of the new right.* Philadelphia: University of Pennsylvania Press.

Klein, F. (Ed.). (1985). *Bisexualities: Theory and research.* New York: Haworth.

Klein, F. (1990). The need to view sexual orientation as a multivariable dynamic process: A theoretical perspective. In D. P. McWhirter, S. A. Sanders, & J. M. Reinisch (Eds.), *Homosexuality/Heterosexuality* (pp. 277–282). New York: Oxford University Press.

Kochanek, K. D. (1991). Induced terminations of pregnancy: Reporting states, 1988. *Monthly Vital Statistics Report, 39,* Hyattsville, MD: National Center for Health Statistics.

Koepke, L., Hare, J., & Moran, P. B. (1992). Relationship quality in a sample of lesbian couples with children and child-free lesbian couples. *Family Relations, 41,* 224–229.

Kohlberg, L. (1976). Moral stages and moralization: The cognitive-developmental approach. In T. Lickona (Ed.), *Moral development and behavior* (pp. 31–53). New York: Holt, Rinehart and Winston.

Kolbert, K. (1988). Developing a reproductive rights agenda for the 1990s. In N. Taub & S. Cohen (Eds.), *Reproductive laws for the 1990s: A briefing handbook* (pp. 7–15). Newark, NJ: State University of New Jersey.

Komarovsky, M. (1985). *Women in college: Shaping new feminine identities.* New York: Basic.

Komter, A. (1989). Hidden power in marriage. *Gender & Society, 3,* 187–216.

Korpi, W. (1990). *The development of the Swedish welfare state in a comparative perspective.* Stockholm, Sweden: The Swedish Institute.

Koss, M. P., Gidycz, C. A., & Wisniewski, N. (1987). The scope of rape: Incidence and prevalence of sexual aggression and victimization in a national sample of higher education students. *Journal of Counseling and Educational Psychology, 55,* 162–170.

Kranichfeld, M. L. (1988). Rethinking family power. In N. D. Glenn & M. T. Coleman (Eds.), *Family relations: A reader* (pp. 230–241). Chicago: Dorsey.

Krestan, J., & Bepko, C. (1980). The problem of fusion in the lesbian relationship. *Family Process, 19,* 277–289.

Krieger, S. (1982). Lesbian identity and community: Recent social science literature. *Signs, 8,* 91–108.

Krieger, S. (1983). *The mirror dance: Identity in a women's community.* Philadelphia: Temple University Press.

LaRossa, R. (1988). Fatherhood and social change. *Family Relations, 37,* 451–457.

LaRossa, R., & LaRossa, M. M. (1989). Baby care: Fathers vs. mothers. In B. J. Risman & P. Schwartz (Eds.), *Gender in intimate relationships* (pp. 138–154). Belmont, CA: Wadsworth.

Laws, J. L., & Schwartz, P. (1977). *Sexual scripts: The social construction of female sexuality.* Hinsdale, IL: Dryden.

Lederer, L. (Ed.). (1980). *Take back the night: Women on pornography.* New York: William Morrow.

Leidholdt, D., & Raymond, J. G. (Eds.). (1990). *The sexual liberals and the attack on feminism.* Elmsford, NY: Pergamon.

Leigh, B. C. (1989). Reasons for having and avoiding sex: Gender, sexual orientation, and relationship to sexual behavior. *The Journal of Sex Research, 26,* 199–209.

Lein, L. (1984). *Families without victims.* Lexington, MA: D. C. Heath.

Lenz, E., & Myerhoff, B. (1985). *The feminization of America.* Los Angeles: Jeremy P. Tarcher.

Lester, G. H. (1991). Child support and alimony: 1989. *Current Population Reports,* (Series P–70, No. 23). Washington, DC: U.S. Government Printing Office.

Levine, J. A., Pleck, J. L., & Lamb, M. E. (1983). The fatherhood project. In M. E. Lamb & A. Sagi (Eds.), *Fatherhood and family policy* (pp. 101–111). Hillsdale, NJ: Lawrence Erlbaum.

Levine, M. P., & Leonard, R. (1984). Discrimination against lesbians in the work force. *Signs*, 9, 700–710.

Lewis, M. I. (1980). Female sexuality in the United States. In M. Kirkpatrick (Ed.), *Women's sexual development: Explorations of inner space* (pp. 19–38). New York: Plenum.

Libby, R. W., & Whitehurst, R. N. (Eds.). (1977). *Marriage and alternatives: Exploring intimate relations.* Glenview, IL: Scott, Foresman.

Lincoln, R., & Kaeser, L. (1988). Whatever happened to the contraceptive revolution? *Family Planning Perspectives*, 20, 20–24.

London, K. A. (1991). *Cohabitation, marriage, marital dissolution, and remarriage: United States, 1988.* Hyattsville, MD: National Center for Health Statistics.

Lopata, H. Z. (1979). *Women as widows: Support systems.* New York: Elsevier.

Lopata, H. Z. (1987). Women's family roles in life course perspective. In B. B. Hess & M. M. Ferree (Eds.), *Analyzing gender* (pp. 381–407). Newbury Park, CA: Sage.

Lorber, J. (1991). Dismantling Noah's ark. In J. Lorber & S. A. Farrell (Eds.), *The social construction of gender* (pp. 355–369). Newbury Park, CA: Sage.

Lorde, A. (1984). *Sister outsider.* Freedom, CA: Crossing Press.

Loth, R. (1992, April 26). Women poised to win in political vacuum. *The Boston Globe*, pp. 1, 28.

Lott, B. (1987). *Women's lives: Themes and variations in gender learning.* Belmont, CA: Wadsworth.

Lugones, M. C., & Spelman E. V. (1983). Have we got a theory for you Feminist theory, cultural imperialism and the demand for "the woman's voice." *Women's Studies International Forum*, 6, 573–581.

Luker, K. (1984). *Abortion and the politics of motherhood.* Berkeley: University of California Press.

Lunneborg, P. (1990). *Women changing work.* New York: Bergin and Garvey.

Maccoby, E. E., & Jacklin, C. N. (1974). *The psychology of sex differences.* Stanford, CA: Stanford University Press.

MacKinnon, C. (1982). Feminism, Marxism, method, and the state: An agenda for theory. *Signs*, 7, 515–544.

MacKinnon, C. A. (1990). Liberalism and the death of feminism. In D. Leidholdt & J. G. Raymond (Eds.), *The sexual liberals and the attack on feminism* (pp. 3–13). Elmsford, NY: Pergamon.

Macklin, E. D. (1987). Nontraditional family forms. In M. B. Sussman & S. K. Steinmetz (Eds.), *Handbook of marriage and the family* (pp. 317–353). New York: Plenum.

Maddock, J. W. (1989). Healthy family sexuality: Positive principles for educators and clinicians. *Family Relations*, 38, 130–136.

Maggiore, D. J. (1988). *Lesbianism: An annotated bibliography and guide to the literature, 1976–1986.* Metuchen, NJ: Scarecrow Press.

Mainardi, P. (1972). The politics of housework. In N. Glazer-Malbin & H. Y. Waehrer (Eds.), *Woman in a man-made world* (pp. 289–292). Chicago: Rand McNally.

Mancini, J. A., & Blieszner, R. (1989). Aging parents and adult children:

Research themes in intergenerational relations. *Journal of Marriage and the Family*, 51, 275–290.

Mansfield, P. K. (1988). Midlife childbearing: Strategies for informed decisionmaking. *Psychology of Women Quarterly*, 12, 445–460.

Marciano, T. D. (1979). Male influence on fertility: Needs for research. *The Family Coordinator*, 28, 561–568.

Marecek, J. (1989). Introduction. *Psychology of Women Quarterly*, 13, 367–377.

Martin, C. S., & Bumpass, L. (1989). Trends in marital disruption. *Demography*, 26, 37–52.

Mascia-Lees, R. E., Sharpe, P., & Cohen, C. B. (1989). The postmodernist turn in anthropology: Cautions from a feminist perspective. *Signs*, 15, 7–33.

Masters, W. H., & Johnson, V. E. (1966). *Human sexual response*. New York: Bantam.

Mattessich, P., & Hill, R. (1987). Life cycle and family development. In M. B. Sussman & S. K. Steinmetz (Eds.), *Handbook of marriage and the family* (pp. 437–469). New York: Plenum.

Matthews, S. H., & Rosner, T. T. (1988). Shared filial responsibility: The family as the primary caregiver. *Journal of Marriage and the Family*, 50, 185–195.

Matthews, S. H., Werkner, J. E., & Delaney, P. J. (1989). Relative contributions of help by employed and nonemployed sisters to their elderly parents. *Journal of Gerontology: Social Sciences*, 44, S36-S44.

McDonnell, K. (1984). *Not an easy choice: A feminist re-examines abortion*. Boston: South End Press.

McGeary, J. (1990, Fall). Challenge in the East. *Time* (Special issue: *Women: The road ahead*), pp. 30–32.

McGill, M. E. (1985). *The McGill report on male intimacy*. New York: Holt, Rinehart and Winston.

McGoldrick, M., Garcia-Preto, N., Hines, P. M., & Lee, E. (1989). Ethnicity and women. In M. McGoldrick, C. Anderson, & F. Walsh (Eds.), *Women in families* (pp. 169–199). New York: W. W. Norton.

McGuire, M., & Alexander, N. J. (1985). Artificial insemination of single women. *Fertility and Sterility*, 43, 182–184.

McKenry, P. C., Price, S. J., Gordon, P. B., & Rudd, N. M. (1986). Characteristics of husbands' family work and wives' labor force involvement. In R. A. Lewis & R. E. Salt (Eds.), *Men in families* (pp. 73–83). Newbury Park, CA: Sage.

McMahon, K. (1990). The *Cosmopolitan* ideology and the management of desire. *The Journal of Sex Research*, 27, 381–96.

McNally, J. W., & Mosher, W. D. (1991). AIDS-related knowledge and behavior among women 15–44 years of age: United States, 1988. *Advance data from vital and health statistics* (No. 200). Hyattsville, MD: National Center for Health Statistics.

McNamara, E. (1989a, June 11). Revived ban on abortion seen creating "Prohibition." *The Boston Globe*, pp. 1, 30–31.

McNamara, E. (1989b, October 3). Fetal endangerment cases on the rise. *The Boston Globe*, p. 1, 11.

McWhirter, D. P., Sanders, S. A., & Reinisch, J. M. (Eds.). (1990). *Homosexuality/heterosexuality.* New York: Oxford University Press.

A measured response: Koop on abortion. (1989). *Family Planning Perspectives, 21,* 31–32.

Melton, G. B. (1989). Public policy and private prejudice: Psychology and law on gay rights. *American Psychologist, 44,* 933–940.

Menaghan, E. G., & Parcel, T. L. (1990). Parental employment and family life. *Journal of Marriage and the Family, 52,* 1079–1098.

Menken, J. (1985). Age and fertility: How late can you wait? *Demography, 22,* 469–483.

Merritt, S., & Steiner, L. (1984). *And baby makes two: Motherhood without marriage.* New York: Franklin Watts.

Miller, B. C., & Moore, K. A. (1990). Adolescent sexual behavior, pregnancy, and parenting: Research through the 1980s. *Journal of Marriage and the Family, 52,* 1025–1044.

Miller, J. B. (1986). *Toward a new psychology of women* (2nd ed.). Boston: Beacon.

Miller, J. B. (1991). Women and power. In J. V. Jordan, A. G. Kaplan, J. B. Miller, I. P. Stiver, J. L. Surrey (Eds.), *Women's growth in connection: Writings from the Stone Center* (pp. 197–205). New York: Guilford.

Miller, P. Y., & Fowlkes, M. R. (1980). Social and behavioral constructions of female sexuality. In C. R. Stimpson & E. S. Person (Eds.), *Women: Sex and sexuality* (pp. 256–273). Chicago: University of Chicago Press.

Miner, V., & Longino, H. (Eds.). (1987). *Competition: A feminist taboo?* New York: Feminist Press.

Minkoff, H. L., & DeHovitz, J. A. (1991). Care of women infected with the human immunodeficiency virus. *Journal of the American Medical Association, 266,* 2253–2258.

Moen, E. W. (1979). What does "control over our bodies" really mean? *International Journal of Women's Studies, 2,* 129–143.

Moen, P. (1985). Continuities and discontinuities in women's labor force activity. In G. H. Elder (Ed.), *Life course dynamics, trajectories and transitions, 1968–1980* (pp. 113–155). Ithaca, NY: Cornell University Press.

Money, J. (1987). Sin, sickness, or status: Homosexual gender identity and psychoneuroendocrinology. *American Psychologist, 42,* 384–399.

Money, J. (1988). *Gay, straight, and in-between: The sexology of erotic orientation.* New York: Oxford University Press.

Moraga, C. (1983). *Loving in the war years.* Boston: South End Press.

Morales, E. S. (1990). Ethnic minority families and minority gays and lesbians. In F. W. Bozett & M. B. Sussman (Eds.), *Homosexuality and family relations* (pp. 217–239). Binghamton, NY: Harrington Park.

More on Koop's study of abortion. (1990). *Family Planning Perspectives, 22,* 35–39.

Morgan, R. (Ed.). (1970). *Sisterhood is powerful.* New York: Randon House.

Morin, R. (1989, September 11–17). Bringing up baby the company way. *The Washington Post National Weekly Edition,* p. 37.

Mott, F. L. (1990). When is a father really gone? Paternal-child contact in father-absent homes. *Demography, 27*, 499–517.

Movius, M. (1976). Voluntary childlessness—the ultimate liberation. *Family Coordinator, 25*, 57–63.

Muro, M. (1991, July 12). Moore's pregnant pose: Is it hip or hype? *The Boston Globe*, pp. 41, 48.

NARAL. (1992). *A state-by-state review of abortion rights.* Washington, DC: The Naral Foundation/NARAL.

National Center for Health Statistics. (1987). Advance report of final natality statistics, 1985. *Monthly vital statistics report, 36*, (Suppl.). Hyattsville, MD: Public Health Service.

National Center for Health Statistics. (1990). Advance report of final natality statistics, 1988. *Monthly vital statistics report, 39*(Suppl.). Hyattsville, MD: Public Health Service.

National Center for Health Statistics (1991a). Advance report of final natality statistics, 1989. *Monthly vital statistics report, 40*(Suppl.). Hyattsville, MD: Public Health Service.

National Center for Health Statistics. (1991b). Advance report of final marriage statistics, 1988. *Monthly vital statistics report, 40*. Hyattsville, MD: Public Health Service.

National Center for Health Statistics. (1991c). Advance report of final divorce statistics, 1988. *Monthly vital statistics report, 39*. Hyattsville, MD: Public Health Service.

Nelson, M. K. (1990). Mothering others' children: The experiences of family day care providers. *Signs, 15*, 586–605.

Nestle, J. (1984). The fem question. In C. Vance (Ed.), *Pleasure and danger* (pp. 232–241). Boston: Routledge & Kegan Paul.

Neuffer, E. (1992, July 2). Senate unit OK's abortion rights. *The Boston Globe*, p. 3.

Newton, E. (1984). The mythic mannish lesbian: Radclyffe Hall and the new woman. *Signs, 9*, 557–575.

Newton, E., & Walton, S. (1984). The misunderstanding: Toward a more precise sexual vocabulary. In C. Vance (Ed.), *Pleasure and danger* (pp. 242–250). Boston: Routledge & Kegan Paul.

Nichols, M. (1990). Lesbian relationships: Implications for the study of sexuality and gender. In D. P. McWhirter, S. A. Sanders, & J. M. Reinisch (Eds.), *Homosexuality/ heterosexuality* (pp. 350–364). New York: Oxford University Press.

Nielsen, J. M. (1990). Introduction. In J. M. Nielsen (Ed.), *Feminist research methods* (pp. 1–37). Boulder, CO: Westview.

Nieva, V. F., & Gutek, B. (1981). *Women and work: A psychological perspective.* New York: Praeger.

Nock, S. L. (1987). The symbolic meaning of childbearing. *Journal of Family Issues, 8*, 373–393.

Noddings, N. (1984). *Caring: A feminine approach to ethics and moral education.* Berkeley: University of California Press.

NOW Legal Defense and Education Fund. (1990). *Facts on reproductive rights:*

Punishing women for conduct during pregnancy. (Fact Sheet 13). New York: NOW.

O'Brien, M. (1981a). Feminist theory and dialectical logic. *Signs, 7*, 144–157.

O'Brien, M. (1981b). *The politics of reproduction.* London: Routledge & Kegan Paul.

O'Bryant, S. L. (1988). Sibling support and older widows' well-being. *Journal of Marriage and the Family, 50*, 173–183.

O'Connell, M., & Bloom, D. E. (1987). *Juggling jobs and babies: America's child care challenge.* Washington, DC: Population Reference Bureau.

Offen, K. (1990). Feminism and sexual difference in historical perspective. In D. L. Rhode (Ed.), *Theoretical perspectives on sexual difference* (pp. 13–20). New Haven, CT: Yale University Press.

Okin, S. M. (1989). *Justice, gender and the family.* New York: Basic.

Okin, S. M. (1990). Thinking like a woman. In D. L. Rhode (Ed.), *Theoretical perspectives on sexual difference* (pp. 145–159). New Haven, CT: Yale University Press.

Opportunity 2000: Creative affirmative action strategies for a changing workforce. (1988). Indianapolis, IN: Hudson Institute.

Osborn, J. E. (1990/91). Women and HIV/AIDS: The silent epidemic? *SIECUS Report, 19*, 1–3.

Palmer, T. (1989). Chantal vs. Jean-Guy: Canada's abortion case. *The Boston Globe*, pp. 1,5.

Pearlman, S. F. (1989). Distancing and connectedness: Impact on couple formation in lesbian relationships. In E. D. Rothblum & E. Cole (Eds.), *Loving boldly: Issues facing lesbians* (pp. 77–88). Binghamton, NY: Harrington Park.

Peplau, L. A. (1982). Research on homosexual couples: An overview. *Journal of Homosexuality, 8*, 3–8.

Peplau, L. A., Cochran, S., Rook, K., & Padesky, C. (1978). Loving women: Attachment and autonomy in lesbian relationships. *Journal of Social Issues, 34*, 2–27.

Peplau, L. A., & Conrad, E. (1989). Beyond nonsexist research. *Psychology of Women Quarterly, 13*, 379–400.

Peplau, L. A., & Gordon, S. L. (1991). The intimate relationships of lesbians and gay men. In J. N. Edwards & D. H. Demo (Eds.), *Marriage and family in transition* (pp. 479–496). Boston: Allyn & Bacon.

Perrucci, C. C., Potter, H. R., & Rhoades, D. L. (1978). Determinants of male family role performance. *Psychology of Women Quarterly, 3*, 53–66.

Peterson, S., & Kelleher, S. (1990, October 23). Surrogate loses child to genetic parents in California. *The Boston Globe*, p. 3.

Pharr, S. (1988). *Homophobia: A weapon of sexism.* Little Rock, AR: Chardon.

Pies, C. (1988). *Considering parenthood* (2nd ed.). San Francisco: Spinsters/Aunt Lute.

Pies, C. A. (1990). Lesbians and the choice to parent. In F. W. Bozett & M. B. Sussman (Eds.), *Homosexuality and family relations* (pp. 137–154). Binghamton, NY: Harrington Park.

Piven, F. F. (1985). Women and the state: Ideology, power, and the welfare state. In A. S. Rossi (Ed.), *Gender and the life course* (pp. 265–287). New York: Aldine.

Pleck, J. H. (1983). Husbands' paid work and family roles: Current research issues. In A. Z. Lopata & J. H. Pleck (Eds.), *Research in the interweave of social roles: Vol. 3. Families and jobs.* Greenwich, CT: JAI.

Pleck, J. H. (1985). *Working wives/Working husbands.* Beverly Hills, CA: Sage.

Plotnick, R. (1989). How much poverty is reduced by state income transfers? *Monthly Labor Review, 112,* 21–26.

Polatnick, M. R. (1983). Why men don't rear children: A power analysis. In J. Trebilcot (Ed.), *Mothering: Essays in feminist theory* (pp. 21–40). Totowa, NJ: Rowman and Allanheld.

Pollitt, K. (1990, March 26). "Fetal rights": A new assault on feminism. *The Nation,* pp. 409–411.

Ponse, B. (1978). *Identities in the lesbian world.* Westport, CT: Greenwood.

Press, A. (1987, January 26). A new family issue. *Newsweek,* pp. 22–24.

Priest, D. (1991, February 18–24). Duty first, but is that to family or country? *The Washington Post National Weekly Edition,* p. 33.

Quinn, S. (1991, February 18–24). Sending American mothers to the Gulf. *The Washington Post National Weekly Edition,* pp. 24–25.

Rafkin, L. (1990). *Different mothers: Sons and daughters of lesbians talk about their lives.* Pittsburgh: Cleis Press.

Rapp, R. (1982). Family and class in contemporary America: Notes toward an understanding of ideology. In B. Thorne & M. Yalom (Eds.), *Rethinking the family: Some feminist questions* (pp. 168–187). New York: Longman.

Raschke, H. J. (1987). Divorce. In M. B. Sussman & S. K. Steinmetz (Eds.), *Handbook of marriage and the family* (pp. 597–624). New York: Plenum.

Reilly, M. E., & Lynch, J. M. (1990). Power-sharing in lesbian partnerships. *Journal of Homosexuality, 19,* 1–30.

Reiss, I. L. (1990). *An end to shame: Shaping our next sexual revolution.* Buffalo, NY: Prometheus.

Reiss, I. L. (1991). Sexual pluralism: Ending America's sexual crisis. *SIECUS Report, 19,* 5–9.

Rhode, D. L. (Ed.). (1990). *Theoretical perspectives on sexual difference.* New Haven, CT: Yale University Press.

Rich, A. (1979). *On lies, secrets, and silence.* New York: W. W. Norton.

Rich, A. (1980). Compulsory heterosexuality and lesbian existence. *Signs, 5,* 631–660.

Rich, A. (1986). *Of woman born* (10th anniv. ed.). New York: W. W. Norton.

Richardson, L. (1989). Secrecy and status: The social construction of forbidden relationships. In B. J. Risman & P. Schwartz (Eds.), *Gender in intimate relationships* (pp. 108–119). Belmont, CA: Wadsworth.

Ricketts, W., & Achtenberg, R. (1990). Adoption and foster parenting for lesbians and gay men: Creating new traditions in family. In F. W. Bozett & M. B. Sussman (Eds.), *Homosexuality and family relations* (pp. 83–118). Binghamton, NY: Harrington Park.

Risman, B. J. (1989). Can men "mother"? Life as a single father. In B. J. Risman

& P. Schwartz (Eds.), *Gender in intimate relationships* (pp. 155–164). Belmont, CA: Wadsworth.

Risman, B. J., & Schwartz, P. (Eds.). (1989). *Gender in intimate relationships.* Belmont, CA: Wadsworth.

Robinson, J. P. (1988). Who's doing the housework? *American Demographics, 10,* 24–27.

Robson, R., & Valentine, S. E. (1990, Fall). Lov(h)ers: *Lesbians as intimate partners and lesbian legal theory.* Philadelphia: Temple University School of Law.

Rollins, J. (1985). *Between women: Domestics and their employers.* Philadelphia: Temple University Press.

Roos, P. A. (1985). *Gender and work: A comparative analysis of industrial societies.* Albany: State University of New York Press.

Rosenfield, A. (1989). RU–486 and the politics of reproduction. *The Female Patient, 14,* 69–74.

Rothblum, E. D. (1989). Introduction: Lesbianism as a model of a positive lifestyle for women. In E. D. Rothblum & E. Cole (Eds.), *Loving boldly: Issues facing lesbians* (pp. 1–12). Binghamton, NY: Harrington Park.

Rothman, B. K. (1989). *Recreating motherhood: Ideology and technology in a patriarchal society.* New York: W. W. Norton.

Rothman, S. M. (1978). *Woman's proper place: A history of changing ideals and practices, 1870 to the present.* New York: Basic.

Rowland, R. (1987). Technology and motherhood: Reproductive choice reconsidered. *Signs, 12,* 512–528.

Rubin, G. (1984). Thinking sex: Notes for a radical theory of the politics of sexuality. In C. Vance (Ed.), *Pleasure and danger* (pp. 267–319). Boston: Routledge & Kegan Paul.

Rubin, L. B. (1976). *Worlds of pain: Life in the working-class family.* New York: Basic.

Rubin, L. B. (1983). *Intimate strangers: Men and women together.* New York: Basic.

Rubin, L. B. (1990). *Erotic wars: What happened to the sexual revolution.* New York: Farrar, Straus & Giroux.

Ruddick, S. (1982). Maternal thinking. In B. Thorne & M. Yalom (Eds.), *Rethinking the family: Some feminist questions* (pp. 76–94). White Plains, NY: Longman.

Ruddick, S. (1989). *Maternal thinking: Toward a politics of peace.* Boston: Beacon.

Ruddick, S. (1990). Thinking about fathers. In M. Hirsch & E. F. Keller (Eds.), *Conflicts in feminism* (pp. 222–233). New York: Routledge.

Rudolph, B. (1990, Fall). Why can't a woman manage more like . . . a woman? *Time* (Special issue: *Women: The road ahead*), p. 53.

Runyan, W. M. (1984). *Life histories and psychobiography.* New York: Oxford University Press.

Russell, D. E. H. (1984). *Sexual exploitation: Rape, child sexual abuse, and workplace harassment.* Newbury Park: CA: Sage.

Russell, D. E. H. (1986). *The secret trauma: Incest in the lives of girls and women.* New York: Basic.

Safilios-Rothschild, C. (1969). Family sociology or wives' family sociology? A cross-cultural examination of decision-making. *Journal of Marriage and the Family, 31*, 290–301.

Saluter, A. (1991). Marital status and living arrangements: March 1989. *Current Populations Report* (Series P20, No. 445). Washington, DC: U.S. Government Printing Office.

Sanday, P. R. (1981). The sociocultural context of rape: A cross-cultural study. *Journal of Social Issues, 37*, 5–27.

Sanders, S. A., Reinisch, J. M., & McWhirter, D. P. (1990). Homosexuality/heterosexuality: An overview. In D. P. McWhirter, S. A. Sanders, & J. M. Reinisch (Eds.), *Homosexuality/heterosexuality* (pp. xix–xxvii). New York: Oxford University Press.

Sandoval, C. (1984). Comment on Krieger's "Lesbian identity and community: Recent social science literature." *Signs, 9*, 725–729.

Sassen, G. (1980). Success anxiety in women: A constructivist interpretation of its source and its significance. *Harvard Educational Review, 50*, 13–24.

Sassoon, A. S. (1987). Introduction: The personal and the intellectual, fragments and order, international trends and national specificities. In A.S. Sassoon (Ed.), *Women and the state: The shifting boundaries of public and private* (pp. 13–42). London: Hutchinson.

Scanzoni, J., Polonko, K., Teachman, J., & Thompson, L. (1989). *The sexual bond: Rethinking families and close relationships*. Newbury Park, CA: Sage.

Scarr, S., Phillips, D., & McCartney, K. (1990). Facts, fantasies and the future of child care in the United States. *Psychological Science, 1*, 26–35.

Schneider, B. (1984). Peril and promise: Lesbians' workplace participation. In T. Darty & S. Potter (Eds.), *Women-identified women* (pp. 211–230). Palo Alto, CA: Mayfield.

Schneider, B. E., & Gould, M. (1987). Female sexuality: Looking back into the future. In B. B. Hess & M. M. Ferree (Eds.), *Analyzing gender* (pp. 120–153). Newbury Park, CA: Sage.

Schwartz, F. (1989, January/February). Management women and the new facts of life. *Harvard Business Review*, pp. 65–76.

Scott, J. W. (1990). Deconstructing equality-versus-difference: Or, the uses of poststructuralist theory for feminism. In M. Hirsch & E. F. Keller (Eds.), *Conflicts in feminism* (pp. 134–148). New York: Routledge.

Sege, I. (1986, October 19). Maternity case splits feminists. *The Boston Globe*, p. 98.

Sevely, J. L. (1987). *Eve's secrets: A new theory of female sexuality*. New York: Random House.

Shanas, E. (1979). The family as a social support system in old age. *The Gerontologist, 19*, 169–174.

Sheffield, C. J. (1987). Sexual terrorism: The social control of women. In B. B. Hess & M. M. Ferree (Eds.), *Analyzing gender* (pp. 171–189). Newbury Park, CA: Sage.

Shelton, B. A., & Firestone, J. (1989). Household labor time and the gender gap in earnings. *Gender and Society, 3*, 105–112.

Sher, G., Marriage, V., & Stoess, J. (1988). *From infertility to in vitro fertilization.* New York: McGraw-Hill.

Sherfey, M. J. (1973). *The nature and evolution of female sexuality.* New York: Random House.

Shuster, R. (1987). Sexuality as a continuum: The bisexual identity. In Boston Lesbian Psychologies Collective (Eds.), *Lesbian psychologies* (pp. 56–71). Urbana: University of Illinois Press.

Sidel, R. (1992). *Women and children last: The plight of poor women in affluent America.* New York: Penguin.

Singer, J. L., & Singer, D. G. (1983). Psychologists look at television: Cognitive, developmental, personality, and social policy implications. *American Psychologist, 38,* 826–834.

Sit, M. (1989, July 11). When family and work collide. *The Boston Globe,* pp. 25, 35.

Skolnick, A. S. (1987). *The intimate environment* (4th ed). Boston: Little, Brown.

Skrzycki, C. (1990, March 5–11). Throwing stones at the glass ceiling. *The Washington Post National Weekly Edition,* p. 21.

Smith, A. D., & Reid, W. J. (1986). *Role-sharing marriage.* New York: Columbia University Press.

Smith, D. (1987). *The everyday world as problematic: A feminist sociology.* Boston: Northeastern University Press.

Smith, E. A. (1989). Butches, femmes, and feminists: The politics of lesbian sexuality. *NWSA Journal, 1,* 398–421.

Smith, R. B. (1988, September 29). Husband to seek review of ruling that OK'd wife's abortion. *The Boston Globe,* p. 7.

Smith, T. W. (1991). Adult sexual behavior in 1989: Number of partners, frequency of intercourse and risk of AIDS. *Family Planning Perspectives, 23,* 102–107.

Smith-Rosenberg, C. (1975). The female world of love and ritual. *Signs, 1,* 1–29.

Snitow, A., Stansell, C., & Thompson, S. (Eds.). (1983). *Powers of desire: The politics of sexuality.* New York: Monthly Review Press.

Spallone, P., & Steinberg, D. L. (1987). *Made to order: The myth of reproductive and genetic progress.* Elmsford, NY: Pergamon.

Spanier, G. B. (1991). Cohabitation: Recent changes in the United States. In J. N. Edwards & D. H. Demo (Eds.), *Marriage and the family in transition* (pp. 94–102). Boston: Allyn & Bacon.

Spanier, G. B., & Furstenberg, F. F., Jr. (1987). Remarriage and reconstituted families. In M. B. Sussman & S. K. Steinmetz (Eds.), *Handbook of marriage and the family* (pp. 419–434). New York: Plenum.

Spanier, G. B., & Thompson, L. (1984). *Parting: The aftermath of separation and divorce.* Beverly Hills, CA: Sage.

Stacey, J. (1986). Are feminists afraid to leave home? The challenge of conservative pro-family feminism. In J. Mitchell & A. Oakley (Eds.), *What is feminism?* (pp. 208–237). New York: Pantheon.

Stacey, J. (1990). *Brave new families: Stories of domestic upheaval in late twentieth century America.* New York: Basic.

Stack, C. B. (1974). All our kin: Strategies for survival in a black community. New York: Harper Colophon.

Stanley, L. (Ed.). (1990). Feminist praxis: Research, theory and epistemology in feminist sociology. London: Routledge.

Staples, R. (1971). Towards a sociology of the black family: A theoretical and methodological assessment. Journal of Marriage and the Family, 33, 119–138.

Staples, R. (1989). Changes in black family structure: The conflict between family ideology and structural conditions. In B. J. Risman & P. Schwartz (Eds.), Gender in intimate relationships (pp. 235–244). Belmont, CA: Wadsworth.

Staples, R., & Mirande, A. (1980). Racial and cultural variations among American families: A decennial review of the literature on minority families. Journal of Marriage and the Family, 42, 887–903.

Stewart, T. A. (1991, December 16). Gay in corporate America. Fortune, pp. 42–46, 50, 54, 56.

Stimpson, C. R. (1988). Where the meanings are: Feminism and cultural spaces. New York: Routledge.

Stimpson, C. R., & Person, E. S. (Eds.). (1980). Women: Sex and sexuality. Chicago: University of Chicago Press.

Stoller, E. P. (1990). Males as helpers: The role of sons, relatives and friends. The Gerontologist, 30, 228–235.

Stone, R., Cafferata, G. L., & Sangl, J. (1987). Caregivers of the frail elderly: A national profile. The Gerontologist, 27, 616–626.

Strober, M. H. (1988). Two-earner families. In S. M. Dornbusch & M. H. Strober (Eds.), Feminism, children and the new families (pp. 161–190). New York: Guilford.

Strong, B., & Devault, C. (1992). The marriage and family experience (5th ed.). New York: West.

Supreme court to review fetal protection policy. (1990). The National Report on Work and Family, 3, 3–4.

Surra, C. A. (1990). Research and theory on mate selection and premarital relationships in the 1980s. Journal of Marriage and the Family, 52, 844–865.

Swedberg, D. (1989). What do we see when we see woman/woman sex in pornographic movies. NWSA Journal, 1, 602–616.

Taggart, M. (1989). Epistemological equality as the fulfillment of family therapy. Journal of Feminist Family Therapy, 1, 85–110.

Tannen, D. (1990). You just don't understand: Women and men in conversation. New York: William Morrow.

Tentler, L. W. (1979). Wage-earning women: Industrial work and family life in the United States, 1900–1930. New York: Oxford University Press.

Thompson, L. (1989, November). Marital responsibility: Contextual and relational morality. Paper presented at the Theory Construction and Research Methodology Workshop, National Council on Family Relations, New Orleans.

Thompson, L. (1991). Family work: Women's sense of fairness. Journal of Family Issues, 12, 181–196.

Thompson, L. (1992). Feminist methodology for family studies. Journal of Marriage and the Family, 54, 3–18.

Thompson, L., & Walker, A. J. (1989). Gender in families: Women and men in marriage, work, and parenthood. *Journal of Marriage and the Family, 51,* 845–871.

Thompson, S. (1990). Putting a big thing into a little hole: Teenage girls' accounts of sexual initiation. *The Journal of Sex Research, 27,* 341–360.

Thorne, B. (1982). Feminist rethinking of the family: An overview. In B. Thorne & M. Yalom (Eds.), *Rethinking the family: Some feminist questions* (pp. 1–24). New York: Longman.

Thorne, B. (1985, November). *Rethinking the family: Some feminist questions.* Paper presented at the annual meeting of the National Council on Family Relations, Dallas, TX.

Thorne, B., & Yalom, M. (Eds.). (1982). *Rethinking the family: Some feminist questions.* New York: Longman.

Thornton, A. (1989). Changing attitudes toward family issues. *Journal of Marriage and the Family, 51,* 873–893.

Tong, R. (1989). *Feminist thought: A comprehensive introduction.* Boulder, CO: Westview.

Torres, A., & Forrest, J. D. (1988). Why do women have abortions? *Family Planning Perspectives, 20,* 169–176.

Trebilcot, J. (Ed.). (1983). *Mothering: Essays in feminist theory.* Totowa, NJ: Rowman and Allanheld.

Tronto, J. C. (1987). Beyond gender difference to a theory of care. *Signs, 12,* 644–663.

Uniform Criminal Reports. (1987). Washington, DC: Federal Bureau of Investigation, U.S. Department of Justice.

U.S. Bureau of the Census. (1986). *Statistical Abstract of the United States.* Washington, DC: U.S. Government Printing Office.

U.S. Bureau of the Census. (1989). Fertility of American women: June 1988. *Current Population Reports* (Series P–20, No. 436). Washington, DC: U.S. Government Printing Office.

U.S. Bureau of the Census. (1990). *Statistical abstract of the United States.* Washington, DC: U.S. Government Printing Office.

U.S. Bureau of the Census. (1991). *Statistical abstract of the United States.* Washington, DC: U.S. Government Printing Office.

U.S. Department of Commerce. (1991). Poverty in the United States: 1990. *Current Population Reports* (Series P–20, No. 175). Washington, DC: U.S. Government Printing Office.

U.S. Department of Labor. (1991). *A report on the glass ceiling initiative.* Washington, DC: U.S. Governement Printing Office.

U.S. Department of Labor Women's Bureau. (1990). *Facts on Working Women,* No. 90–1. Washington, DC: U.S. Government Printing Office.

Ussher, J. M. (1989). *The psychology of the female body.* New York: Routledge.

Vance, C. (Ed.). (1984). *Pleasure and danger: Exploring female sexuality.* Boston: Routledge & Kegan Paul.

Vannoy-Hiller, D., & Philliber, W. W. (1989). *Equal partners: Successful women in marriage.* Newbury Park, CA: Sage.

Vargo, S. (1987). The effects of women's socialization on lesbian couples. In

Boston Lesbian Psychologies Collective (Eds.), *Lesbian psychologies* (pp. 161–173). Urbana: University of Illinois Press.

Vaughan, D. (1986). *Uncoupling: How relationships come apart.* New York: Random House.

Veevers, J. E. (1976). Voluntarily childless wives: An exploratory study. *Sociology and Social Research, 57,* 356–366.

Veevers, J. E. (1979). Voluntary childlessness: A review of issues and evidence. *Marriage and Family Review, 2,* 1–26.

Veevers, J. E. (1980). *Childless by choice.* Toronto: Butterworth.

Voydanoff, P. (1988). Women, work, and family: Bernard's perspective on the past, present, and future. *Psychology of Women Quarterly, 12,* 269–280.

Walker, A. J. (1992). Conceptual perspectives on gender and family caregiving. In J. W. Dwyer & R. T. Coward (Eds.), *Gender, families and elder care* (pp. 34–46). Newbury Park, CA: Sage.

Walker, A. J., & Allen, K. R. (1991). Relationships between caregiving daughters and their elderly mothers. *The Gerontologist, 31,* 389–396.

Walker, A. J., Martin, S. S. K., & Thompson, L. (1988). Feminist programs for families. *Family Relations, 37,* 17–22.

Walker, A. J., Pratt, C. C., Shin, H., & Jones, L. L. (1990). Motives for parental caregiving and relationship quality. *Family Relations, 39,* 51–56.

Walker, A. J., & Thompson, L. (1984). Feminism and family studies. *Journal of Family Issues, 5,* 545–570.

Wallerstein, J. S., & Blakeslee, S. (1989). *Second chances: Men women, and children a decade after divorce.* New York: Ticknor & Fields.

Walsh, D. L. (1986). What women want. *American Demography, 8,* 60.

Walter, C. A. (1986). *The timing of motherhood.* Lexington, MA: D. C. Heath.

Watkins, S. C., Menken, J. A., & Bongaarts, J. (1987). Demographic foundations of family change. *American Sociological Review, 52,* 346–358.

Wattenberg, B. (1987, June 22). The birth dearth: Dangers ahead? *U.S. News and World Report,* 56–65.

Weeks, J. (1987). Questions of identity. In P. Caplan (Ed.), *The cultural construction of sexuality* (pp. 31–51). London: Tavistock.

Weinberg, M. S., & Williams, C. J. (1988). Black sexuality: A test of two theories. *The Journal of Sex Research, 25,* 197–218.

Weitzman, L. J. (1988). Women and children last: The social and economic consequences of divorce law reforms. In S. M. Dornbusch & M. H. Strober (Eds.), *Feminism, children, and the new families* (pp. 212–248). New York: Guilford.

Welter, B. (1966). The cult of true womanhood, 1820–1860. *American Quarterly, 18,* 151–174.

Westkott, M. (1979). Feminist criticism of the social sciences. *Harvard Educational Review, 49,* 422–430.

Weston, K. (1991). *Families we choose: Lesbians, gays, kinship.* New York: Columbia University Press.

Weston, K. M., & Rofel, L. B. (1984). Sexuality, class, and conflict in a lesbian workplace. *Signs, 9,* 623–646.

White, S. (1991). *Political theory and postmodernism.* Cambridge, Eng.: Cambridge University Press.

Wiley, J. L. (1989, April 30). "My body, myself" is a costly view. *The Boston Globe*, p. 76.

Wilkie, J. R. (1981). The trend toward delayed parenthood. *Journal of Marriage and the Family, 43,* 583–591.

Wilkinson, D. (1987). Ethnicity. In M. B. Sussman & S. K. Steinmetz (Eds.), *Handbook of marriage and the family* (pp. 183–210). New York: Plenum.

Willwerth, J. (1991, May 13). Should we take away their kids. *Time*, pp. 62–63.

Wilson, W. J. (1987). *The truly disadvantaged: The inner city, the underclass, and public policy.* Chicago: University of Chicago Press.

Wismont, J. M., & Reame, N. E. (1989). The lesbian childbearing experience: Assessing developmental tasks. *IMAGE: Journal of Nursing Scholarship, 21,* 137–141.

Witherell, C., & Noddings, N. (Eds.). (1991). *Stories lives tell: Narrative and dialogue in education.* New York: Teachers College Press.

Wolfe, L. (1981). *The Cosmo report.* New York: Arbor House.

Wright, H. (1959). *The sex factor in marriage.* London: Williams and Norgate.

Yllo, K., & Bograd, M. (Eds.). (1988). *Feminist perspectives on wife abuse.* Newbury Park, CA: Sage.

Yogev, S. (1981). Do professional women have egalitarian marital relationships? *Journal of Marriage and the Family, 43,* 865–871.

Zabin, L. S., Hirsch, M. B., & Emerson, M.R. (1989). When urban adolescents choose abortion: Effects on education, psychological status and subsequent pregnancies. *Family Planning Perspectives, 21,* 248–255.

Zimmerman, B. (1984). The politics of transliteration: Lesbian personal narratives. *Signs, 9,* 663–682.

Zimmerman, M. (1989). Experiencing abortion as a crisis: The impact of social context. In B. J. Risman & P. Schwartz (Eds.), *Gender in intimate relationships* (pp. 132–137). Belmont, CA: Wadsworth.

Zinn, M. B. (1990). Family, feminism, and race in America. *Gender & Society, 4,* 68–82.

Index

diversity in, 63
and early experiences in adolescence, 87–88
and education programs, 99–100,
141
feminist vision of, 98–101
four-component model of, 66–67
gender inequality in, 65
historical analysis of, 65, 94–97
lack of research attention, 61–62
male dominance in, 82–84
physiologic responses in, 68–69
pleasure and danger in, 87–90
pluralistic approach to, 98–99
politics of, 65–66
postmodern feminist perspective on,
63
renaming of terminology in, 66
resistance to research in, 64–65
and risk of AIDS, 89–90
and social construction of sexual
scripts, 69–70
modifications of, 79–81
and tensions about dominance and
equality, 90–92
Social construction of difference, 14–
17, 154
Social norms, and sexual behavior, 69–
70
Socialization of women, 31–33, 58
Standpoint theories, feminist, 9–10
Strategies for change, 21–23
Subordination, and caregiving by
women, 160–164
Surrogate mothering, 134–135
Surrogate sisters, 31
Sweden, social policy in, 228–229

T

Traditional family ideology, 1, 6, 20,
25, 106, 146–147, 149, 178, 223
Transactional approach, 5–6

U

Uncoupling process
in lesbian couples, 55–56
in married couples, 53–55
*United Auto Workers v. Johnson Con-
trols Inc.*, 193–194

V

Violence against women
in lesbian relationships, 53
in marriage, 52–53
rates of, 52
redefining reality of, 20
and sexual assaults by husbands, 83–
84

W

Webster v. Reproductive Health Services,
119–120, 125
Woman-centered life, 92–93
Women of color, variations among, 7,
9, 19, 28–29, 30–31, 32, 63, 88,
89, 103, 126, 139, 144, 146, 161,
176, 179, 191, 224
Work cutback, mandatory, suggested
for new parents, 173–174, 198–
199
Work women do, 176–217
as caregivers. *See* Caregiving by
women
and decisions about motherhood,
108, 110–111
deconstruction of, 176
and feminist vision for change, 213–
217
in household work, 205–213. *See
also* Household work
in military service, 195
in paid employment, 178–205
barriers to corporate advancement
in, 185–187
changing patterns of, 178–182
commitment to permanence in,
181–182
conflicting demands of work and
family, 180, 197–200
employment rates, 176, 183
and gender gap in income, 183–
184
gender stratification in, 177, 182,
196–200
and governmental neglect of family policy, 200–202
and heterosexism, 187–190
and household work, 208–211
and importance of child care,
202–203